DEVELOPMENTAL NUTRITION

DEVELOPMENTAL NUTRITION

LUCILLE S. HURLEY
University of California, Davis

Prentice-Hall, Inc., *Englewood Cliffs, New Jersey 07632*

Library of Congress Cataloging in Publication Data

Hurley, Lucille S
Developmental nutrition.

Includes bibliographies and index.
1. Fetal malnutrition—Complications and sequelae.
2. Pregnancy—Nutritional aspects. 3. Children—
Nutrition. I. Title.
RG627.6.M34H87 618.3′2 78-26152
ISBN 0-13-207639-X

Printed in the United States of America

10 9 8 7 6 5 4 3 2 1

Prentice-Hall International, Inc., *London*
Prentice-Hall of Australia Pty. Limited, *Sydney*
Prentice-Hall of Canada, Ltd., *Toronto*
Prentice-Hall of India Private Limited, *New Delhi*
Prentice-Hall of Japan, Inc., *Tokyo*
Prentice-Hall of Southeast Asia Pte. Ltd., *Singapore*
Whitehall Books Limited, *Wellington, New Zealand*

to my teachers
and my students
and
to Kenneth

Contents

Preface

With the increasing awareness that development of the mammalian organism may be permanently affected by its nutritional state, there has in recent years been a significant augmentation of research in this subject. Research findings not only have provided new factual information but have led to conceptual revisions as well. This book was written to present this subject matter, the influence of nutrition on development, which I have termed *developmental nutrition.*

The major emphasis of the book is on the prenatal period. After a discussion of the principles of growth and development, and a brief summary of morphogenesis and placental function, the principal portion of the volume is devoted to the relationship of nutrition to prenatal development. Finally, nutritional aspects of development in infants, young children, and adolescents are considered.

The subject matter of developmental nutrition borders on the disciplines of embryology, biochemistry, physiology, genetics, and teratology, as well as that of nutrition. Although this volume includes a brief summary of morphological development and placental function, complete background material in these subjects cannot, of course, be presented. The book is written with the assumption that the reader has some knowledge of biochemistry and nutrition.

It is a pleasure to acknowledge the contributions of my husband, Kenneth Thompson, whose help in editing, proofreading, and indexing was invaluable. I also thank Drs. Peter Dallman and Judith Stern for reading portions of the text, and Mrs. Jeanne Miller Falkenham for her expert and cheerful typing of the manuscript.

LUCILLE S. HURLEY

1

Introduction

Developmental nutrition is concerned with the role of nutritional factors in the development of an organism. The term *nutritional factors* encompasses metabolic or genetic effects on the quantities of essential nutrients or their function, as well as those related to diet. By *development* we mean the irreversible changes undergone by an individual from the fertilized ovum to maturity. Some investigators include aging as part of the developmental process, but we shall not do so in this book. A fuller explanation of the term development is given in Chapter 2. As developmental biology is the biology of the developmental process, developmental nutrition concerns the relationship of nutrition to development.

This book, then, is concerned with the influence of nutrition on development, the effects of nutritional deficiencies and excesses, and the relationship of essential nutrients to the morphogenetic or biochemical processes that take place during the course of development. As one of the manifestations of perturbation of normal development, current information on birth defects resulting from nutritional insult is discussed in some detail.

Although embryologists and developmental biologists use many lower forms as models, this book considers only studies of mammalian species, primarily rats, mice, some ruminants, and humans. The reasons are twofold. First, our ultimate concern is the relation of this subject matter to human problems, and, certainly for the embryo and the suckling at least, the mammalian form is the most appropriate model. Another reason for limiting the subject matter to mammals is that for the periods of development that are the major concern of the book, most of the research has been done with these species.

The span of the life cycle with which this book is concerned ranges from the fertilized egg stage through adolescence, with its biological capability of initiating a new cycle. Not all of the stages of this developmental span will, however, be stressed equally. The major emphasis is on the influence of nutrition on prenatal development. This focus is indicated because a current and thorough synthesis of the subject is not available in book form. Only a relatively small portion of the volume is devoted to nutrition of infants and children, including adolescents. Excellent books are available on these subjects, and the reader is urged to consult them for more understanding and detailed information.

I

Growth and Development

2

Principles of growth and development

In order to have some understanding of the influence of nutrition or nutritional factors on growth and development, it is necessary to be acquainted with the characteristics of developmental phenomena.

What is meant by growth and development? It is important to distinguish between the two terms. Growth refers to increase in size,[1] while development can occur without any change in overall size. Development will be considered first.

DEVELOPMENT

The changes in the body shape of humans from the fetus to the adult individual show that development involves alterations in body proportions. In Figure 2–1, to emphasize these changes, the body shapes are drawn in such a way that the total body length is the same for all the figures, from the two-month-old fetus to the 25-year-old man. In the fetus, half of the total body length comes from the head, while in the adult the head is only one-eighth the total body length. These alterations in body proportions are in themselves not changes of size (growth) but are developmental changes.

This is only one example of a developmental change. All the way through life changes occur, from the fertilized egg through the embryo stage to the young individual and the adult, until, finally, degenerative changes take place leading to death.

Development is the sequence of the orderly changes from the fertilized egg to the adult. The changes are progressive and irreversible; they occur in a regular sequence with little variation, and each change leaves the organism different from and unable to return to its previous state. These

[1]But again, there is a difference between true growth and increases in body weight caused by water retention or fat deposition.

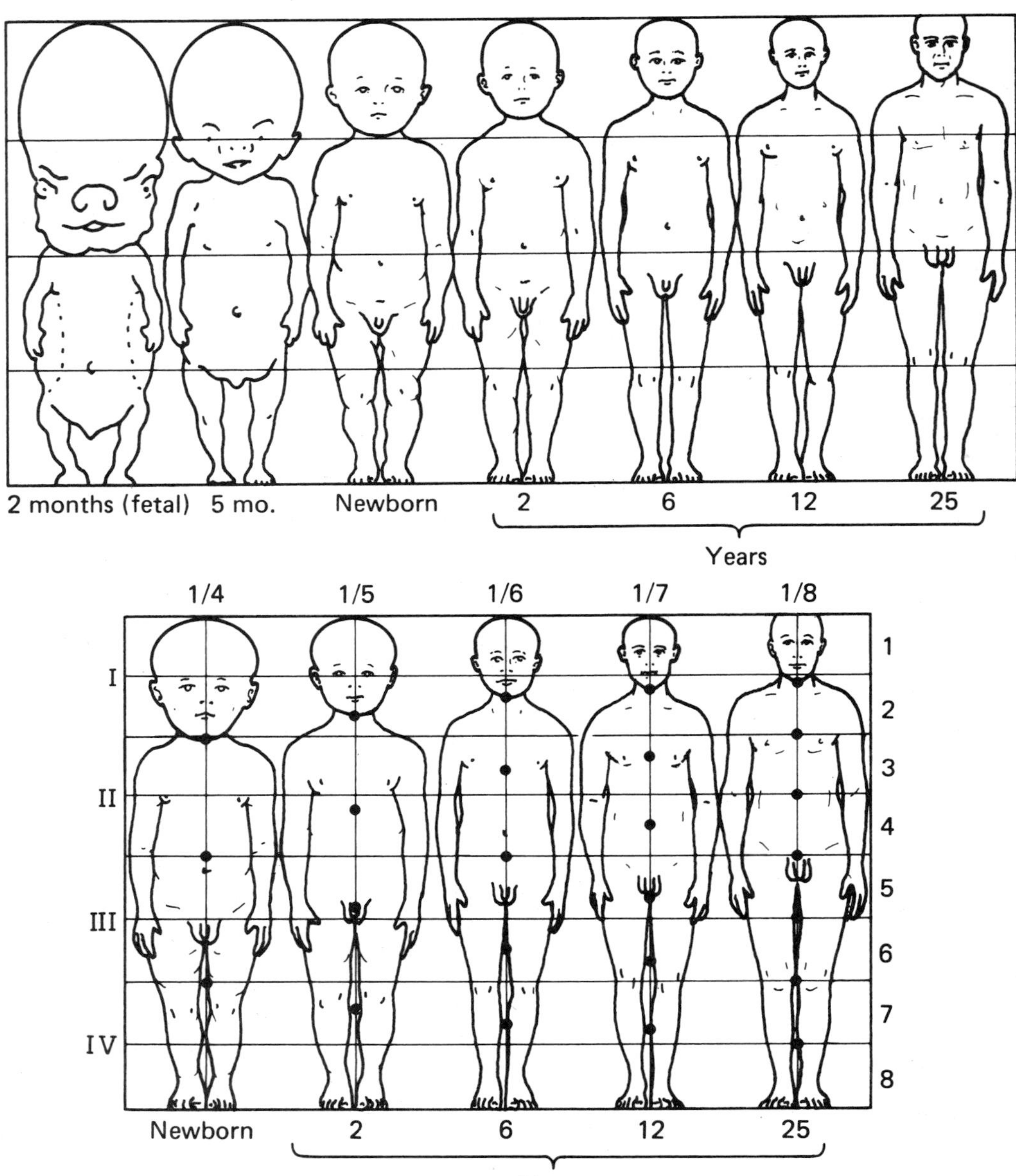

From Scammon, 1927.

Figure 2–1 Diagram illustrating the changes in the proportions of the human body during growth. Prenatal and postnatal changes are compared in the upper diagram. Changes in proportion are expressed in head length in the lower diagram. In the newborn, the length of the head is approximately one-fourth of the total length of the body; in the adult it is only one-eighth. Conversely, the legs are comparatively much shorter in the baby than in the adult. The proportions of the adult human are established in the way that the head grows relatively slower and the legs faster than the rest of the body. Thus, differences in relative growth rates, i.e., the ratio of growth rates of the various parts of the body, lead to changes in proportion and represent an important morphogenetic factor.

changes constitute the life cycle of the organism, because as part of the developmental process, the new adult becomes capable of producing the eggs or sperm that will give rise to the next generation. All of these changes are changes in development. Single cells and unorganized populations of cells also undergo developmental progression.

There are three major aspects of development: one is *growth.* Growth, which differs from development but is one aspect of it, is a basic phenomenon which has been extensively studied in many different ways for a long time. One of the important questions concerning growth is the mechanism of initiation. We know that various hormones are required to initiate growth and also that nutrients are necessary to the phenomenon. In fact almost any nutritional deficiency will influence growth. More is known about how growth starts than about how or why it stops. Regulatory mechanisms must be involved in the initiation and the cessation of growth as well as in its maintenance.

The second major aspect of development is *differentiation.* This refers to the differentiation of specialized cells from one original fertilized cell. From the fertilized ovum, which is one single cell, there is developed a multicellular organism with cells of many different types, varying both in structure and in function. Important questions concerning differentiation are: what are the processes in the differentiation of cells and what regulatory mechanisms control these processes? Of interest is not only the control of the type of cell, but also control of the numbers of each cell type. This is a basic problem in cancer research. If the mechanisms that controlled the numbers of cell types were known, the development of cancer, in which the production of a particular cell type is excessive, would be better understood.

The third aspect of development is *morphogenesis.* This process includes the growth and development of the anatomical structure of the organism. It involves the establishment of specific patterns of structural form and is the process whereby the adult assumes its final shape. However, development is functional as well as morphological. Functional development is an important aspect of the fetal and neonatal period.

STAGES OF DEVELOPMENT

Table 2–1 shows the periods of life before maturity in the human. In the first trimester of prenatal life, the embryonic period, there is rapid differentiation and establishment of systems and organs. The early fetal stage occurs during the second trimester. This stage is characterized by accelerating growth, elaboration of structures, and early functional activities. This is also a period of biochemical development. In the late fetal stage there is considerable biochemical change and activity. The parturient period is the time of labor and delivery, and the neonatal period is the first month of postnatal life. Recently a new term has come into use, the perinatal period, literally, the period around the time of birth. This term refers to the late fetus and the early newborn stage. The next stages are the infant, the late infant, the preschool child, the school child, and the adolescent. With sexual maturity comes the capacity to reproduce, and the cycle begins again.

TABLE 2–1 AGE PERIODS OF LIFE BEFORE MATURITY

Name of Period	*Ages Represented (approximate)*	*Some Characterizing Features*
Embryonic	First trimester of prenatal life	Rapid differentiation Establishment of systems and organs
Early fetal	Second trimester of prenatal life	Accelerated growth Elaboration of structures Early functional activities
Late fetal	Third trimester of prenatal life	Rapid increase in body mass Completion of preparation for postnatal experience
Parturient	Period of labor and delivery	Risk of trauma and anoxia Cessation of placental function
Neonatal and early infancy	First month of postnatal life	Postnatal adjustments in circulation Initiation of respiration and other functions
Middle infancy	1 month to 1 year	Rapid growth and maturation Maturation of functions, especially of nervous system
Late infancy	1 to 2 years	Decelerating growth Progress in walking and other voluntary motor activities and in control of excretory functions
Childhood:		
Preschool	2 to 6 years	Slow growth Increased physical activity Further coordination of functions and motor mechanisms Rapid learning

TABLE 2–1 (cont.)

Name of Period	*Ages Represented (approximate)*	*Some Characterizing Features*
School	Girls: 6 to 10 years Boys: 6 to 12 years	Steady growth Developing skills and intellectual processes
Adolescent		
Prepubertal (late school or early adolescent)	Girls: 10 to 12 years Boys: 12 to 14 years	Accelerating growth Rapid weight gain Early adolescent endocrine and sex organ changes
Pubertal (adolescence proper)	Girls: 12 to 14 years Boys: 14 to 16 years	Secondary sex character maturation
Postpubertal	Girls: 14 to 18 years Boys: 16 to 20 years	Maximum postnatal growth increase Decelerating and terminal growth Rapid muscle growth and increased skills Rapid growth and maturing functions of sex organs Need for self-reliance and independence

From Timiras, 1972.

GROWTH

CURVE OF GROWTH

All things that grow have one thing in common, the S-shaped curve of growth. If mass is plotted against time, an S-shaped curve results that has three stages: (1) the lag phase where no growth occurs, (2) the exponential phase where growth occurs at an exponential rate, and (3) the stationary phase [Figure 2–2(a)]. The lag phase occurs because it takes time for growth to begin. The nutrient supply influences the length of the lag phase, as well as the number of cells present. The physiological state of the cells also contributes to the length of the lag phase. Enzyme systems required for growth must be synthesized. Cells have to multiply before the organisms can grow.

During the exponential phase there occurs a doubling of the number of cells at each division. This is because the more cells there are, the more there can be, and a straight-line relationship results. The same phenomenon occurs in human populations. Exponential growth takes place where most of the organisms are reproducing, and the generation times are constant. The stationary phase begins as the nutrient supply becomes exhausted (in a cell population), or the environment becomes toxic. If another nutrient supply is added at this time, another S-curve will result.

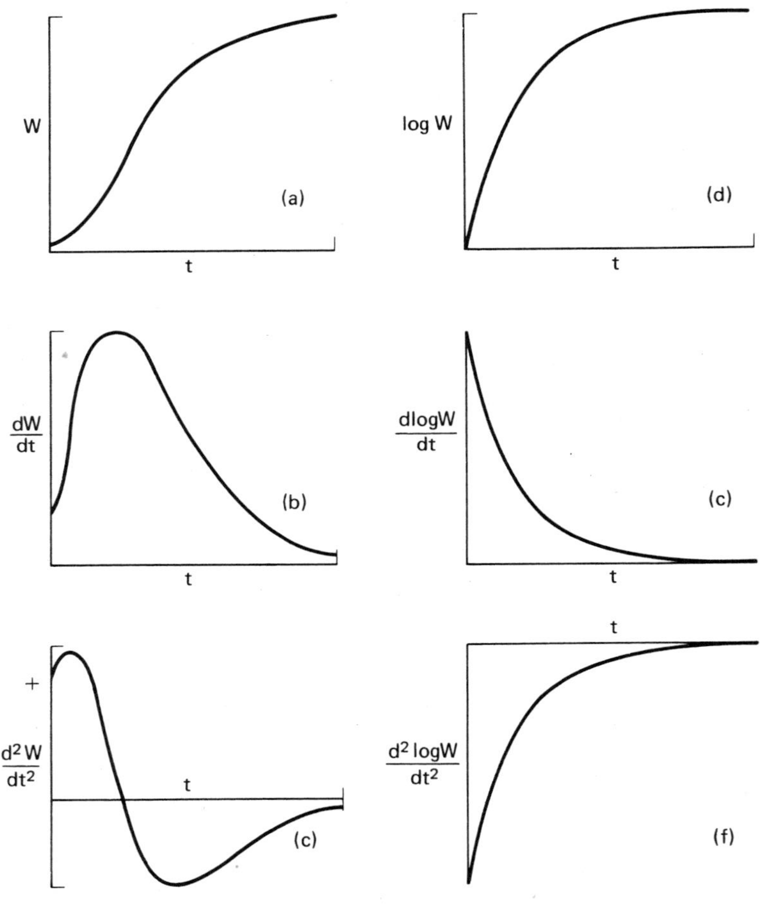

From Medawar, 1945.

Figure 2–2 (a) The curve of growth, (b) of growth rate, (c) of acceleration; (d) the curve of *specific* growth, (e) of specific growth rate, (f) of specific acceleration. The curves have been plotted from an equation for the Gompertz function, but the scales of the ordinates have been so adjusted as to make the height of each graph uniform.

Although all growth systems show the S-shaped curve of growth, the rate of growth varies among different species. This may be seen by the differences in time required to double their mass: *E. coli*, 20 minutes; fly larva, 13 hours; the rabbit at birth, 6 days; the pig at birth, 6 to 7 days; the guinea pig, 18 days; the horse, 60 days; and man, 180 days.

In the growth of a multicellular organism, all the parts of the body do not grow at the same rate, but still the total follows the S-curve. Similarly, all of the parts do not stop growing simultaneously. Once maturity has been reached, the overall body size remains relatively constant. Another characteristic of growth in a multicellular organism is that the growth of one part of the body is controlled by other parts of the body. For instance, growth of the skeleton is controlled by the pituitary gland, which must produce the necessary hormones. There is an integrating interaction among the parts that maintains the body's proportions.

LIMITATION OF SIZE AND FORM

Another aspect of growth is the limitation of size and form. In multicellular organisms, factors are involved in addition to those that govern cell cultures. The genetic constitution of the individual is a consideration, since hereditary factors will influence the organism's size and form. The supply of available nutrients or the presence of toxic factors will also limit size and affect form. More fundamental in the limitation of size is the body's ratio of surface area to volume. With an increase in body size, the volume of the body increases much faster than its surface area. This is very important for warm-blooded animals because of the functions of heat dissipation and maintenance of body temperature, which have to be accomplished through the body surface area. The ratio of body surface area to volume therefore represents a very basic limitation on body size.

RATE OF GROWTH

If, instead of plotting increased weight against time for a growing entity, we use change in weight (dW/dt), the resulting curve shows the *rate* of growth [Figure 2–2(b)]. The curve of growth rate is the inverse of the curve of growth. The rate of growth is highest at the point of inflection of the growth curve and declines thereafter, even though maximum absolute growth has not been attained. In the curve of *acceleration* of growth (d^2W/dt^2), the intersection with the time axis, where acceleration is zero, corresponds to the inflection point of (a) and the peak of (b) [Figure 2–2(c)]. The curve of *specific growth* [Figure 2–2(d)] provides a record of the multiplication of body substance. The *specific growth rate* $(dW/dt)(1/W)$ against time indicates that the percentage increment in weight decreases steadily with time [Figure 2–2(e)]. The curve of *specific acceleration* is shown in Figure 2–2(f).

CELLULAR GROWTH

Another way of looking at growth in a multicellular organism is to consider increases in the number or size of cells. Actually the growth of an organism (which is an increase in mass) occurs in two different ways. One is an increase in the *number* of cells (hyperplasia), the other an increase in the *size* of the cells (hypertrophy). The number of cells can be estimated by measuring the amount of DNA in various organs and tissues. If the amount of DNA in each cell nucleus is known and the total amount of DNA in an organ is measured, the number of cells in that organ can be calculated. The number of nuclei in the organ is equal to the total amount of DNA divided by the DNA per nucleus, and, of course, the number of nuclei is (usually) equivalent to the number of cells.

In order to determine the DNA per nucleus, the amount of DNA in a particular sample of tissue is measured, and by histological methods the number of cells for which that amount of DNA is equivalent is established. Thus,

$$\text{number of nuclei} = \frac{\text{total DNA}}{\text{DNA/nucleus}} = \text{number of cells (?)}$$

Also,

$$\frac{\text{total organ weight}}{\text{number of nuclei}} = \text{weight per nucleus} = \text{cell size}$$

Such calculations depend upon two assumptions: (1) that the DNA per nucleus is constant and (2) that cells have only one nucleus per cell. The amount of DNA per nucleus is species-specific.

These principles were first applied by Enesco and Leblond in a classic work demonstrating the changes in cell number and cell size that occur during growth of various organs of the male rat. In Figure 2–3, growth of the whole body in rats is compared to the increase in DNA from ten days before birth to 90 days after birth. There is a rapid increase in the total amount of DNA, but it stops accumulating before the body weight stops increasing. Therefore, the total amount of DNA remains constant, even though the body weight of the animal increases. The body weight per nucleus (cell size) increases for two days during the prenatal period and rises steadily during most of the postnatal period, beginning at seven days after birth.

Phases of cellular growth. From these studies Enesco and Leblond showed that there are three phases of growth. The first is a period of rapid cell proliferation, during which there is little or no change in the cell size. In the rat this

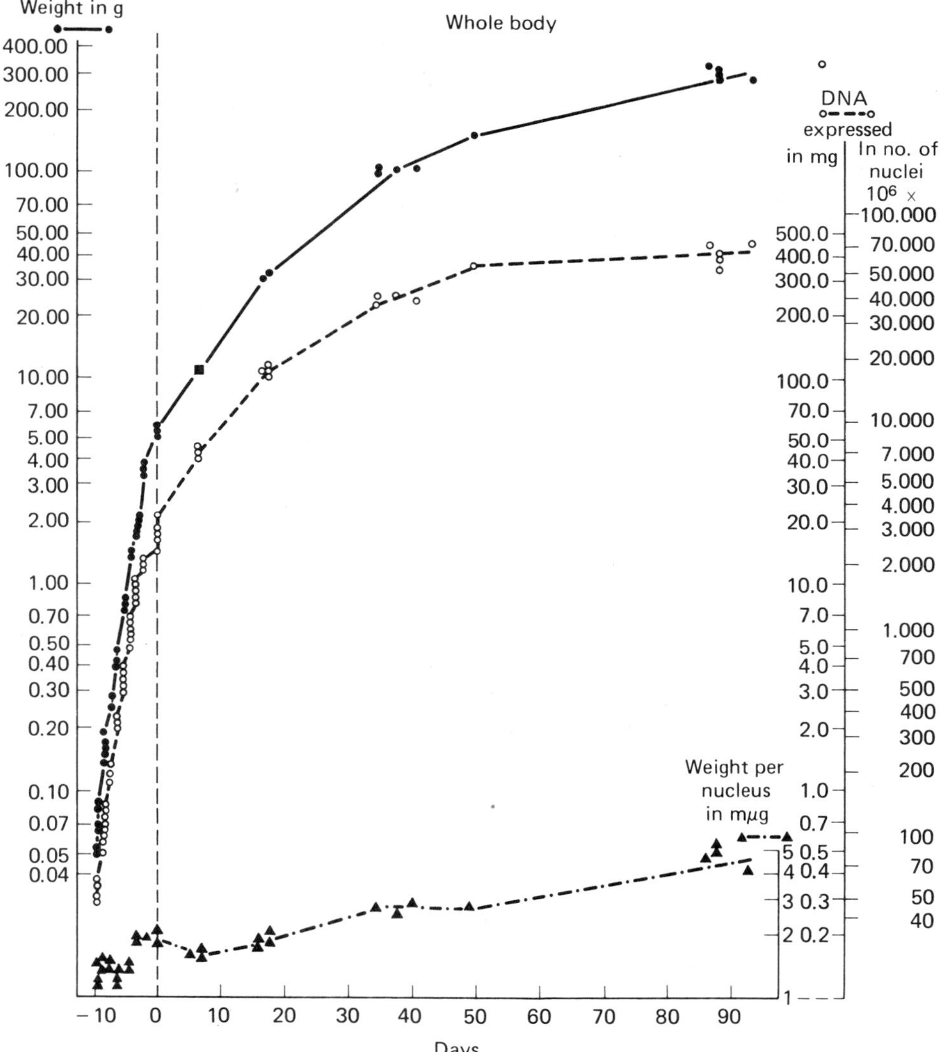

From Enesco and Leblond, 1962.
Reprinted by Permission of Cambridge University Press.

Figure 2–3 Semilogarithmic plot of the whole-body weight in grams (dots), DNA in mg (circles), and weight per nucleus in mμg (triangles) versus the age in days. The DNA results are not only expressed in mg, but also converted into millions of nuclei (scale at right). The time of birth is indicated by the vertical broken line at 0 day. Weight and DNA curves rise in parallel until a few days before birth, and then diverge more and more with age. Both, however, rise less and less steeply as the animals become older. The weight per nucleus increases for only two days during the prenatal period and, starting from the seventh day after birth, rises steadily through most of the postnatal period.

period extends to about day 17 of postnatal life. This phase varies from organ to organ and cannot be recognized on a whole-body basis.

During the second phase, cell proliferation slows down, but cell size increases rapidly. In the rat this period takes place from about day 17 to day 48 postnatal. In the third phase there is almost no cell proliferation, but there is a rapid increase in cell size.

Another way to show these changes is to measure relationships among protein, DNA, and RNA. This was first done by Winick and Noble in a series of investigations that led to important research on the influence of undernutrition on development. Winick and Noble delineated the parameters of cellular growth in rats and showed in detail that DNA synthesis or cell proliferation varies with different organs (Figure 2–4). They also showed that in most organs in the rat, RNA is proportional to DNA during the first few months of postnatal life, resulting in a constant value for RNA per nucleus. Thus, the ratio RNA/DNA is constant for each organ. Tissues with active protein synthesis, such as liver, heart, and muscle, have high RNA/DNA ratios.

The organs in which DNA synthesis stops first are the lung and the brain; these are also the organs in which the first period of rapid cell proliferation first ends. This happens in the rat at about nine days after birth. In the kidney the phase of rapid cell proliferation does not stop until about day 39, and in the heart, about day 49. The various organs of the body thus have different rates of DNA synthesis and different time sequences for the various phases of growth. This is important in terms of nutritional effects on development, because it appears that if malnutrition affects the developing individual at the stage of rapid cell proliferation, the number of cells is decreased and cannot be reversed even by supplementary feeding at a later time.

This elucidation of cellular growth is an important contribution because it enables evaluation of the effects of malnutrition at the various stages of cellular growth.

FACTORS AFFECTING GROWTH

Some factors in addition to nutrition that affect growth of the fetus can be seen in Figure 2–5. One is the effect of twinning. The growth curve of a twin deviates from the normal curve. Low socioeconomic level of the parents also correlates with decreased growth rate of the fetus. Fetuses whose parents are of Swedish ancestry have a growth rate higher than average, presumably because of genetic characteristics.

Maternal size can also influence the size of the offspring at birth. This was shown experimentally by transplanting fertilized eggs from dwarf sows into normal sows and fertilized eggs from normal sows into dwarf sows. The body weights of the piglets at birth clearly demonstrated the influence of maternal size on growth of the fetus (see Table 2–2).

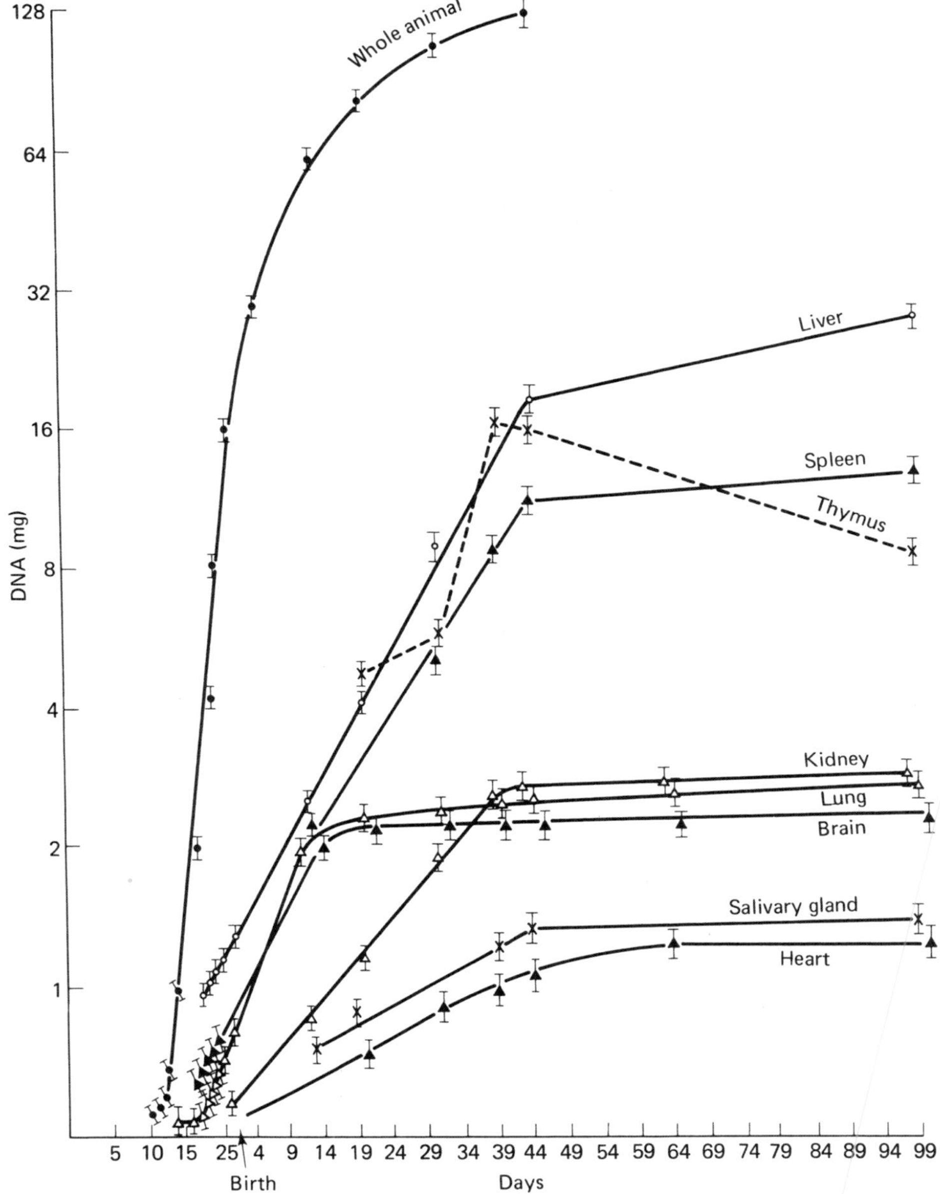

From Winick and Noble, 1965.

Figure 2–4 DNA (mg) during normal growth in the rat. Points represent mean values for at least ten animals or organs. I represents range.

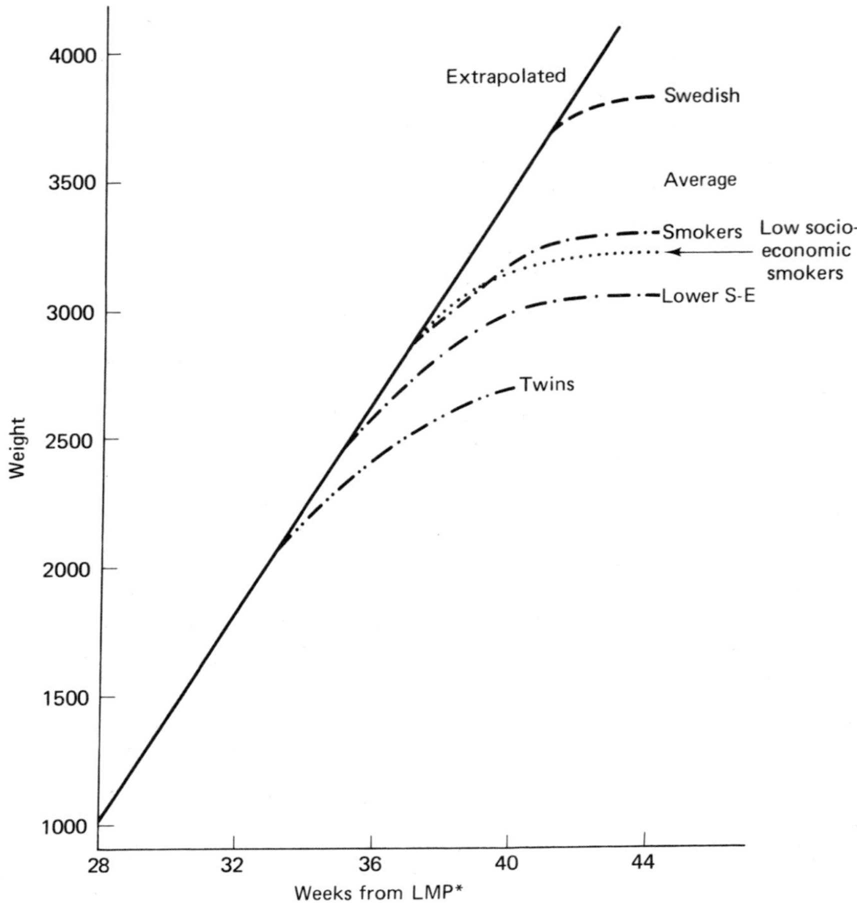

* Last menstrual period

From Gruenwald, 1966.

Figure 2–5 Semidiagrammatic presentation of fetal growth (determined from birth weight) of several population groups. Depending on the time when limitation of supplies to the fetus begins, the curves depart from the straight, extrapolated course at different times in gestation.

TABLE 2–2 INFLUENCE OF MATERNAL SIZE ON BIRTH WEIGHT IN PIGS

Group	*Birth Weight, g*
Egg of *normal* pig developed in *normal* sow	1488
Egg of *normal* pig developed in *dwarf* sow	744
Egg of *dwarf* pig developed in *normal* sow	835
Egg of *dwarf* pig developed in *dwarf* sow	418

From Smidt et al., Mschr. Kinderheilk. 115: 533, 1967, in Giroud, 1970.

GROWTH PATTERNS OF VARIOUS SPECIES

Although all growing systems show the S-shaped curve of growth, specific patterns of the growth curve differ among various species (Figure 2–6). In the growth of the human fetus there is a decline in the rate of growth just before birth, which can be correlated with a drop in the rate of placental transfer of sodium. This decreased placental transfer (presumably of all nutrients, not only sodium) seems to be related to the aging of the placenta at that period. Thus, the decline in fetal growth rate at this time may be attributed to decreased effectiveness of placental transfer. At birth (or at hatching in the chick) there are problems connected with the processes of birth and the physiological adjustment of the newborn to its new environment, all of which bring about a decrease in the growth rate. After this period the growth rate rises again. In the pig, however, the curve of growth is continuous and is even more rapid after birth than before birth.

Differences in growth patterns among various species are also very evident in rates of growth before birth, as shown in Table 2–3.

TABLE 2–3 RATE OF GROWTH OF NINE SPECIES BEFORE BIRTH

Species	*Length of Gestation, days*	*Weight at Birth, g*	*Mean Growth Rate, g/day*
Mouse	21	2	0.09
Rat	21	5	0.24
Cat	63	100	1.6
Dog	63	200	3.2
Pig	120	1,500	4.2
Man	280	3,500	12.5
Elephant	600	114,000	190
Hippopotamus	240	50,000	240
Blue whale	330	3,000,000	9,000

From Widdowson, 1968.

RELATIVE GROWTH

The growth curves shown in Figure 2–6 represent absolute growth, but there are also important changes in relative growth. Body proportions are greatly altered during development, which means that different parts of the body must grow at different rates. As shown in Figure 2–1, the head of the individual becomes progressively relatively smaller as the legs become progressively relatively longer. The same applies to the arms and the trunk. These are changes in the proportion of the length of the head and of the

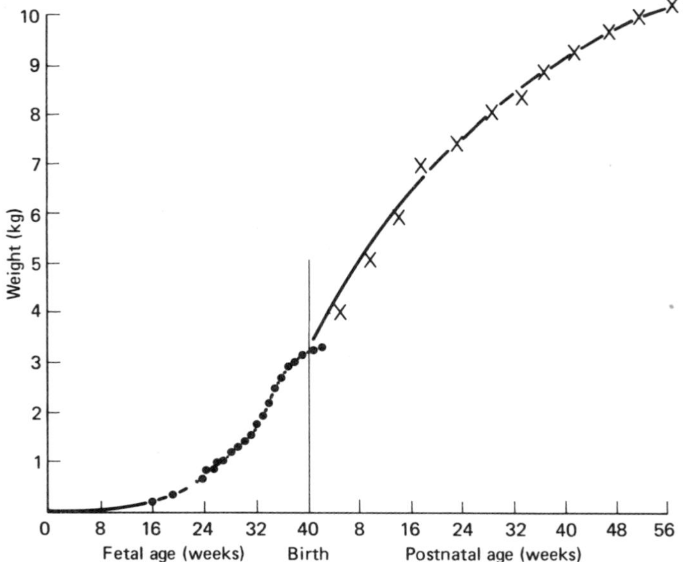

(*a*) *From Widdowson, 1968.*

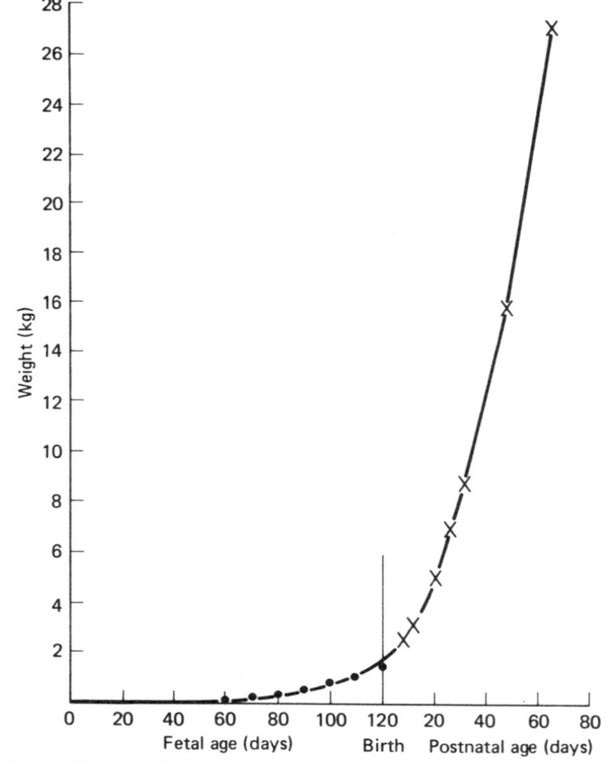

(*b*) *From Widdowson, 1968.*

Figure 2–6 Differences in growth curve among species. (a) Growth of human fetus and baby. (b) Growth of pig before and after birth. (c) Growth of chick before and after hatching. (d) Growth of guinea pigs before and after birth.

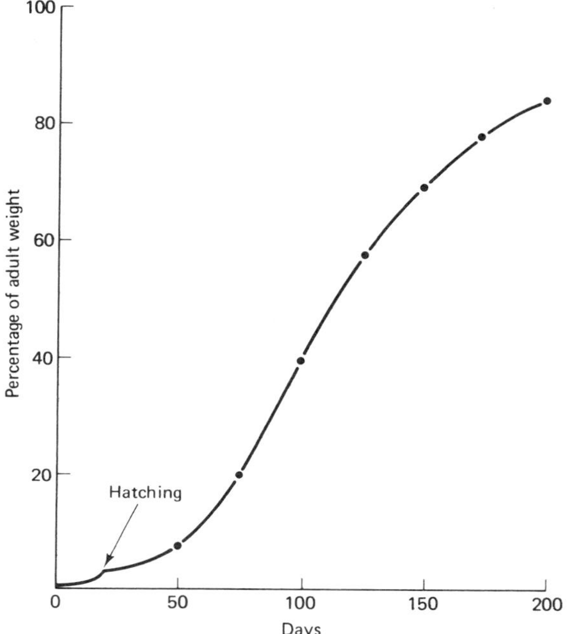

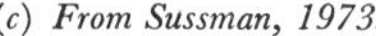
(*c*) *From Sussman, 1973.*

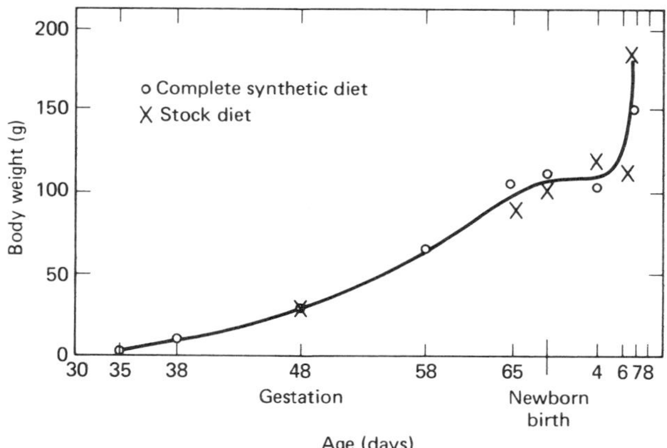

(*d*) *From Hurley and Volkert, 1965.*

limbs to the total body length, so that in the adult human the head is a relatively small proportion of the total length and the legs are relatively long.

Another aspect of proportional growth is seen by examining the contributions of various organs and tissues to the total body weight at different ages (Table 2–4). The brain is the same proportion of the body weight in the

TABLE 2-4 CONTRIBUTION OF ORGANS AND TISSUES TO THE BODY WEIGHT OF MAN AT DIFFERENT AGES[a]

Tissue	*Fetus, 20–24 Weeks*	*Full-Term Baby*	*Adult*
Skeletal muscle	25	25	13
Skin	13	15	7
Skeleton	22	18	18
Heart	0.6	0.5	0.4
Liver	4	5	2
Kidneys	0.7	1	0.5
Brain	13	13	2

[a]Values are given as a percentage of the body weight.

From Widdowson, 1968.

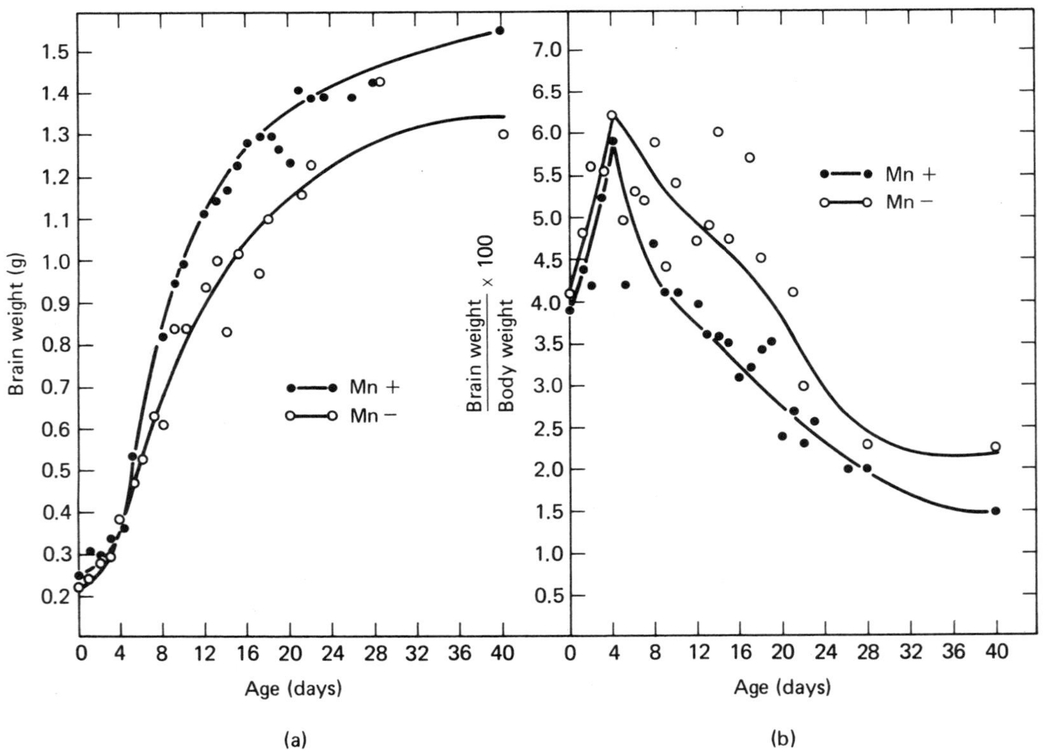

From Hurley et al., 1961b.

Figure 2–7 Brain weight in offspring of manganese-deficient and manganese-supplemented female rats. Each point represents the mean of from three to 15 animals. (a) Absolute brain weight. (b) Brain weight relative to body weight.

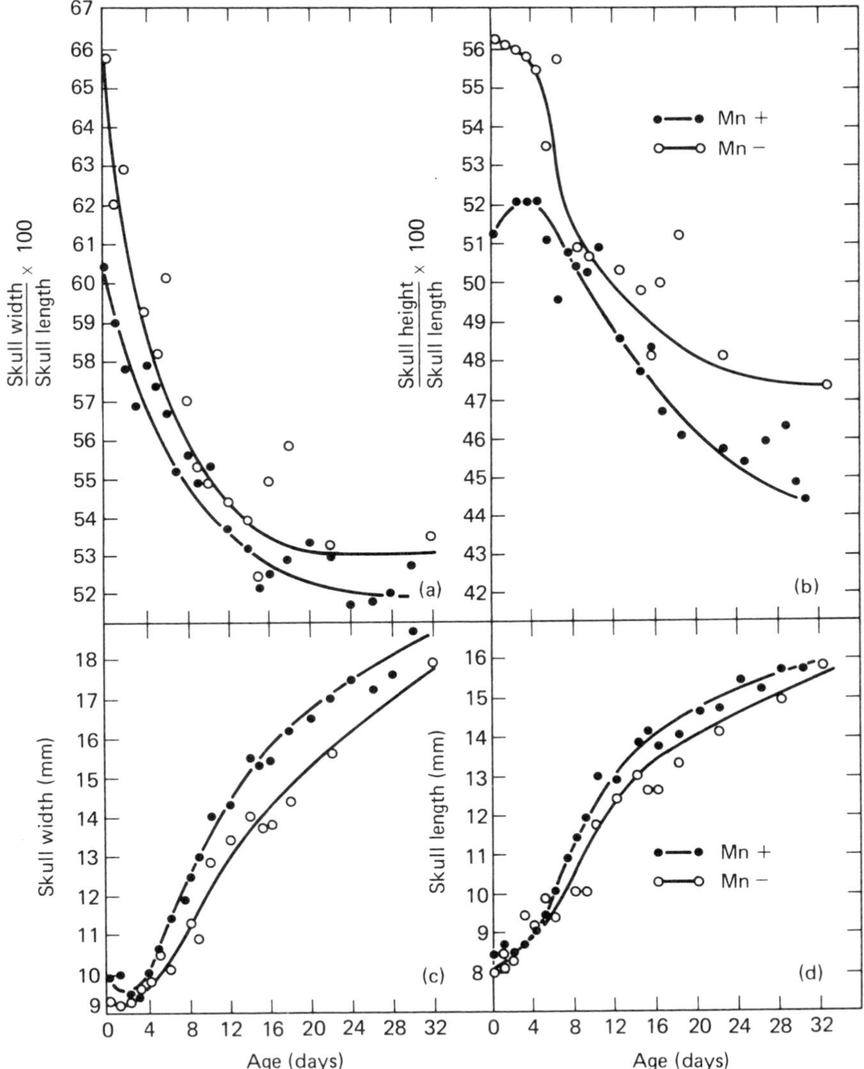

From Hurley et al., 1961b.

Figure 2–8 Skull width and height in offspring of manganese-deficient and manganese-supplemented female rats. Each point represents the mean of from three to 30 animals (in most cases, five to seven). (a) Skull width relative to skull length. (b) Skull height relative to skull length. (c) Absolute skull width. (d) Absolute skull height.

fetus and the full-term infant, but it is a smaller proportion of the total body weight in the adult. This comes about because at the time of birth the brain has almost reached its final size and does not grow very much postnatally, although the rest of the body grows considerably. Thus, the brain becomes proportionally smaller. The muscles are just the opposite; they form a much

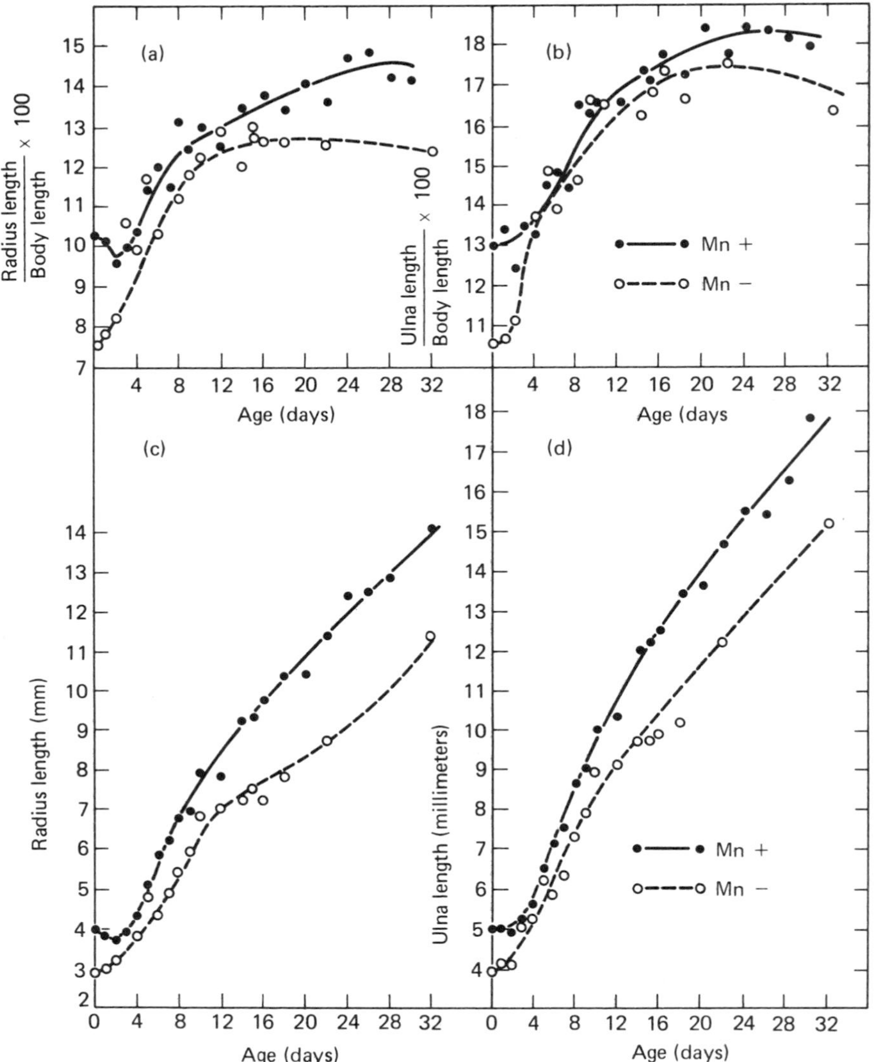

From Hurley et al., 1961a.

Figure 2–9 Growth of radius and ulna in offspring of manganese-deficient and manganese-supplemented female rats. Each point represents the mean of from three to 33 animals. (a) Radius length relative to crown-rump length. (b) Ulna length relative to crown-rump length. (c) Absolute radius length. (d) Absolute ulna length.

more important part of the body in the adult than they do in the fetus or the infant.

Another example of differential brain growth is from a study of growth of the brain in manganese-deficient and normal rats from birth to age 40 days (Figure 2–7). The total body size of the manganese-deficient animals was small. Their brains were smaller than those of the control rats, but their bodies were also smaller. When brain weight was related to body weight, brain weight was actually larger in the deficient animals than in the controls. This figure also shows that the proportion of brain weight to total body weight is smaller in the adult animal than in the young animal because the brain does not grow as much or as rapidly as the rest of the body.

The same kind of proportionate growth is seen in the skeleton. Figure 2–8 shows the growth of the skull in length from the experiment cited above. The manganese-deficient rats have a smaller absolute skull size, as is to be expected. If, however, skull width and skull height in relation to skull length are compared, it is seen that the manganese-deficient animals have skulls that are both wider and higher in proportion to their length than do normal animals. In the normal animal, it is apparent that as the skull grows, the proportions change; the width becomes smaller in relation to the length, and the same is true of the height. The manganese-deficient animals were thus retaining body proportions that were immature for their chronological age.

Similar proportional changes take place in the long bones as well (Figure 2–9). The radius grows at a more rapid rate than overall body length. Manganese-deficient animals have disproportionately shorter bones in relation to total body length. This is also true for the long bones of the leg, so that by the time the manganese-deficient animal is an adult, there is a very marked difference in the proportionality of the long bones to the skeleton, as compared with normal animals. Exactly the same principles apply to the animals during their fetal growth as well, and chondrodystrophy (the condition in which the arms and legs are short in relation to total body length, the head is disproportionate in its dimensions, and there is curvature of the spine) has been produced in chick embryos by manganese deficiency. Chondrodystrophy also occurs in human beings, but the connection, if any, between chondrodystrophy and manganese metabolism is unknown.

References and Supplementary Readings

Enesco, M., and C. P. Leblond. "Increase in cell number as a factor in the growth of the organs and tissues of the young male rat." *J. Embryol. Exp. Morph.* **10**: 530–562 (1962).

Gruenwald, P. "Growth of the human fetus. I. Normal growth and its variation." *Am. J. Obstet. Gynec.* **94**: 1112–1119 (1966).

Hurley, L. S., G. J. Everson, E. Wooten, and C. W. Asling. "Disproportionate growth in offspring of manganese-deficient rats. I. The long bones." *J. Nutrition* **74**: 274–281 (1961a).

Hurley, L. S., E. Wooten, and G. J. Everson. "Disproportionate growth in offspring of manganese deficient rats. II. Skull, brain and cerebrospinal pressure." *J. Nutrition* **74**: 282–288 (1961b).

Hurley, L. S., and N. E. Volkert. "Pantothenic acid and coenzyme A in the developing guinea pig liver." *Biochim. Biophys. Acta* **104**: 372–376 (1965).

MEDAWAR, P. B. "Size, shape, and age." In: W. E. LE GROS CLARK AND P. B. MEDAWAR, eds., *Essays on Growth and Form.* New York: Oxford University Press, 1945.

SCAMMON, R. E. "The first seriatim study of human growth." *Am. J. Phys. Anthropol.* **10**: 329 (1927).

SMIDT ET AL., in GIROUD, A., *The Nutrition of the Embryo.* Springfield, Ill.: Charles C Thomas, Publisher, 1970.

SUSSMAN, M. *Developmental Biology: Its Cellular and Molecular Foundations,* Part Two, "The Growth of Cells and Cell Populations," pp. 61–101. Englewood Cliffs, N.J.: Prentice-Hall, Inc., 1973.

TIMIRAS, P. *Developmental Physiology.* New York: Macmillan, 1972. Copyright © 1972 by Paola S. Timiras.

WIDDOWSON, E. M. "Growth and composition of the fetus and newborn," pp. 1–6 in N. S. ASSALI, ed., *Biology of Gestation,* Vol. II. New York: Academic Press, 1968.

WINICK, M., AND A. NOBLE. "Quantitative changes in DNA, RNA and protein during prenatal and postnatal growth in the rat." *Dev. Biol.* **12**: 451–466 (1965).

3

Biochemical maturation: changes in body composition and biochemical function

As the embryo, fetus, and young individual develop, important changes occur in both overall size (absolute growth) and body proportions (relative growth), as discussed in Chapter 2. Other important changes take place in body composition and biochemical function.

CHANGES IN BODY COMPOSITION

As the individual grows in total size, many chemical components simply increase in amount. Overall increases in the nitrogen, calcium, and phosphorus content of the body during the prenatal life of a human being are very marked. However, probably more important than the absolute increases are the changes in *relative* concentrations of chemical substances that occur with development.

CHANGES IN RELATIVE CONCENTRATIONS

These changes are exemplified by Table 3–1, where the changes in chemical composition of the human taking place in development are set off against those due to simple increase in size. There is a continual decline in the concentration of water during development. The baby has more nitrogen than the fetus in proportion to its body size, and the adult has proportionately more nitrogen than the baby. The baby has proportionately more calcium than the fetus, and the man shows a very large increase in his proportion of calcium as compared to the baby. Phosphorus also increases much more than does total body size. Since the bone salt is calcium phosphate, it would be expected that calcium and phosphorus would increase together as the skeleton grows and becomes progressively more calcified. Iron and copper are proportionately somewhat lower in concentration in the man than in the baby, since the newborn has a relatively high concentration of these elements.

TABLE 3–1 CHANGES TAKING PLACE IN DEVELOPMENT, SET OFF AGAINST THOSE DUE TO A SIMPLE INCREASE IN SIZE

	Water, kg	*Total N, g*	*Na, m-equiv.*	*K, m-equiv.*	*Cl, m-equiv.*	*Ca, g*	*Mg, g*	*P, g*	*Fe, mg*	*Cu, mg*	*Zn, mg*
A fetus weighing 175 g contains	0.154	2.45	18.2	7.4	13.7	0.60	0.024	0.42	9.25	0.575	3.50
This fetus × 20 would contain	3.08	49	364	148	274	12.0	0.48	8.4	185	11.5	70
A baby weighing 3.5 kg contains	2.4	66	243	150	160	28.2	0.76	16.2	262	13.7	53
This baby ×20 would contain	48	1,320	4,860	3,000	3,200	564	15.2	324	5,240	274	1,060
A man weighing 70 kg contains	42	2,000	5,150	4,050	2,940	1,320	27.4	740	4,350	100	1,640

From McCance and Widdowson, 1961.

The same kind of relationships can be seen in Table 3–2, which shows the concentration of nitrogen in human organs and tissues as an index of their chemical maturation. Nitrogen does not occur in the various tissues in the same concentration in the fetus, the newborn, and the adult. The concentration of nitrogen is higher in the newborn than in the fetus, and highest of all in the adult.

TABLE 3–2 CHEMICAL MATURATION OF THE ORGANS AND TISSUES AS INDICATED BY THE CONCENTRATION OF NITROGEN IN THEM[a]

Tissue	*Fetus, 20–24 Weeks*	*Full-term Newborn*	*Adult*
Skeletal muscle	1.48	2.07	3.08
Skin	1.19	2.65	5.30
Heart	1.40	1.96	2.29
Liver	2.21	2.26	2.82
Kidneys	1.42	1.92	2.45
Brain	0.84	0.93	1.71

[a]In g/100 g fresh tissue.

From Widdowson, 1968.

A change takes place also in the percentages of fat and water in the human fetus in relation to fetal age (Figure 3–1). The concentration of water continues to decrease through the latter part of gestation and diminishes even further after birth. Fat concentration, however, rises during the latter part of the prenatal period. There are also differences in concentrations of extracellular and intracellular water with age (Figure 3–2). During the development of the fetus, the proportion of extracellular water decreases while that of intracellular water increases.

SPECIES DIFFERENCES

Such changes in body composition vary in different species. The newborn human and guinea pig have higher levels of body fat than do the pig and the rat (Table 3–3). The guinea pig has a very high concentration of fat in the liver just before birth, but it decreases rapidly after birth (Figure 3–3). This characteristic is probably related to the maturity of the guinea pig at birth. Similar changes can be seen in the glycogen content of the liver. The amount of glycogen in the human liver increases markedly before birth and then falls rapidly after birth (Figure 3–4), being used up quickly when the neonate has to depend on it for energy. This has also been found in the pig.

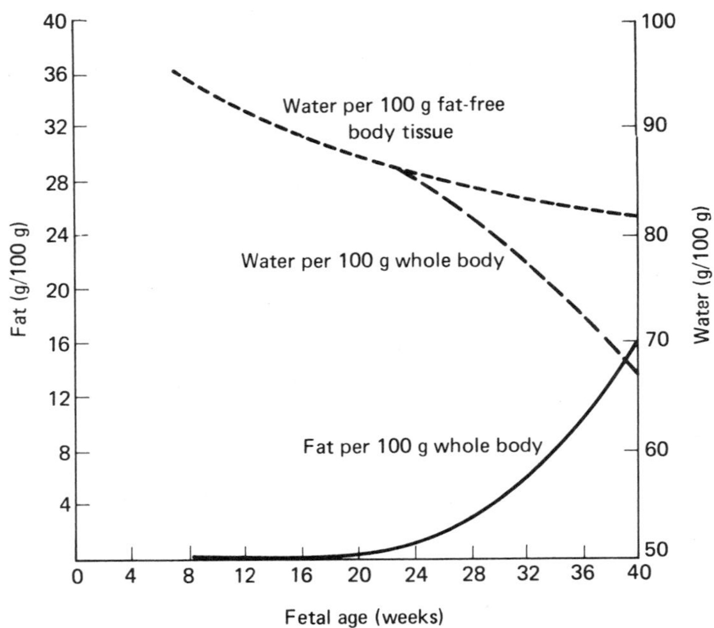

From Widdowson, 1968.

Figure 3–1 Percentages of fat and water in the human fetus in relation to fetal age.

Figure 3–2 Extracellular and intracellular water in the fat-free body tissue of the fetus.

From Widdowson, 1968.

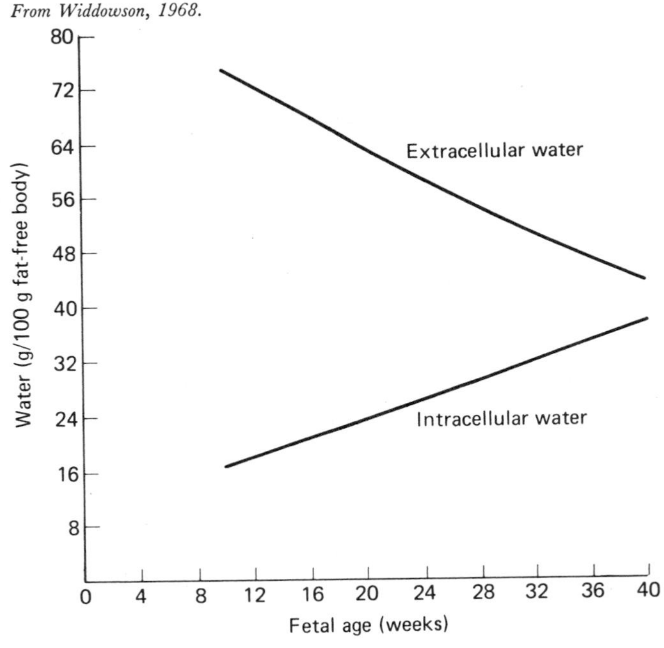

TABLE 3–3 MEAN PERCENTAGE OF FAT IN THE BODIES OF NEWLY BORN MAMMALS

Species	*Fat, g/100 g*
Human	16
Guinea pig	10
Grey seal	9
Rabbit	4.0
Mouse	2.1
Cat	1.8
Dog	1.4
Pig	1.1
Rat	1.1

From Widdowson, 1968.

The chemical composition of the body and its alterations during development are of interest not only in themselves and because they help to elucidate the nature of development, but also because they provide a framework upon which the influence of nutrition upon development can be tested. This concept will become increasingly evident as we examine the effects of malnutrition in general and of specific nutrient deficiencies or excesses on the developing organism.

Figure 3–3 Liver fat concentration in developing guinea pigs. Each point represents the mean of from two to ten animals (in most cases, five); each mean represents animals born in from two to six litters. Open circles indicate stock diet; closed circles, complete purified diet.

From Hurley et al., 1965.

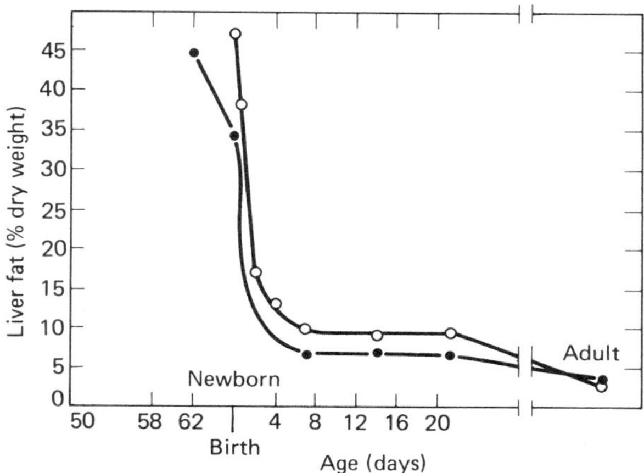

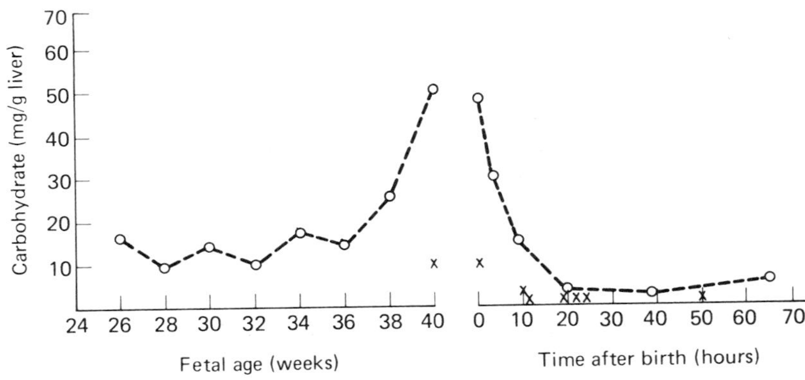

From Shelley and Neligan, Br. Med. Bull. 22: 34–39, 1966.

Figure 3–4 Glycogen in human liver before and after birth. ○ = Babies of normal birth weight for period of gestation; × = individual babies of low birth weight for period of gestation.

CHANGES IN BIOCHEMICAL FUNCTION

The alterations described above in body composition during development are undoubtedly related in part to differences in biochemical function, which of course also changes throughout development of the embryo, fetus, and suckling. Such changes, termed *functional differentiation*, are examined through studies of functional activity. Changes in concentration or activity of enzymes or coenzymes have been studied to elucidate the principles of biochemical or functional maturation.

PANTOTHENIC ACID AND COENZYME A

Pantothenic acid and coenzyme A were studied in livers of guinea pigs during development (Figure 3–5). The concentrations of free and bound pantothenic acid and coenzyme A remained almost stationary from the 33rd to the 58th days of gestation, when a sharp rise in bound pantothenic acid and in coenzyme A occurred which reached its maximum four days after birth. Thus the perinatal period appears to be critical for the guinea pig with respect to pantothenic acid and coenzyme A, as appears also to be the case for liver glycogen. These changes in coenzyme A activity may also be related to the abrupt decline in liver fat level seen during this period (Figure 3–3).

When pregnant guinea pigs were given a pantothenic acid-deficient diet during the tenth (last) week of pregnancy, the period of increase in coenzyme

A activity, their newborn young had higher fat and lower pantothenic acid concentrations than did controls (Figure 3–6). With a maternal dietary deficiency of pantothenic acid during the ninth, seventh, or sixth weeks, newborns had normal liver fat but low liver pantothenic acid levels.

ENZYMIC DIFFERENTIATION

The development of enzymes and the changes in enzyme activity that occur during development are interesting because of their relationship to biochemical maturation. In addition, knowledge of enzymic differentiation may provide information on the mechanism of gene control. In recent years a considerable quantity of data has accumulated on the changes in enzyme activities according to age in various organs of several species. When an enzyme is quantified as a function of age, the developmental history of that enzyme is apparent.

Richter has classified changes in activity of different types of enzymes during development into three groups (Figure 3–7). He postulates that enzymes concerned primarily with growth are most active in the early embryo and produce activity curves of type A. As the embryo develops, enzymes concerned with function give rise to activity curves of type B. Morphological and other changes associated with processes of maturation

Figure 3–5 Pantothenic acid (PA) and coenzyme A in livers of developing guinea pigs from females receiving the complete synthetic diet. Each point represents the mean of from two to nine fetuses or young guinea pigs, in most cases, five.

From Hurley and Volkert, 1965.

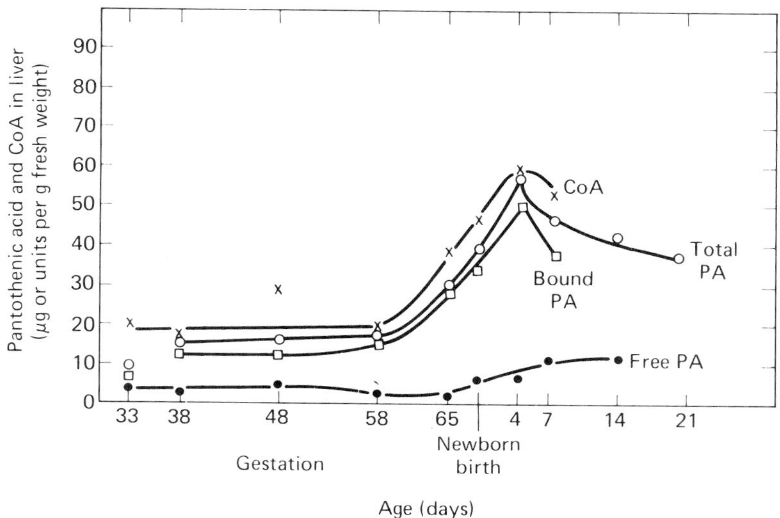

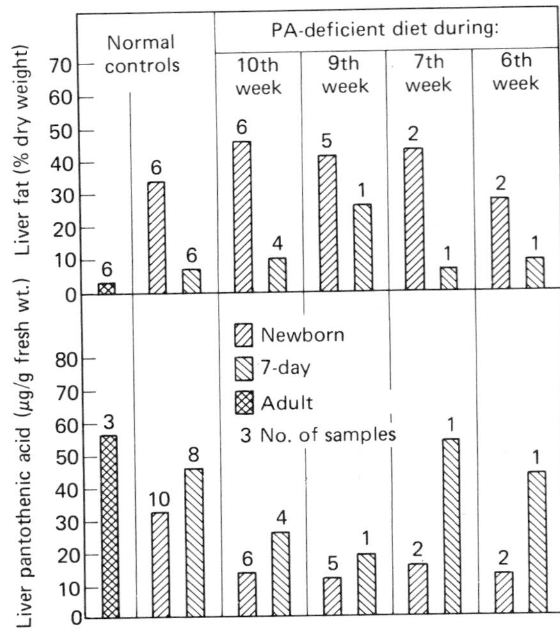

From Hurley et al., 1965.

Figure 3–6 Effect upon the offspring of a transitory dietary deficiency during gestation in guinea pigs. Each bar represents the mean of several samples, the number of which is shown above the bars.

Figure 3–7 Changes in enzymic activity during development. Curves of type A are obtained for enzymes concerned mainly with growth. Curves of type B are given by enzymes concerned in functional activity. Curves of type C are obtained for enzymes concerned with processes of maturation.

From Richter, 1961.

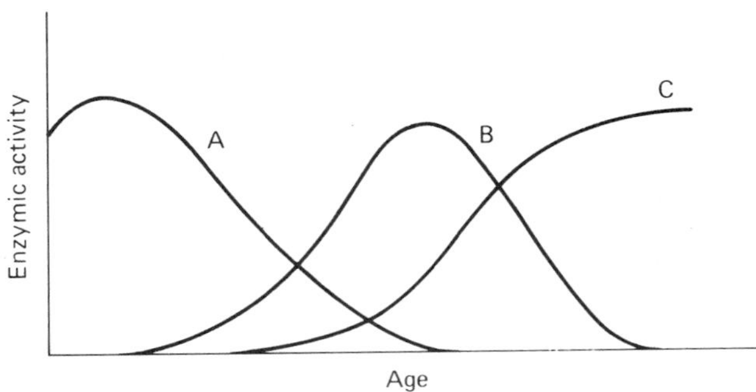

give rise to enzymes whose activity curves may be classified as curve C. Thus, according to this scheme, changes in metabolism during development may be considered to be indicated by ascending and descending curves of enzymic activity, which gradually changes from one metabolic pattern to the next.

The developmental history of enzymes of the liver is better known than that of other tissues. Greengard has pointed out two important features of these developmental histories of liver enzymes in the rat. First, enzyme levels do not increase evenly during development, but all or most of the adult level accumulates suddenly within hours or days. Second, the appearance of new enzymes or the increased activity of enzymes previously present does not occur throughout the developmental period, but rather takes place in clusters. In rat liver the appearance of new enzyme activity can thus be classified into four periods: the enzymes of cluster I, an early period, appear to be mandatory for growth, are present in all early fetal tissues, and decrease in amount towards the end of gestation. Cluster II occurs during late fetal life (the 16th to 22nd day of gestation), cluster III on the first day after birth, and cluster IV in the third postnatal week. Greengard has called the enzymes that emerge during these last three periods the "late fetal," "neonatal," and "late suckling" clusters (Figure 3–8).

Greengard has also studied the control of enzymic differentiation. Certain enzymes of the neonatal cluster could be evoked prematurely by the injection of glucagon (Figure 3–9) on the 20th or 21st day of gestation. These

Figure 3–8 Typical enzymes of the late fetal, neonatal and late suckling cluster of rat liver: (a) UDPG-glycogen glucosyltransferase; (b) phosphoenolpyruvate carboxylase; (c) tryptophan oxygenase; 0: birth. The broken line refers to protein concentration.

From Greengard, 1971.

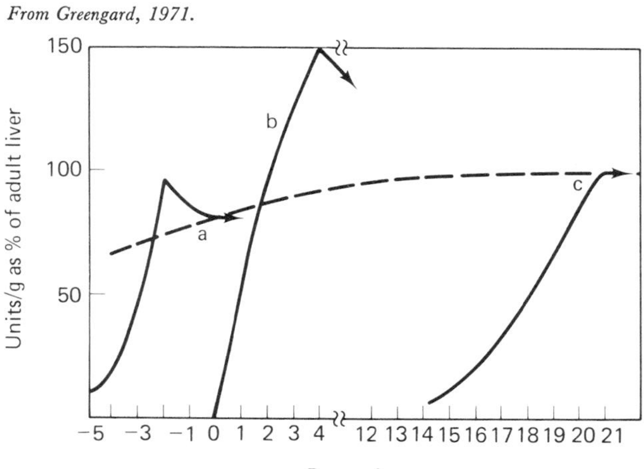

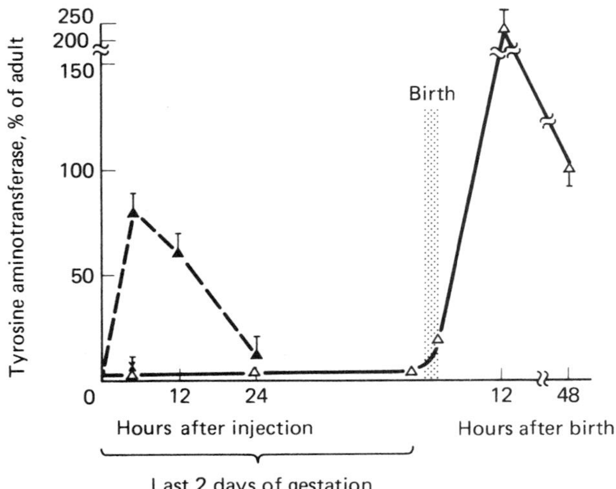

From Greengard, 1971.

Figure 3–9 The premature evocation of tyrosine aminotransferase. Rats were untreated (—△—) or injected with glucagon (—▲—) or with glucagon plus actinomycin (X).

observations suggest that the normal hypoglycemia of the newborn causes release of glucagon which then triggers the appearance of certain enzymes in the normal neonate. Hormonal stimulation may also be involved in the emergence of enzymes in the late fetal cluster and in the late suckling cluster.

Another line of investigation that has demonstrated the changing en-

Figure 3–10 Changing population of LDH molecules in developing heart muscle of the mouse. The numbers in the abscissa refer to days before or after birth.

From Markert and Ursprung, 1971.

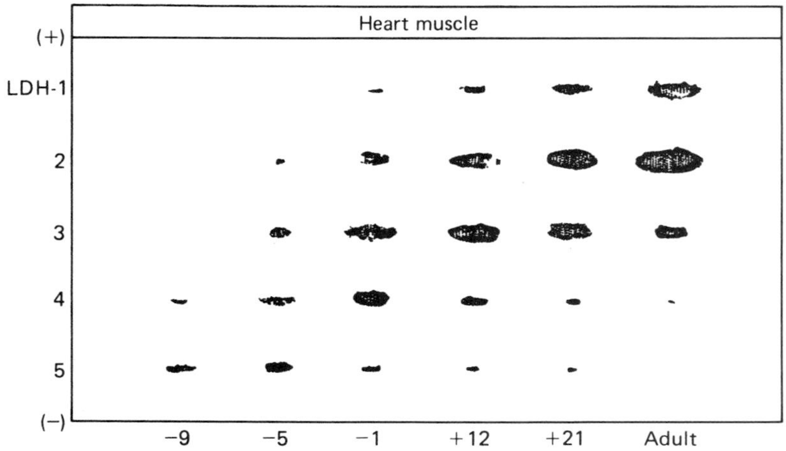

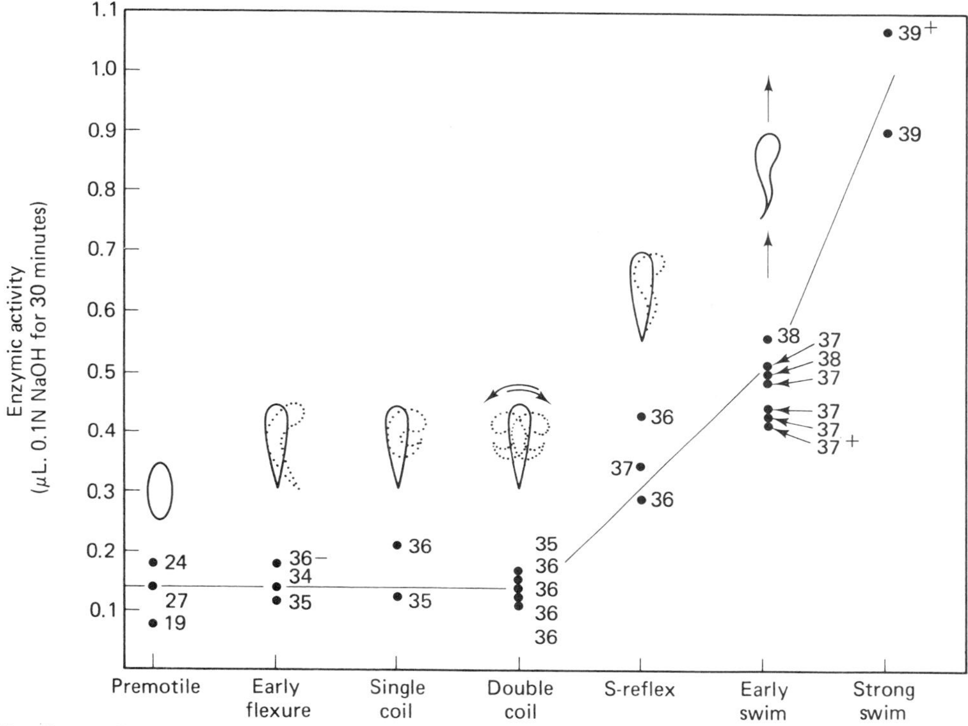

From *Sawyer, 1943.*

Figure 3–11 The relation between development of cholinesterase and neuromuscular activity in *Amblystoma punctatum*. Ordinate denotes enzyme activity; abscissa, sequence of behavioral manifestations.

zyme patterns in the developing animal comes from studies of isozymes, especially those of lactic dehydrogenase. Figure 3–10 shows the electrophoretic pattern of LDH isozymes from developing heart muscle according to age.

The relationship between enzyme differentiation and function has been studied in many systems; for example, urea cycle enzymes were studied in the rat and pig and the relationship to function was attempted. Likewise, numerous studies have been made of the development of enzymes of carbohydrate metabolism. One of the earliest studies demonstrating the relationship of enzyme activity and function showed a correlation between increasing cholinesterase activity and neuromuscular function in *Amblystoma punctatum* (Figure 3–11). In recent intensive studies of the development of rat pancreas, morphological development was correlated with biochemical function in appearance and activity of pancreatic enzymes and hormones (Rutter et al.).

References and Supplementary Readings

Greengard, O. "Enzymic differentiation in mammalian tissues." *Essays Biochem.* **7**: 159–205 (1971).

Hurley, L. S., and N. E. Volkert. "Pantothenic acid and coenzyme A in the developing guinea pig liver." *Biochim. Biophys. Acta* **104**: 372–376 (1965).

Hurley, L. S., N. E. Volkert, and J. T. Eichner. "Pantothenic acid deficiency in pregnant and non-pregnant guinea pigs, with special reference to effects on the fetus." *J. Nutrition* **86**: 201–208 (1965).

Markert, C. L., and H. Ursprung. *Developmental Genetics.* Englewood Cliffs, N.J.: Prentice-Hall, Inc., 1971.

McCance, R. A., and E. M. Widdowson. "Mineral metabolism of the fetus and newborn." *Brit. Med. Bull.* **17**: 132–136 (1961).

Richter, D. "Enzymic development during early development." *Brit. Med. Bull.* **17**: 118–121 (1961).

Rutter, W. J., R. L. Pictet, and P. W. Morris. "Toward molecular mechanisms of developmental processes." *Ann. Rev. Biochem.* **42**: 601–646 (1973).

Sawyer, C. H. "Cholinesterase and the behavior problem." *J. Exp. Zool.* **92**: 1–29 (1943).

Widdowson, E. M. "Growth and composition of the fetus and newborn." In: N. S. Assali, ed., *Biology of Gestation.* Vol. II. *The Fetus and Neonate,* pp. 1–49. New York: Academic Press, 1968.

4

Differentiation and morphogenesis

Development of a new individual begins with the fertilization of an ovum by a spermatozoon. The resulting union of the male and female chromosomal material marks the beginning of pregnancy and of prenatal development. In this chapter we will consider in an abbreviated and synoptic manner some aspects of differentiation and embryogenesis, using the human as a model.

After ovulation, the ovum may be fertilized within 12 to 24 hours. Spermatozoa may be viable for three to four days in the female reproductive tract, but after the first day the chance of fertilization diminishes. Fertilization takes place in the distal third of the Fallopian tube. Spermatozoa arrive there about 10 hours after coitus.

Fertilization and the subsequent union of the two germ cells has immensely important consequences for the new individual besides initiation of its life cycle. Reconstitution of the diploid number of chromosomes occurs, doubling the number that is contained in each of the gametes (the ovum and the sperm). In the human, the diploid cell contains 46 chromosomes as compared with half that number in each of the two haploid germ cells. Fertilization also results in sex determination. The sex of the embryo is determined by the type of sperm that fertilizes the ovum—either an X-bearing sperm, which in combination with the X-bearing ovum develops into a female, or a Y-bearing sperm producing an XY zygote, which develops into a male. Fertilization also forms the basis of an inheritance from two parents, since half the chromosomes come from the mother and the other half from the father. This mechanism results in variability of the new individuals. Finally, fertilization activates the ovum and initiates development by stimulating a series of rapid cell divisions called cleavage.

Through cleavage, the fertilized ovum reaches the morula (from the Latin for mulberry) stage (Figure 4–1). This occurs about the fourth day. The morula is composed of 12 to 16 cells called blastomeres. Fluid passes from the uterine cavity into the morula, and as the fluid increases, it separates the cells into an outer layer, the trophoblast, and a group of cells called the inner cell mass or embryoblast. Soon a fluid-filled central cavity is formed;

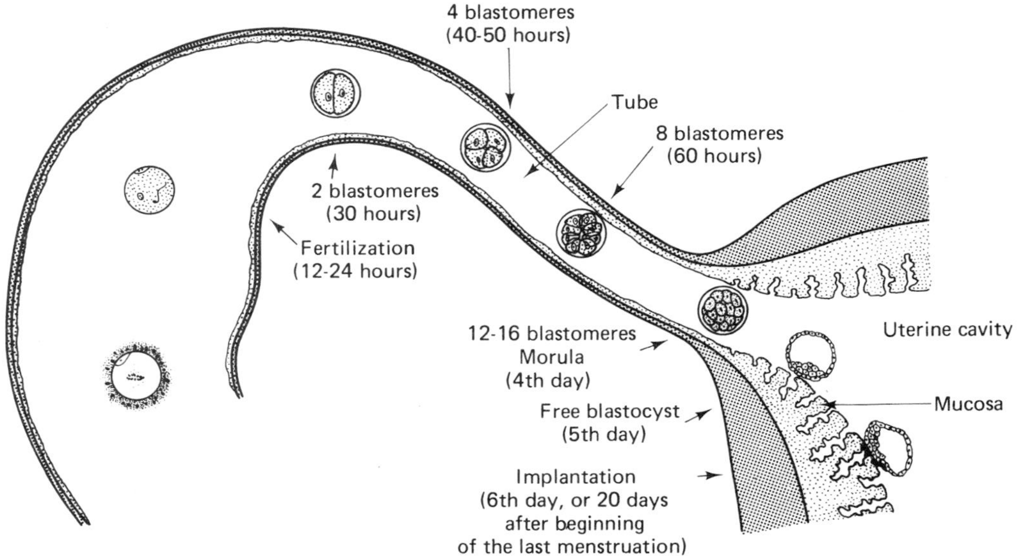

From Tuchmann-Duplessis et al., 1972.

Figure 4–1 Movement of the egg in the Fallopian tube in the human.

the egg is now called a blastocyst. The blastocyst lies free in the uterine secretions for about two days.

From the unfertilized ovum through the morula stage, there is no increase in volume of the egg; there is simply cell division, so that the volume of the cells composing the young embryo decreases as division occurs. On the sixth day, or 20 days after the beginning of the last menstruation, the blastocyst begins to implant into the uterine mucosa (Figure 4–2).

During the second week of prenatal life in the human, together with the beginning of placentation (see Chapter 5), the blastocyst undergoes development with differentiation of the endoderm and then the ectoderm (Figure 4–3). These two layers form the embryonic disc.

The formation of the third layer of the embryo, the mesoderm, takes place through the process of gastrulation, which occurs at the beginning of the third week. The mesoderm is formed through a process of cellular migration. Ectodermal cells glide downward and grow into the cavity of the embryo, differentiating into the mesoderm as they spread out. The primitive streak, which is seen along the longitudinal axis of the embryo, is the morphologic indication characteristic of gastrulation; it is the result of the movement of these cells.

The ectoderm, the mesoderm, and the endoderm are the three basic layers of the embryo from which all of its organs and structures are formed. Table 4–2 shows the derivatives of the three germ layers in the adult body.

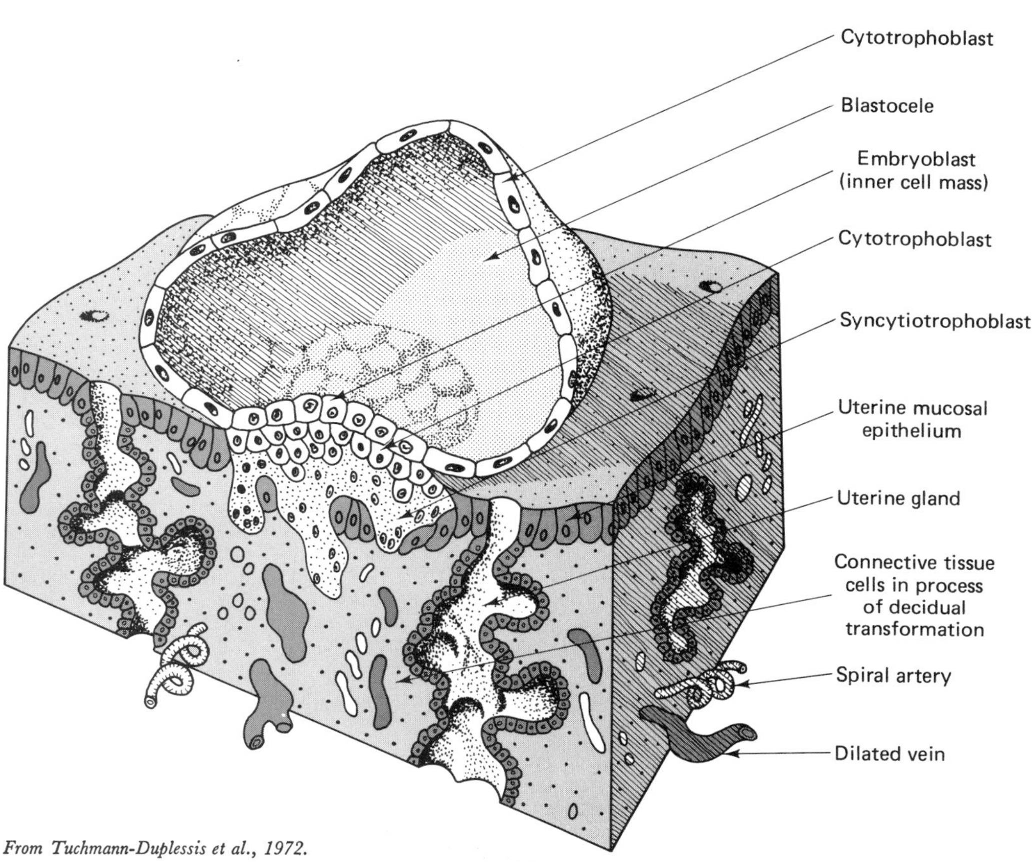

From Tuchmann-Duplessis et al., 1972.

Figure 4–2 Diagrammatic relief representation of the blastocyst in process of implantation in the uterine mucosa.

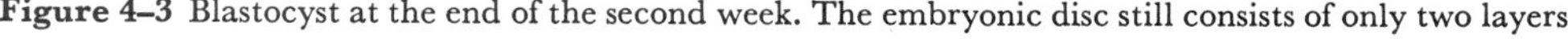

Figure 4–3 Blastocyst at the end of the second week. The embryonic disc still consists of only two layers.

From Tuchmann-Duplessis et al., 1972.

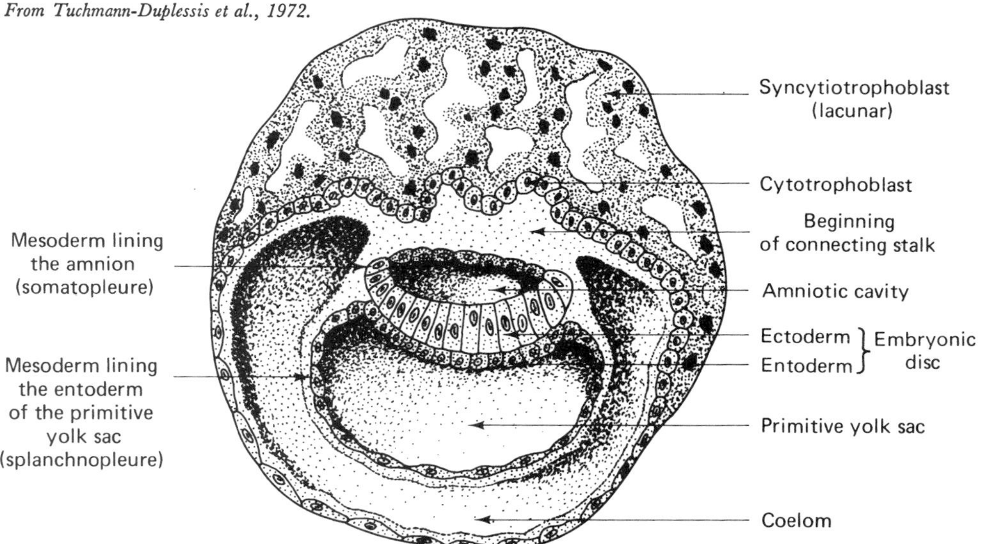

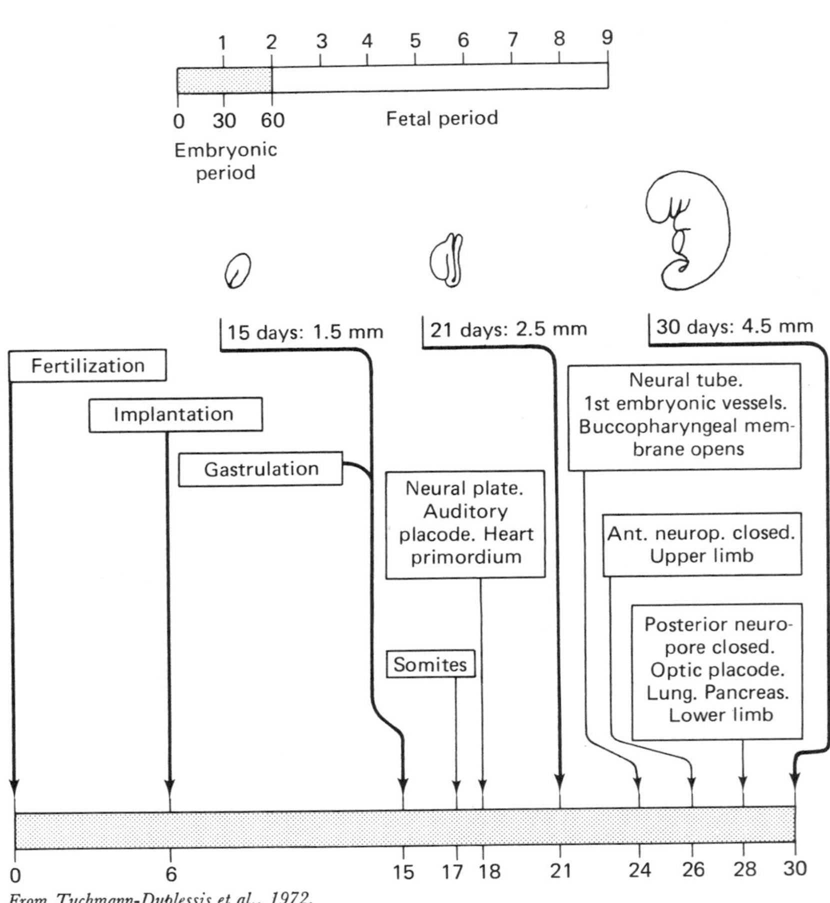

From Tuchmann-Duplessis et al., 1972.

Figure 4–4 Stages of embryonic development, fertilization to 30 days.

TABLE 4–1 AVERAGE SIZE OF EMBRYO AND FETUS IN CROWN-RUMP LENGTH

Age	*Length, mm*
2 weeks	1.5
3 weeks	2.5
4 weeks	5
5 weeks	8.5
7 weeks	20
2 months	33
3 months	95
4 months	135
6 months	230
9 months	335[a]

[a]500 mm for crown-heel length at 9 months.

From Tuchmann-Duplessis et al., 1972.

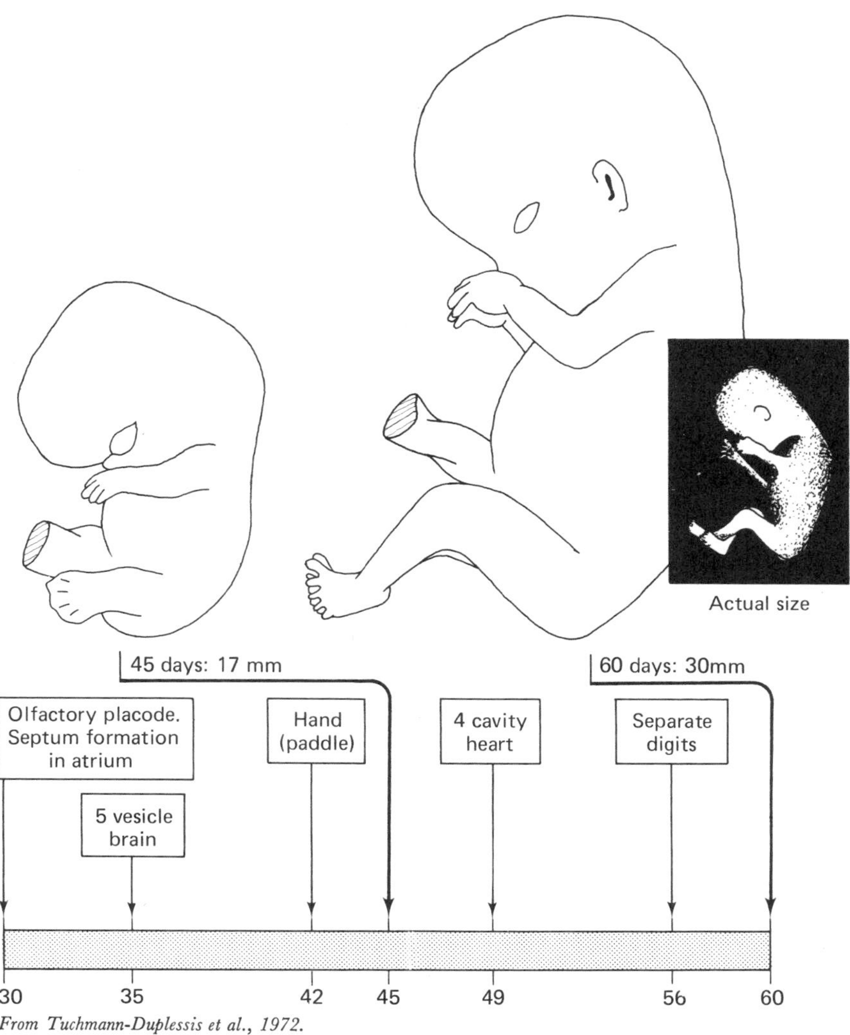

From Tuchmann-Duplessis et al., 1972.

Figure 4–5 Stages of embryonic development, 30 to 60 days.

Shortly after formation of the three germ layers, the notochord is formed. This structure serves as the primary skeleton of the three-layer embryo and eventually disappears as the definitive skeleton is formed.

The stages of embryonic development are illustrated diagrammatically in Figures 4–4 and 4–5. Figure 4–6 shows photographs of actual human embryos at six stages of development, and Figure 4–7 shows a photograph of a human fetus at 3½ months of gestation. To put the size of these embryonic and fetal stages in perspective, the crown-rump length of human embryos and fetuses from two weeks of gestation to term is shown in Table 4–1. Comparative development of various species is summarized in Table 4–3 and Figure 4–8.

TABLE 4–2 CHANNELS OF DEVELOPMENT OF THE VERTEBRATE EMBRYO

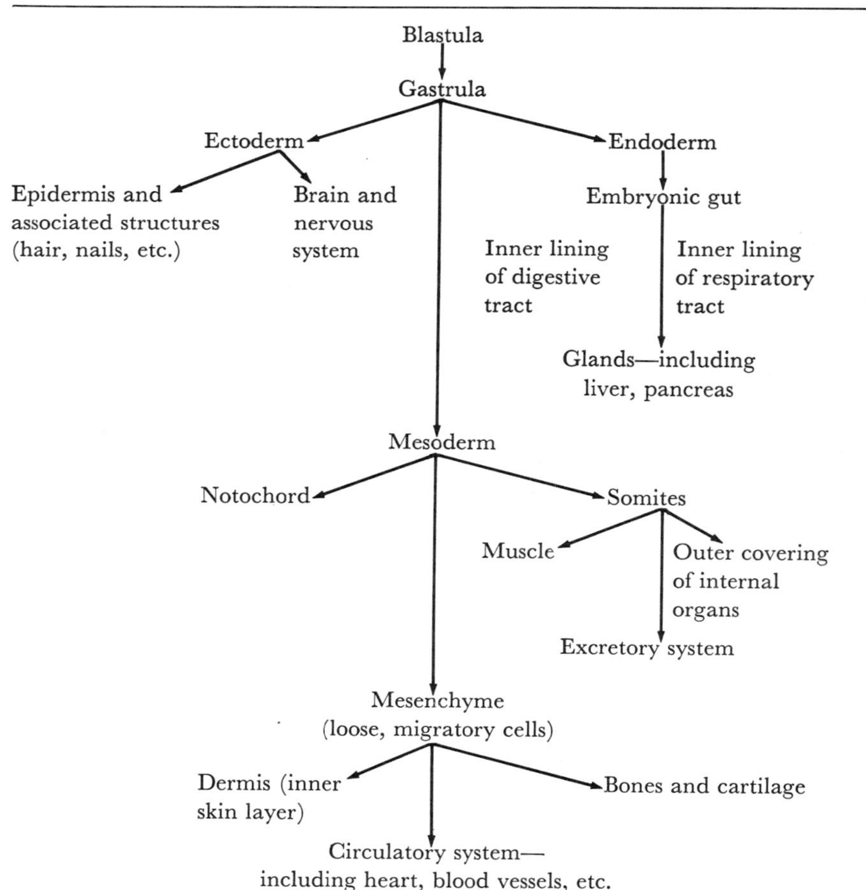

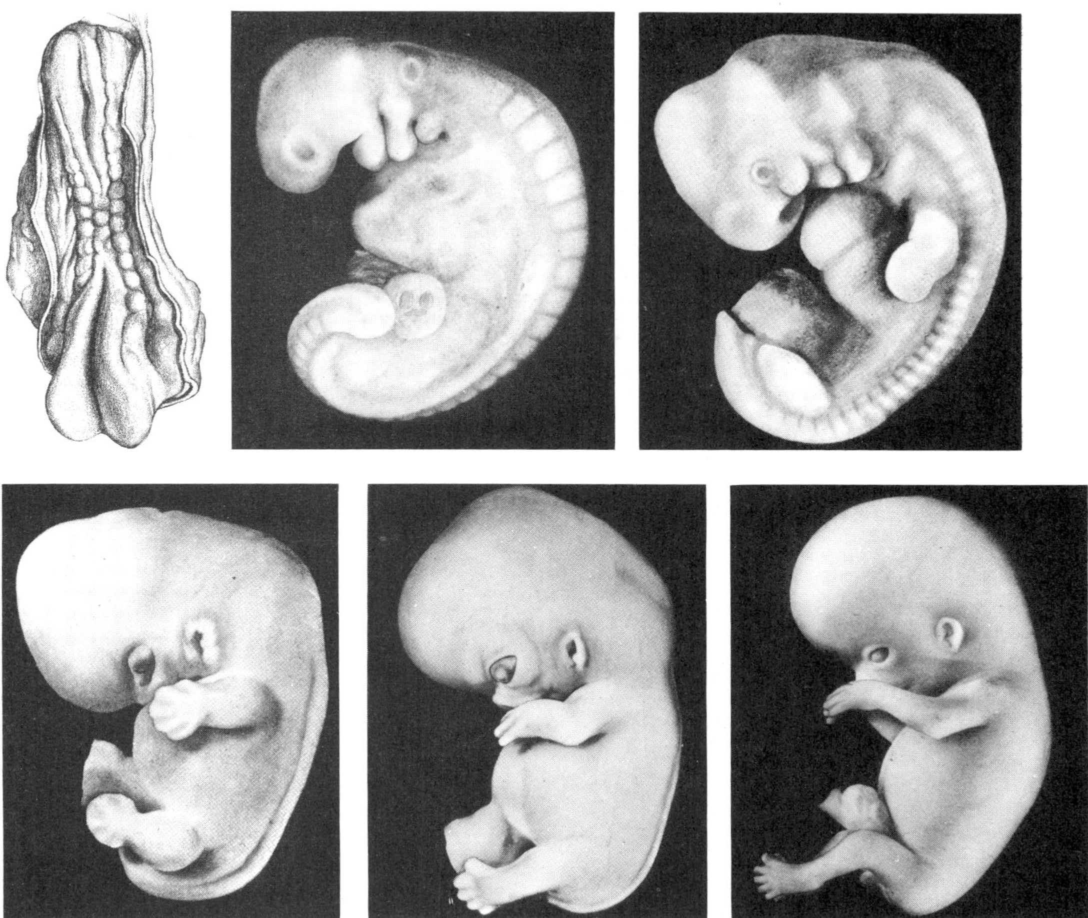

From Wilson, 1973.

Figure 4–6 Human embryonic development. (a) Stage X: 22–24 days; 1.5–3.5 mm; 4–12 somites. Neural tube begins closure, optic sulcus present, otic placode forms, first branchial arch visible, first and second aortic arches seen, bilateral cardiac primordia unite in single tube, first heart movement (?), pleural and peritoneal cavities begin, oral pit and pharynx indicated, hind gut begins, first pronephroi (redrawn surface view of Payne embryo, Payne, 1925). (b) Stage XII: 27–29 days; 3–5 mm; 21–29 somites. Third branchial arch appears, third aortic arch forms, arm bud appears, posterior neuropore closing, yolk stalk constricting, thyroid and laryngotracheal buds evaginate, dorsal pancreas appears, common bile duct and gall bladder form, mesonephric tubules and ducts begin, blood circulation begins, body axis C-shaped (after embryo No. 5923, Streeter, 1942). (c) Stage XV: 36–37 days; 6–9 mm. Lens vesicle closes, olfactory pits develop, cerebral evagination seen, aortopulmonary septal ridges forming, atrioventricular endocardial cushions forming, sixth aortic arch and pulmonary artery appear, secondary bronchi indicated, ventral pancreas seen, midgut loop projects ventrally, caecum dilates, musculoskeletal condensations in arm buds, hand plate evident (after embryo No. 3512, Streeter, 1948). (d) Stage XVIII: 42–43 days; 12–16 mm. Facial primordia united, lids begin, auricular hillocks forming auricle, digital rays of foot appear, semicircular ducts forming, primary cardiac partitioning complete, Mullerian ducts begin, renal collecting ducts appear, active proliferation within gonads, urorectal septum complete, genital tubercle prominent, muscles identifiable in arm (after embryo No. 7007, Streeter, 1948). (e) Stage XX: 46–47 days; 17–22 mm. Optic fibers reach brain, choroid plexus begins, tail regressing, palate folds present beside tongue, future ossification centers indicated by clearing of cartilage, anal membrane ruptures (after embryo No. 8157, Streeter, 1951). (f) Stage XXIII: 52–53 days; 24–30 mm. Palatal closure begins, diaphragm forms, secretory tubules appear in kidney, ciliary body forming in eye, genital ducts undergoing sexual differentiation, midgut hernia may be withdrawn from umbilical cord, first marrow in humerus (after embryo No. 4570, Streeter, 1951).

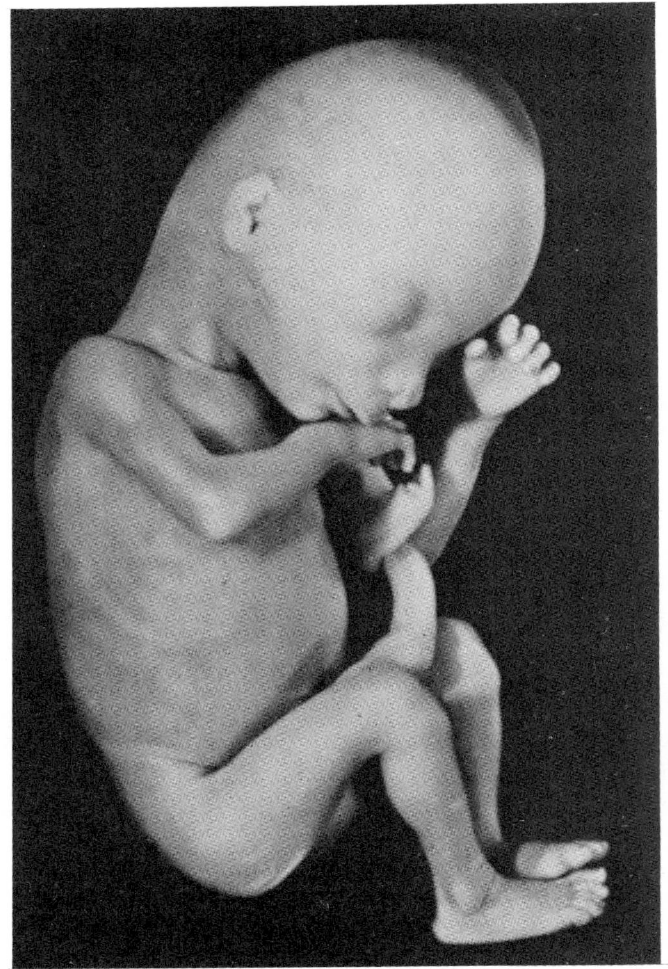

From Tuchmann-Duplessis et al., 1972.

Figure 4–7 Human fetus, 12 cm ($3\frac{1}{2}$ months). Actual size.

In order to compare development of different species, we need some idea of the time periods during gestation at which similar stages occur. Witschi divided prenatal development of vertebrate embryos into 36 standard stages. Streeter similarly classified development of human embryos into a series of 23 "horizons," which can be correlated with Witschi's stages. Figure 4–8 shows these stages for man and for two commonly used laboratory animals, the rat and chick.

TABLE 4–3 ORGANOGENESIS AND RELATED EVENTS DURING INTRAUTERINE DEVELOPMENT OF SEVERAL MAMMALS[a,b]

Species	*Implantation Begins*	*Primitive Streak Established*	*Organogenesis* Primordia Beginning	*Organogenesis* Largely Completed[c]	*Usual Time of Delivery*
Hamster	4.5–5	6	7	14	16–17
Mouse	4.5–5	7	7.5	16	20–21
Rat	5.5–6	8.5	9	17	21–22
Rabbit	7	6.5	7	20	30–32
Guinea pig	6	10	11	25	65–68
Pig	10–12	11	12	34	110–116
Sheep	10	13	14	35	145–152
Ferret	10–12	13	14	—[d]	40–43
Cat	12–13	—[d]	—[d]	30	60–65
Dog	13–14	13	14	30	60–65
Rhesus monkey	9	18	20	45	164–170
Baboon	9	19	22	47	172–178
Man	6.5–7	18	20	55	260–280

[a]From various sources.

[b]Timing is in estimated days after fertilization.

[c]For want of a more definite end point, closure of the palate was taken as the criterion of completed organogenesis, but it should be noted that such organs as the brain and the genitalia undergo appreciable structural change after this time.

[d]Little information available.

From Wilson, 1973.

NUTRITIONAL ASPECTS OF EMBRYOGENESIS

Before implantation of the embryo into the uterus, the only nutrient sources available are its reserves and the secretions of the Fallopian tube and the uterus. In mammalian ova, however, which have very little yolk, the nutrient reserves are small. Although few studies have been made, there is some evidence that maternal nutrition may influence the preimplantation embryo through alterations in the composition of uterine fluid (see the section on zinc in Chapter 15).

During the second and third weeks of gestation, while placental circulation is becoming established, the yolk sac (see Figure 4–9) apparently plays a role in the transfer of nutrients to the embryo. The yolk sac is also important as the site of hematopoiesis from the third week of gestation until the sixth

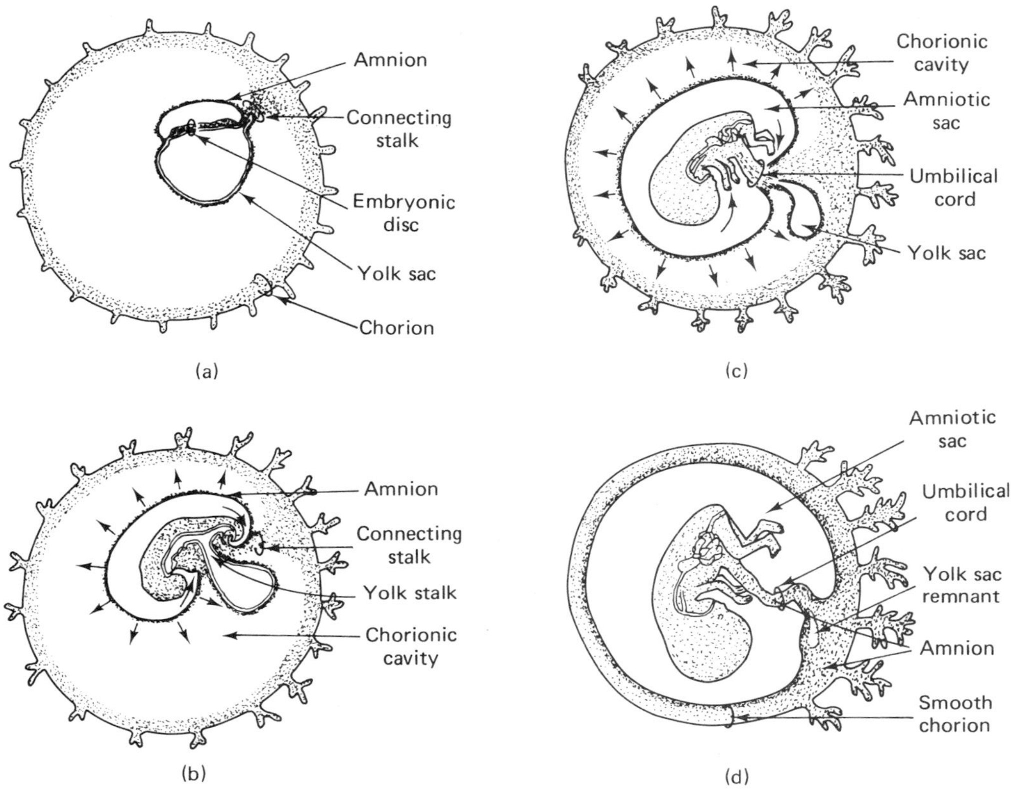

From Monie, 1965.

Figure 4–8 Comparative development of various species.

week, when blood formation begins in the liver. In the fourth week, part of the yolk sac is incorporated into the embryo as the primitive gut, eventually forming the digestive tract.

The most important mechanism for nutrition of the embryo and fetus is, of course, placental transfer (see Chapter 5), in terms of both its duration during pregnancy and the amount of nutrients transferred. In addition to the placenta and the yolk sac, however, there is a third source of nutrition for the developing individual, the amniotic fluid. The embryo floats freely in the amniotic fluid, which fills the amniotic cavity. This fluid performs several mechanical functions. It prevents the gelatinous embryo from sticking to the amnion, maintains a constant temperature for the embryo, and provides a cushion for physical jolts from the exterior. In addition, it allows the young fetus to move freely.

Most of the amniotic fluid is derived from maternal blood, but the fetus

Gestation stages

Stand.		7-8		12		16		18		25		35-36	Witschi stages
Horiz.		III-IV		VIII		XI		XII		XIV		XXIII +	Streeter horizons
Rat	←6→	6	←2.5→	8.5	←2→	10.5	←1→	11.5	←1→	12.5	←9.5→	22	Days
Chick	←1.5→			1.5	←1.5→	3	←0.25→	3.25	←1.75→	5	←16→	21	Days
Man	←6.5→	6.5	←12.5→	19	←8→	27	←2→	29	←7→	36	←231→	267	Days
	Fertilization	Implantation		Prim. Streak		Neurula		Tail bud		End of emb. phase		Birth	

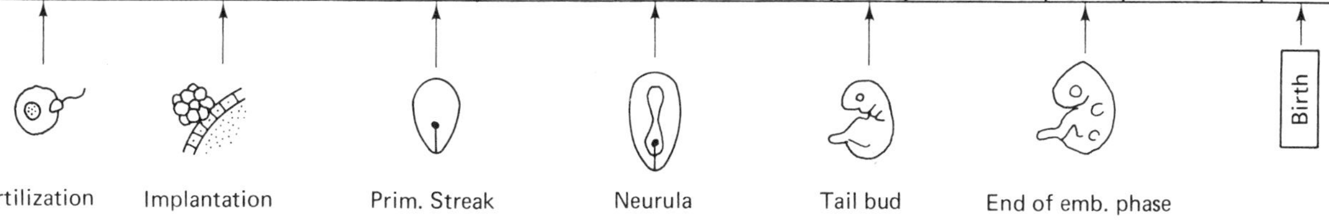

From Moore, 1977.

Figure 4–9 Drawings illustrating how the amnion becomes the outer covering of the umbilical cord and how the yolk sac is partially incorporated into the embryo as the primitive gut: (a) three weeks, (b) four weeks, (c) 10 weeks, (d) 20 weeks.

also contributes to it by its excretion of urine. The volume of amniotic fluid varies from about 30 ml at 10 weeks to 350 ml at 20 weeks, and is maximal at about 1000 ml at term. There is a large and rapid exchange of fluid in both directions between the fetal and maternal circulations. The contribution of fetal components to the amniotic fluid is the basis of its use in fetal diagnosis. Amniocentesis, the removal of a sample of amniotic fluid and its analysis, is used to diagnose a number of conditions such as abnormal chromosomes (or even normal ones—the sex of the fetus), genetic diseases such as enzyme defects, and certain congenital malformations.

Amniotic fluid may also be significant as a source of fetal nutrition. It is swallowed by the fetus (up to 400 ml/day) and absorbed by the gastrointestinal tract. Very little is known, however, regarding the nutrients involved and their magnitude or importance to the fetus. Figure 4–9 illustrates the relationships of the embryo and fetus to the yolk sac and amniotic fluid in the amniotic sac.

References and Supplementary Readings

BALINSKY, B. I. *An Introduction to Embryology.* Philadelphia: W. B. Saunders, 1970.

MONIE, I. W. "Comparative development of rat, chick and human embryos." *Proc. Teratol. Workshop, 2nd, Berkeley, Calif.* 1965.

MOORE, K. L. *The Developing Human, Clinically Oriented.* Philadelphia: W. B. Saunders, 1977.

SHERMAN, M. T. *Concepts in Mammalian Embryogenesis Embryology*, 2nd ed., Cambridge: The MIT Press, 1977.

TUCHMANN-DUPLESSIS, H., G. DAVID, AND P. HAEGEL. Translated by L. S. HURLEY. *Illustrated Human Embryology.* Vol. I: *Embryogenesis.* New York: Springer-Verlag, 1972.

WILSON, J. G. *Environment and Birth Defects.* New York: Academic Press, 1973.

5

The placenta and placental transfer

THE PLACENTA

PLACENTAL MORPHOLOGY

The placenta is a transitory oval or discoid spongy structure that acts to transport substances between the tissues of the mother and those of the embryo. The placenta has two components. One, the fetal portion, develops from the trophoblast, and the other, the maternal portion, is formed from the endometrium. The placenta, in combination with the fetal membranes (the chorion, the amnion, the yolk sac, and the allantois) is responsible for the protection, nutrition, respiration, and excretion of the embryo and fetus. At parturition (birth) the fetal membranes and the placenta are separated from the uterus and are expelled.

The placenta develops from the trophoblast, which first appears at the blastocyst stage of embryonic development, about five days after fertilization in the human embryo (see Chapter 4). On the sixth day after fertilization the blastocyst attaches itself to the endometrial epithelium. Implantation of the embryo into the endometrial wall begins when the trophoblastic cells invade the endometrial epithelium by means of their proteolytic activity. By this time the trophoblast has differentiated into two layers, an inner cellular layer called the cytotrophoblast (cellular trophoblast) and an external syncytiotrophoblast, which consists of a multinucleated layer in which intercellular boundaries are lacking. The fingerlike projections of the syncytiotrophoblast penetrate the endometrial epithelium as the blastocyst "burrows" into the wall of the uterus. By seven days after fertilization the blastocyst is implanted in the endometrial lining of the uterus (see Figure 5–1).

As the trophoblast cells invade the endometrium, they tap uterine blood vessels, creating lacunae (spaces), which become filled with maternal blood from ruptured capillaries. The lacunae expand and eventually join to become

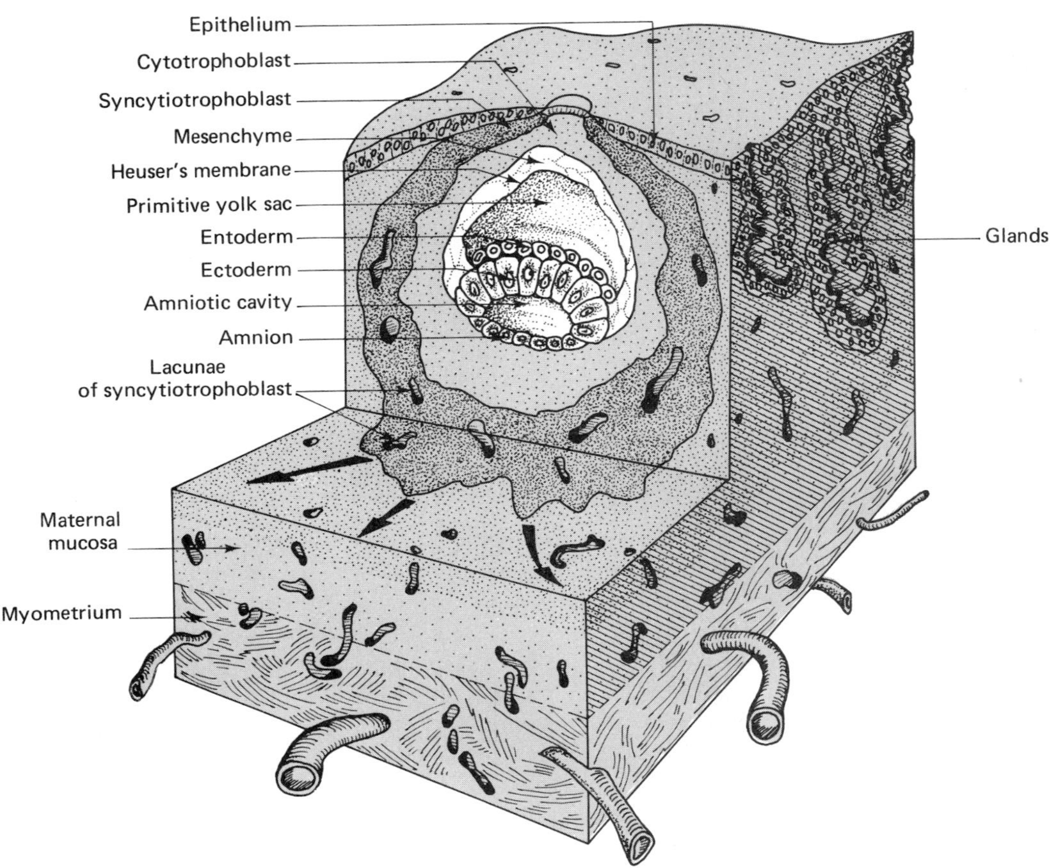

From Tuchmann-Duplessis et al., 1972.

Figure 5–1 Penetration of the blastocyst in the mucosa. Proliferation and progression of the trophoblast.

a complicated labyrinth separated by columns of trophoblastic tissue known as villi. The villi begin to appear about the 13th day. A villus consists of a mesenchymal core surrounded by a double layer of cyto- and syncytiotrophoblast. In the middle of the mesenchyme, vascular islets appear, the beginning of the future fetal circulation. In contrast, the lacunae, which are now intervillous spaces, are already sites of intense maternal circulation. The villus develops a treelike form (Figure 5–2). Some branches of the villi make contact with the maternal tissue, and are called anchoring villi; others remain free in the intravillous spaces, floating villi. There are 20 to 30 large villous trunks or trees, which correspond to lobes seen on the maternal side of the placenta. Each tree with its branches floats in the space partitioned laterally by the placental septa (Figure 5–3).

The blood of the mother and the embryo never mix, since they are always separated by the placental membrane (see below). The blood is carried to and from the site of placental transfer by the umbilical veins and arteries (see Figure 5–4). The structure of the placenta is intimately related to its function. Although the uterine and embryonic tissues are distinctly separate, they are extremely interdigitated, which increases the surface area for the maximum amount of transfer of nutrients from the mother to the fetus.

TYPES OF PLACENTAS

The type of placental connection between the mother and the fetus varies with different species. The human placenta is of the hemochorial type. The fetal tissue (chorion) is directly in contact with the maternal blood. In the hemochorial type of placenta, the placental membrane consists of only three layers, the syncytiotrophoblast, connective tissue, and vascular fetal

Figure 5–2 Placental villus from second to fourth month.

From Tuchmann-Duplessis et al., 1972.

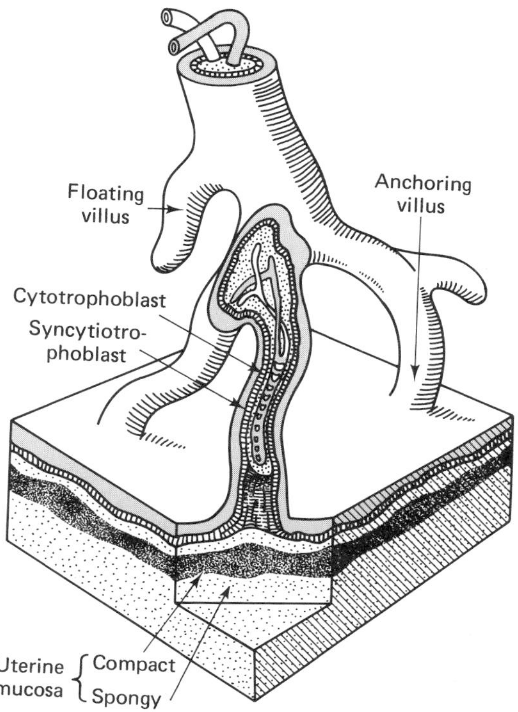

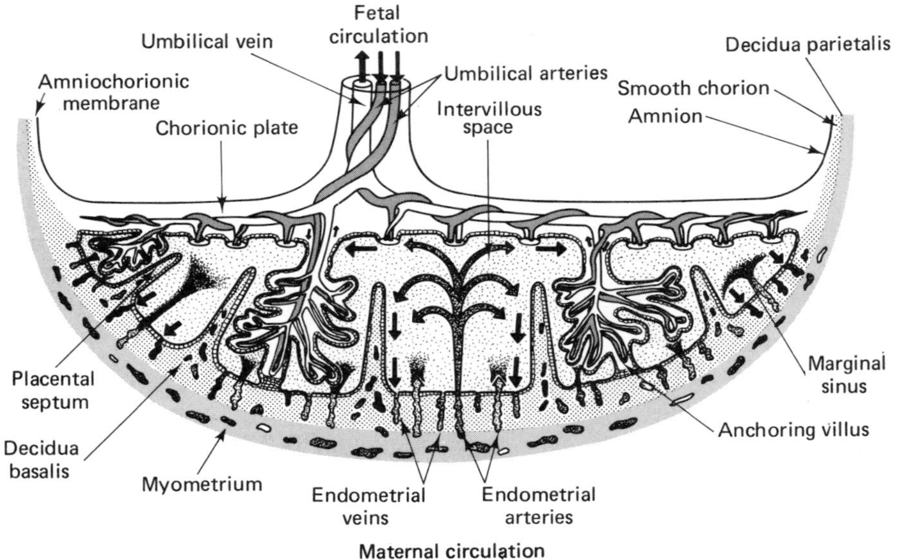

From Moore, 1977.

Figure 5–3 Schematic drawing of a section through a mature placenta, showing (1) the relation of the villous chorion (fetal placenta) to the decidua basalis (maternal placenta), (2) the fetal placental circulation, and (3) the maternal placental circulation. Maternal blood is driven into the intervillous space in funnel-shaped spurts, and exchanges occur with the fetal blood as the maternal blood flows around the villi. The inflowing arterial blood pushes venous blood out into the endometrial veins, which are scattered over the entire surface of the decidua basalis. Note that the umbilical arteries carry deoxygenated fetal blood to the placenta and that the umbilical vein carries oxygenated blood to the fetus.

Figure 5–4 Diagrammatic illustration of placental transfer.

From Moore, 1977.

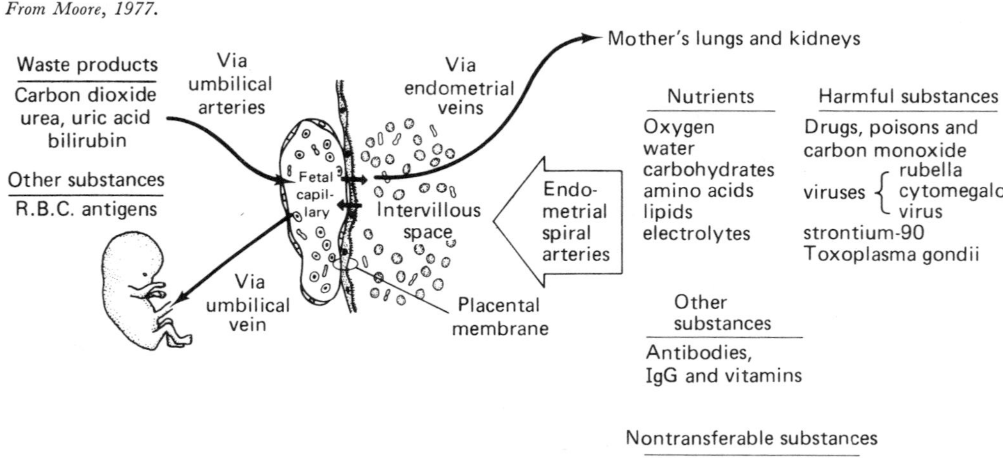

TABLE 5–1 TYPES OF PLACENTAS AND THEIR LAYERS

	Type of Placentas			
Layer	*Hemo-chorial*	*Endothelio-chorial*	*Syndesmo-chorial*	*Epithelio-chorial*
Endothelium of a fetal blood vessel	+	+	+	+
Connective tissue of villus	+	+	+	+
Trophoblast	+	+	+	+
Endothelium of a maternal vessel	–	+	+	+
Connective tissue of the maternal mucosa	–	–	+	+
Epithelium of the maternal mucosa	–	–	–	+

+ = layer present
– = layer absent

endothelium (the endothelial wall of the fetal blood vessels). This type of placenta also occurs in the rat and rabbit.

In the endotheliochorial placenta (found in the cat and dog, for example), the syndesmochorial placenta (in sheep and other ruminants), and the epitheliochorial placenta (in the pig and the horse), the placental membrane is much thicker and consists of more layers than the hemochorial type (see Table 5–1 and Figure 5–5). The intensity of exchange across the placental membrane is related to the type of placenta. Placental transfer is more rapid in the hemochorial placenta than in the other types, and the rate depends upon the thickness of the membrane.

PLACENTAL TRANSFER

The placenta has three major functions: (1) transfer of nutrients and gases to the fetus and waste products from the fetus to the mother, (2) metabolism, and (3) endocrine secretion. In relation to the influence of nutrition on the embryo and fetus, placental transfer is probably the most important single placental activity. However, many of the metabolic functions of the placenta are probably necessary for its transport function as well.

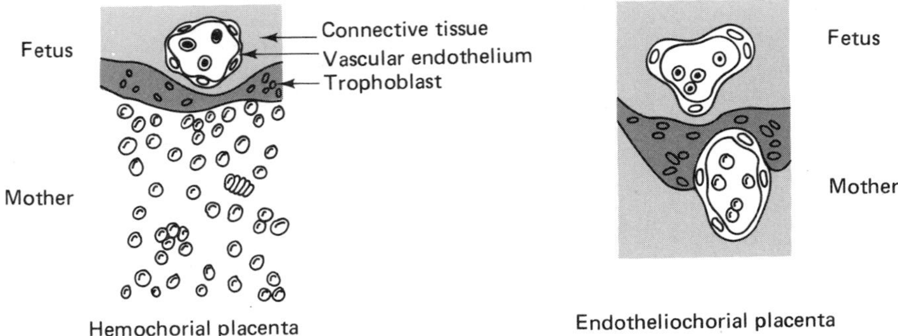

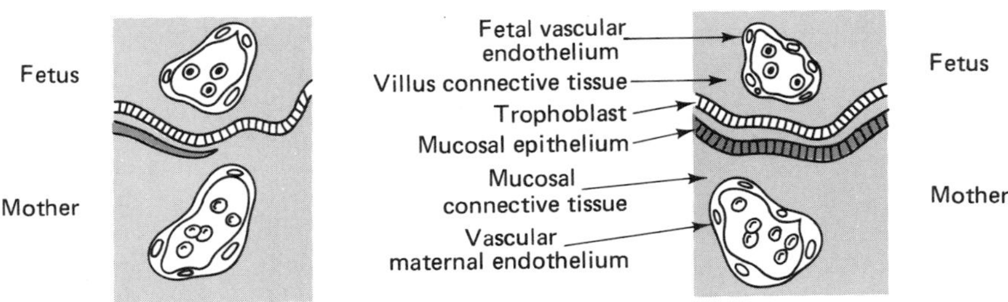

From Tuchmann-Duplessis et al., 1972.

Figure 5–5 Types of placentas: (a) hemochorial placenta, (b) endotheliochorial placenta, (c) syndesmochorial placenta, (d) epitheliochorial placenta.

PHYSIOLOGIC TRANSFER MECHANISMS

Placental transfer, as with transport across other biologic membranes, occurs through several basic mechanisms: simple diffusion, facilitated diffusion, active transport, pinocytosis, and bulk flow. Simple diffusion occurs by random thermal motion from an area of high concentration to one of low concentration. In general, substances of smaller molecular size diffuse more rapidly than do large molecules. Electrical charge and lipid solubility also influence the rate of transfer. Simple diffusion is a passive process involving no energy or work by the membrane, and it continues "downhill" until uniform concentration or electrochemical equilibrium is reached.

Facilitated diffusion differs from simple diffusion in that the rate of transfer is faster than would be predicted simply on a physical chemical basis. Facilitated diffusion does not occur against a gradient and does not require energy. The mechanism of facilitated diffusion is not established, but it is thought that a carrier in the membrane is involved.

Active transport is the transfer of molecules by processes requiring metabolic energy, and it is usually "uphill" against a gradient.

In pinocytosis, invaginations of the cell membrane engulf droplets of solute and water, cross the cell, and discharge their contents on the other side. Although the rate of transfer by pinocytosis may be slow, the process may be important over a long period for the transfer of large proteins or drugs.

Bulk flow or ultrafiltration refers to the process by which hydrostatic or osmotic pressure gradients cause a transfer of water molecules. The water movement carries dissolved particles, resulting in a more rapid rate of transfer of both water and solute than would be predicted on the basis of simple diffusion. The magnitude of the maternal blood flow in the placenta (about 500 ml/minute) and the pressure differences of placental hemodynamics probably account for the rapid movement of water between amniotic fluid, fetus, and mother by bulk flow or ultrafiltration (Figure 5–6).

Breaks in placental villi may also function to permit the transfer of substances. For example, the passage of fetal erythrocytes into the maternal

Figure 5–6 Placental hemodynamics. The numbers show pressures in mm/Hg.

From Tuchmann-Duplessis et al., 1972.

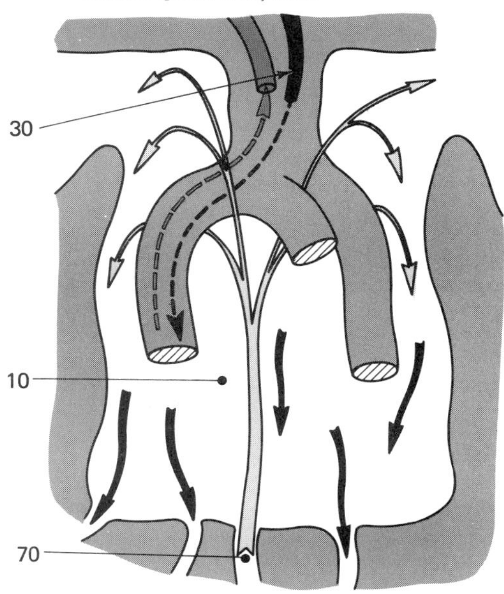

circulation may occur in this manner. Finally, the transfer of materials from maternal to fetal blood may occur by several processes simultaneously.

PLACENTAL TRANSPORT OF NUTRIENTS

An important consideration in evaluating studies concerning placental transfer is the factor of fetal and placental metabolism. Since the placenta is capable of metabolizing most nutrients, and the fetus also has some metabolic capabilities, the interpretation of the results is not always simple. Table 5–2 illustrates the problems involved by showing the possible interpretations of equal maternal and fetal concentration of a nutrient.

TABLE 5–2 POSSIBLE INTERPRETATIONS OF EQUAL MATERNAL AND FETAL NUTRIENT CONCENTRATIONS

[Maternal] = [Fetal]	
(1) No transport	
(2) Unobstructed transport (equilibrium)	
(3) M———active————→	transport with fetal consumption
(4) F ———active————→	M transport with maternal consumption
(5) M———partial————→	F transport with fetal production
(6) F ———partial————→	M transport with maternal production
(7) Combinations of the above	

From Robertson and Karp, 1976.

Glucose. Glucose is the major metabolic fuel of the fetus. The placenta transfers about 6 mg glucose/min/kg of fetal weight or about 18 mg/min near term. Variations in maternal glucose levels are reflected in the fetal levels with a high correlation (Figure 5–7). The usual maternal-fetal ratio is about 3 to 2. Placental uptake of glucose and its transport are affected primarily by maternal glucose levels and the amount of oxygen available to the placenta. Glucose is not simply transported across the placental cell, however. It is also used by the placenta to produce glycogen. Glycogenolysis occurs as well, with the production of lactate, and glucose is metabolized to pyruvate, lactate, and then to CO_2 in placental tissue (Figure 5–8).

Amino acids. Amino acids are generally transferred across the placenta by an active transport mechanism. The fetal-maternal amino acid ratio is above 1.0 for most amino acids, suggesting transplacental transport against a gradient. The concentration of amino acids in placental tissue is higher than in either maternal or fetal plasma; thus the active transport may occur between the maternal plasma and the placenta, while the transfer from the placenta to fetal plasma may not be by active transport. Amino acids

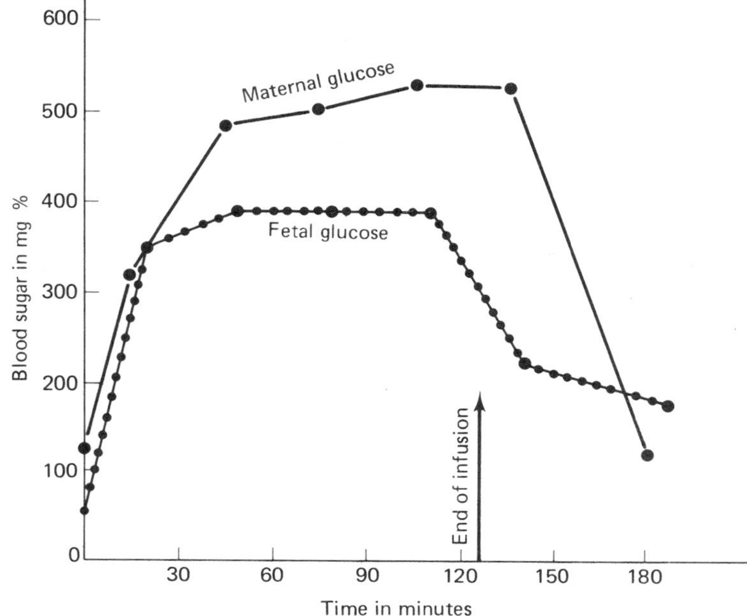

From Davies, J., Am. J. Physiol. 181: *532–538, 1955.*

Figure 5–7 Elevation of maternal blood glucose in rabbit for a prolonged period by infusions. Fetal glucose remains at lower level.

Figure 5–8 Placental transport and metabolism of glucose and lactate.

From Robertson and Karp, 1976.

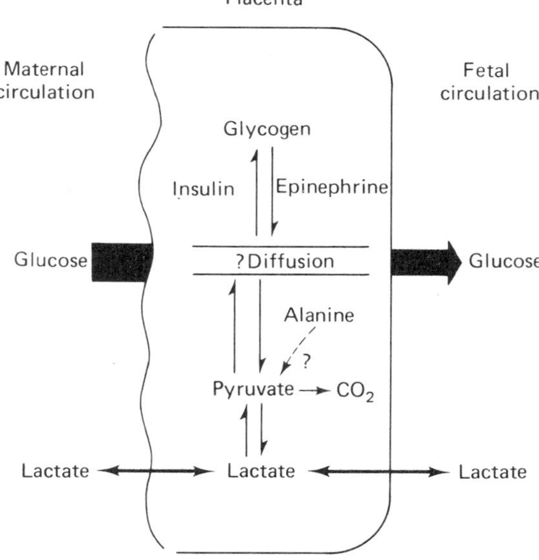

transported into the placental cell may be used for protein synthesis or, since the placenta contains proteolytic enzymes, may be degraded to free amino acids. The placenta may also transaminate amino acids, and it is possible that the keto acids could then be used for oxidation (Figure 5–9).

Fatty acids. Essential fatty acids cross the placenta to the fetus, but the mechanism of transport is unknown. The high placental concentration of free arachidonic acid has led to the speculation that the placenta may function as a fetal store for this essential fatty acid. Free fatty acids in the placenta may be converted to triglycerides, phospholipids, and cholesterol esters, or oxidized to CO_2. Fetal fat is probably derived from free fatty acids from placental transfer as well as from fetal synthesis from carbohydrate and acetate.

Ketone bodies also cross the placenta readily, as indicated by the high correlation between maternal and fetal levels. Probably less than 10% of the fetal caloric needs are supplied by ketones, but there is evidence that large amounts of β-hydroxybutyrate are converted to CO_2 by the fetal brain in early gestation. The respiratory quotient (RQ) of the newborn is also consistent with ketone oxidation. Thus ketone bodies may provide another source of energy for the fetus and the newborn and may be related to the apparent resistance of newborn infants to hypoglycemia. Glycerol, on the other hand, is transported across the placenta only minimally. Figure 5–10 summarizes placental transport and metabolism of fatty acids and ketones.

Figure 5–9 Placental transport and metabolism of amino acids.

From Robertson and Karp, 1976.

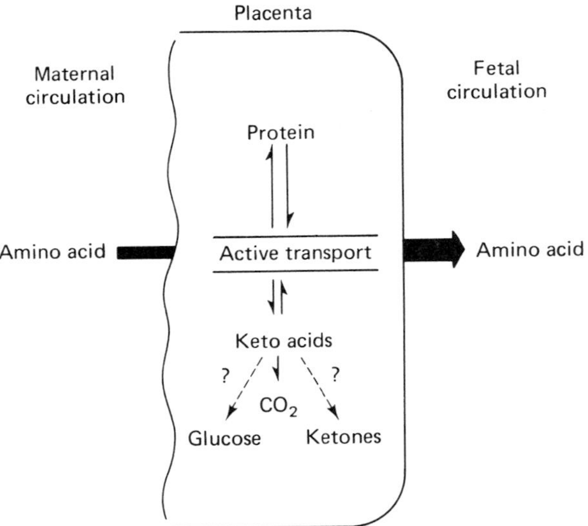

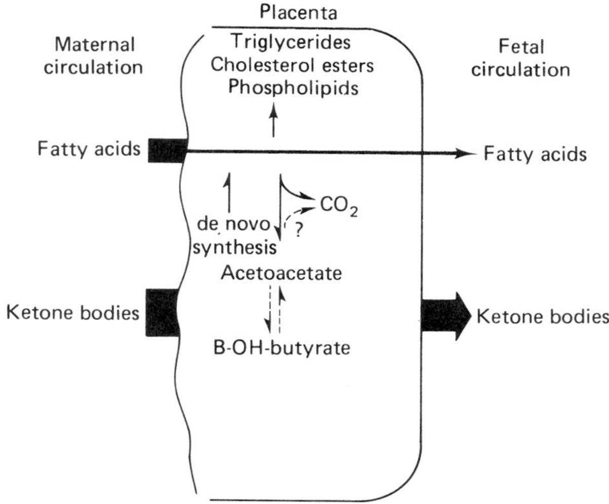

From Robertson and Karp, 1976.

Figure 5–10 Placental transport and metabolism of fatty acids and ketone bodies.

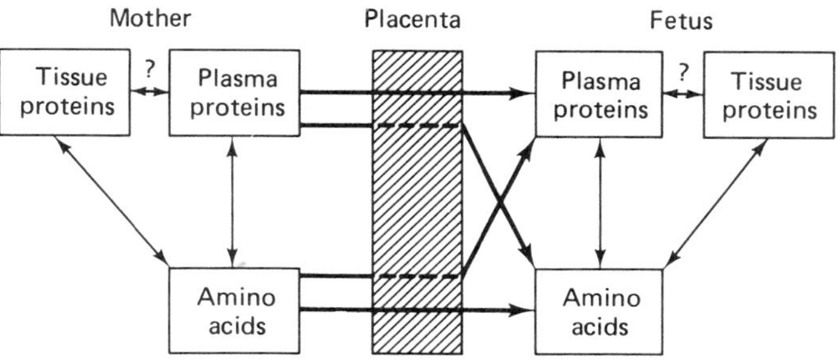

From Dancis and Shafran, J. Clin Invest. 37: *1093, 1958.*

Figure 5–11 Diagrammatic representation of possible precursors of fetal protein.

Cholesterol crosses the placenta only slowly and is lower in fetal than in maternal blood.

Proteins. The fetus probably synthesizes most of its protein from amino acids received from the maternal circulation. However, there is evidence for transplacental transfer of protein as such, as well as of amino acids. The sources of fetal protein and their possible precursors have been summarized diagrammatically by Dancis (Figure 5–11). When radioactive iodine-labeled plasma proteins were prepared from guinea pigs and injected into pregnant guinea pigs, radioactivity was found in the fetal plasma proteins. The results were not the same as those obtained when radiosulfur-labeled amino acids were injected, and the evidence suggested direct transfer of protein.

Another type of evidence for the transport of proteins across the placenta is the transfer of immunity from mother to fetus, which has been known for a long time. In man, monkey, rabbit, and guinea pig, passive immunity is not increased significantly after birth. In rats, mice, dogs, ruminants, and horses, most of this transmission or all of it occurs by way of the milk and the gut of the young animal after birth. Experimental studies show that transmission of antibodies is a highly selective process, since not all antibodies are transmitted equally readily.

Vitamins. There is a major difference in the rate of transfer across the placenta between the water-soluble vitamins and the fat-soluble vitamins. Fat-soluble vitamins are found in low concentration in cord blood, apparently reflecting a low rate of transport. Water-soluble vitamins are often found in higher concentration in cord blood than in maternal blood.

The presence of water-soluble vitamins in higher concentration in fetal than in maternal blood has led to the idea that these vitamins are actively transported by the placenta, but the evidence for active transport is not conclusive. Metabolism in the placenta may affect the concentrations that are measured.

Villee and his coworkers have studied the placental transfer of riboflavin and its coenzyme forms, FAD and FMN. Table 5–3 shows the riboflavin

TABLE 5–3 RIBOFLAVIN CONTENT OF HUMAN MATERNAL AND FETAL SERUM[a]

	Maternal	*Fetal*
Free riboflavin	0.55 ± 0.12	2.14 ± 0.18
Flavin adenine dinucleotide (FAD)	2.48 ± 0.18	1.29 ± 0.16
Riboflavin mononucleotide (FMN)	0.09 ± 0.10	0.28 ± 0.15
Total riboflavin	3.07 ± 0.20	3.70 ± 0.29

[a]The mean ± standard error of 12 analyses expressed as μg/100 ml of serum.

From Villee, 1960.

content of human maternal and fetal serum. FAD was found to be higher in the maternal circulation, but free riboflavin was higher in the fetal circulation, suggesting that the placenta is relatively impermeable to both compounds. Incubation of FAD with minced placental tissue produced increased concentration of FMN and free riboflavin, suggesting that the placenta could break down FAD into free riboflavin. It is thus possible that the FAD in fetal serum is produced from free riboflavin by fetal metabolism.

Mineral elements. Sodium and other electrolytes cross the placenta very readily. Other essential elements must, of course, also be transferred from the mother to the fetus.

PLACENTAL CHANGES DURING GESTATION

Both the structure and the function of the placenta change during the course of pregnancy. Changes are apparent in the morphology of the placenta, depending on the period of pregnancy. As the placenta ages, there is a progressive increase in the number and the surface area of the villi exposed to the maternal blood in the intervillous spaces. There is a corresponding increase in the fetal capillaries, as well as a decrease in thickness of the trophoblast. The gross morphological changes that take place with the maturation of the placenta, such as the development of the septa, have already been described. It is apparent that the increased surface area of the villi and the other changes are such as to increase the efficiency of transport between the maternal and the fetal circulation.

Cellular growth of the placenta follows the same pattern as that of the brain and other organs. There is a hyperplastic phase of cell division followed by a hypertrophic phase in which the cells are enlarging their size but not their number (see Chapter 2). In humans, hyperplasia of the placenta lasts about 36 weeks of the total 40-week period, while in rats this phase of growth occurs in the first 17 days of the 21-day gestation period. Although total RNA and protein content continue to increase throughout pregnancy, the rate of synthesis of these two substances decreases with age (Figure 5–12). There is also a continuous reduction in the overall metabolic rate of the placenta, which is reflected in a progressive decline in the rate of oxygen consumption. Furthermore, glucose utilization, production of pyruvate and lactate, and glycogen concentration also decrease during the course of gestation (Figure 5–12).

Changing placental function. In addition to the alterations in morphology and metabolism of the placenta during the course of gestation, there are also changes in its transport function. The transfer of sodium as related to gestational age has been carefully studied in humans (Figure 5–13). The permeability of the placenta to sodium increases considerably during nine-tenths of the total period of gestation, then decreases to term. This pattern of placental transfer rates for sodium occurs in most animals, including the rat. A similar pattern is observed in the rat for placental transfer of glucose and a test amino acid, α-aminoisobutyric acid (AIB), a nonmetabolizable amino acid (Figure 5–14).

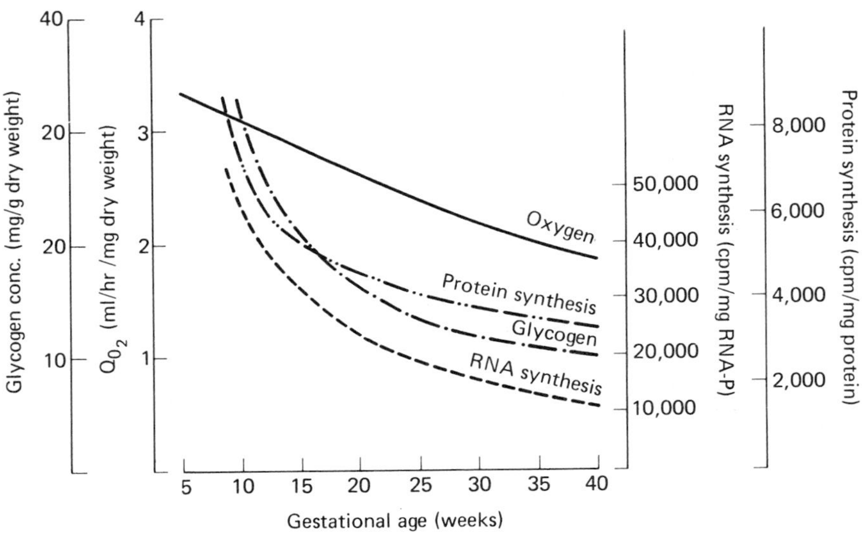

From Rosso, 1976.

Figure 5–12 Changes in oxygen consumption, glycogen content, and rate of RNA and protein synthesis in human placenta during normal gestation.

Figures 5–12 and 5–13 illustrate the paradox that a placenta at its lowest metabolic level is providing the peak of its transfer function with presumably a concomitant energy need for the transport mechanisms required. The increased rate of transfer between day 14 and day 21 corresponds to a period of rapid fetal growth, during which there is approximately a 30-fold increase in fetal body weight. At the end of gestation, however, the fetus, which is growing at a very rapid rate, is subject to a placenta whose capacity to

Figure 5–13 Variation of rate of transfer of sodium related to gestational age in human.

From Flexner et al., 1948.

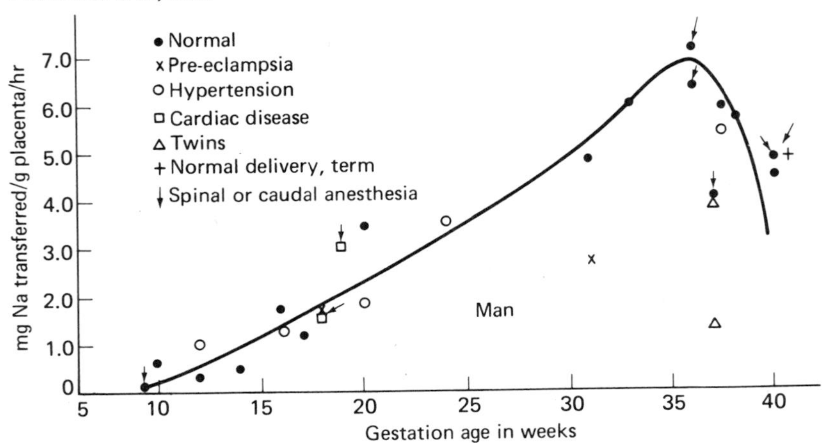

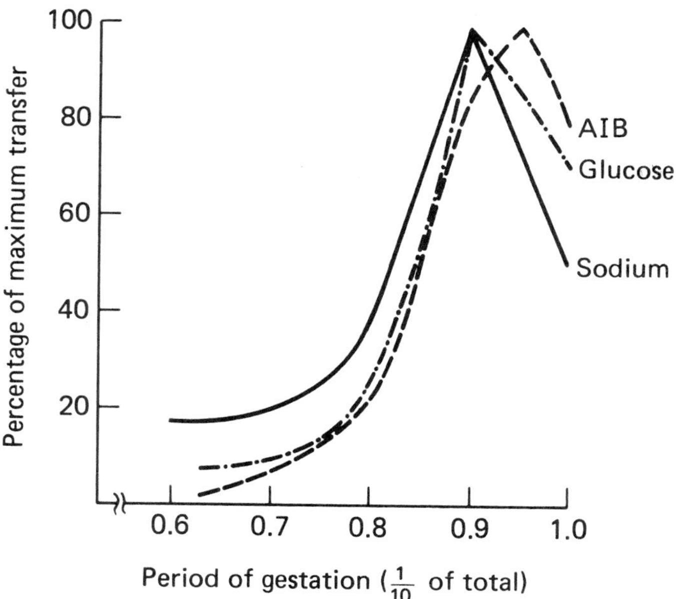

From Rosso, 1976.

Figure 5–14 Changes in the rate of transfer of AIB, glucose, and sodium across the rat placenta per gram of placental tissue during normal gestation.

transfer nutrients seems to decline. Thus, when the absolute requirements of the fetus are highest, there is a reduced capacity of placental transfer. This decline in placental capacity may explain the decreased rate of fetal growth that occurs before birth and is recovered postnatally in many animals (see Chapter 2). When gestation continues beyond the normal time, spontaneously in man or hormonally induced in experimental animals, the fetuses are retarded as compared with the postnatal growth of neonates delivered at term.

The effects of maternal malnutrition on the placenta and its function have been studied only to a very limited extent. Some of the changes in the placenta brought about by maternal malnutrition in the rat are similar to those of prolonged gestation. It is possible therefore that malnutrition may have a synergistic effect on the normal changes of aging in the placenta. The possible significance of such alterations on placental function and on development of the fetus remains to be investigated.

References and Supplementary Readings

Dancis, J., and Shafran, M. *J. Clin. Invest.* **37**: 1093 (1958).

Davies, J. *Am. J. Physiol.* **181**: 532 (1955).

FLEXNER, L. B., COWIE, D. B., HELLMAN, L. M., WILDE, W. S., AND VOSBURGH, G. I.: "The permeability of the human placenta to sodium in normal and abnormal pregnancies and the supply of sodium to the human fetus as determined with radioactive sodium." *Am. J. Obstet. Gynecol.* **55**: 469–480, 1948.

LONGO, L. D. "Placental transfer mechanisms—an overview." *Obstet. Gynec. Ann.* **1**: 103–131 (1972).

MOORE, K. L., *The Developing Human*, Clinically Oriented Embryology, 2nd ed., Philadelphia: W. B. Saunders, 1977.

ROBERTSON, A. F., AND W. B. KARP. "Placental transport of nutrients." *Southern Medical J.* **69**: 1358–1362 (1976).

ROSSO, P. "Placenta as an aging organ." In: M. WINICK, ed., *Nutrition and Aging*. New York: Academic Press, 1976.

TUCHMANN-DUPLESSIS, H., G. DAVID, AND P. HAEGEL. Translated by L. S. HURLEY. *Illustrated Human Embryology*, Vol. I. *Embryogenesis*. New York: Springer-Verlag, 1972.

FOUNDATION FOR CHILD DEVELOPMENT. *The Placenta and Fetal Membranes*. Edited by C. A. Villee. New York: The Williams and Wilkins Co., 1960.

II

Nutritional Influences on Embryonic and Fetal Development

6

History and significance of congenital abnormalities

CRITERIA OF ABNORMAL DEVELOPMENT

How do we know that an embryo or fetus is affected by nutrition—or indeed by any other factor? The most extreme indication of an abnormal event during prenatal life is embryonic or fetal death. Prenatal death in the human and in certain other species can take two forms: if it happens very late in pregnancy or during birth, then the infant is stillborn; if the fetus dies at an earlier time, then it is expelled. This process, the expulsion of the dead embryo, is called *abortion* or miscarriage. In other species, such as the rat, the dead conceptus is not aborted, but its tissue is broken down and absorbed back into the mother's circulation. This process is called *resorption.*

A second criterion of abnormal development is congenital abnormality. This term is synonymous with the term *birth defect. Congenital* means that the condition exists at birth, whether it is caused by genetic or environmental factors. Birth defects are defined as structural or metabolic disorders present at birth due to genetic or environmental factors occurring during prenatal life. The terms "birth defect" or "congenital anomaly" thus include functional abnormalities as well as grossly visible congenital malformations.

Often congenital anomalies are not apparent at birth, but defects are discovered later in life because they produce functional problems. Congenital heart disease, for example, is very commonly discovered after birth as heart function becomes abnormal. The study of congenital abnormalities and their etiology is called *teratology.*

A third index of nutritional influence on prenatal development is low birth weight (see Chapter 7). Finally, premature birth or other complications of pregnancy may be indications of possible problems in embryonic or fetal development.

There are two general ways in which a mammalian embryo can be affected by environmental factors, including nutrition: (1) by a direct effect on the embryo itself or (2) indirectly through an effect on the mother.

SIGNIFICANCE OF CONGENITAL DEFECTS

In recent times the causation of infant death has changed greatly (see Figure 6–1). In 1910, the percentage of infant deaths due to congenital malformations was quite low, about 5%, while 30% of deaths during the first year of life were caused by enteritis, diarrhea, and other infectious diseases. As methods of infant care and hospital sanitation improved, and especially as antibiotics and other such drugs became available, infant deaths due to these and other infectious diseases declined. By 1952, death due to infectious diseases was down to about 5%, and as these deaths declined, the proportion of deaths due to congenital malformations increased. By 1964, 19% of infant deaths were caused by congenital malformations. The absolute incidence of congenital malformations has probably not changed, but they become more and more important as other causes of infant death are removed, owing to improved medical knowledge and care.

CONGENITAL DEFECTS AS A PUBLIC HEALTH PROBLEM

The significance of congenital defects as a public health problem was examined by Apgar and Stickle. These authors defined the term birth defect as a structural or metabolic disorder present at birth, whether deter-

Figure 6–1 Comparison of trends of deaths from diarrhea and enteritis with deaths from congenital malformations (expressed as percent of all deaths in the United States under one year of age).

From Warkany, 1957.

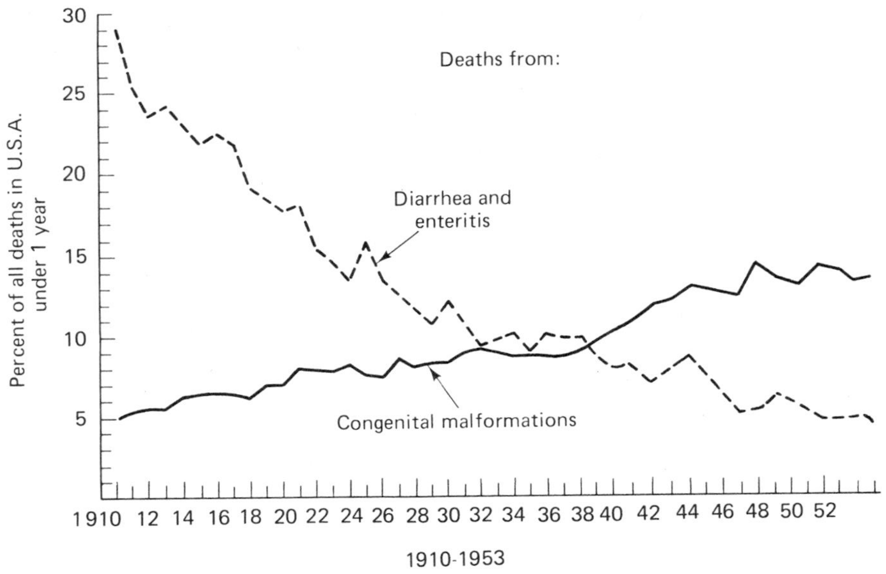

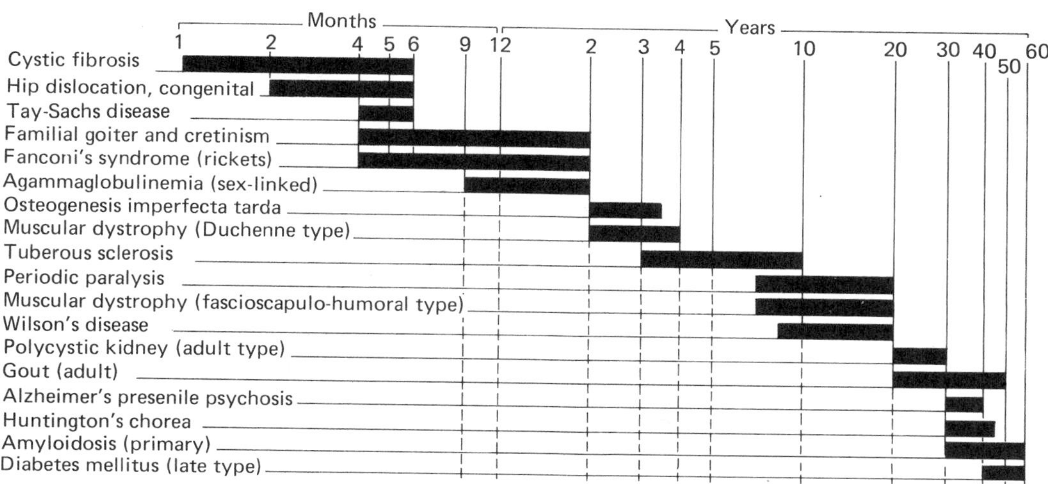

From Apgar and Stickle, 1968.

Figure 6–2 Age range of victims at onset of late-appearing birth defects.

mined genetically or by environmental influences during embryonic or fetal life, and they included metabolic defects such as phenylketonuria, hemophilia, sickle cell anemia, and diabetes. According to their search of the U. S. vital statistics for 1964, congenital defects were the largest single cause of infant death (during the first year of life). They also found that at least 62,000 deaths at any age each year may be attributed to congenital defects (Table 6–1 and Figure 6–2). This figure includes older ages, as well as infant deaths since many defects are not apparent until later in life.

The number of living people suffering from congenital defects was also analyzed. Analysis of prospective studies involving the outcome of over 21,000 pregnancies indicated that at least 7% of all infants born have structural or functional defects of prenatal origin that are detectable in infancy or early childhood. Fewer than one-half of these defects are evident at birth. When statistics related to the total population were examined, it was estimated conservatively that 15 million persons in the United States have one or more congenital defects that affect their daily lives. The occurrence of congenital defects thus constitutes an important public health problem.

Another aspect of the significance of congenital defects is the special care required for infants and children with perinatal handicaps (Table 6–2). Such children include premature infants, low-birth-weight infants, those with severe physical handicaps, the mentally retarded, and those for whom special education is needed. For the year 1967, it was estimated that 474,650

TABLE 6–1 DEATHS FROM CONGENITAL CONDITIONS IDENTIFIABLE FROM SEVENTH REVISION OF INTERNATIONAL CLASSIFICATION OF DISEASES, UNITED STATES, 1965

Cause of Death	*Number of Deaths*
Congenital syphilis	34
Neoplasms, under 28 days only	91
Myxedema and cretinism	342
Diabetes mellitus	33,174
Cystic fibrosis	610
Lipidosis (disturbance of lipid metabolism)	158
Amyloidosis	171
Other metabolic diseases	672
Familial acholuric jaundice	130
Sickle cell anemia	358
Hemophilia	59
Mongolism	267
Hernia of abdominal cavity	3,277
Inborn defect of muscle	689
Congenital malformations	19,512
Neonatal disorders arising from certain diseases of the mother during pregnancy	717
Hemolytic disease of newborn (erythroblastosis)	1,485
Hemorrhagic disease of newborn	477
Other congenital conditions	8
Total	62,231

From Apgar and Stickle, 1968.

children required special care. The magnitude of the care required represents a serious social problem. A large human loss can also be seen in estimates of prenatal and perinatal deaths (Table 6–3).

CAUSES OF CONGENITAL DEFECTS

In most cases of infants with congenital defects, the cause of the abnormal development cannot be established. As shown in Table 6–4, known causes of congenital defects account for only 30 to 35% of the cases, and include genetic transmission, chromosomal aberrations, radiation, rubella and other infectious viruses, diabetes, drugs, and environmental chemicals. It has been estimated by Wilson that 65 to 70% of all human congenital defects are of unknown cause. It is thus possible that nutrition is involved in some of that unknown group, either in itself or in interaction with some of the other factors that are known to affect development (for discussion of interacting factors, see Chapter 15).

HISTORY OF IDEAS ABOUT CONGENITAL MALFORMATIONS

The most striking indication of abnormal embryonic development is congenital malformation. It is therefore not surprising that congenital malformations have been recognized for thousands of years and have apparently

TABLE 6–2 ESTIMATED NUMBER OF CHILDREN WITH PERINATAL HANDICAPS REQUIRING SPECIAL CARE: UNITED STATES, 1967

Type of Care	*Estimated Number of Children*
Short-term:	
Low-birth-weight and preterm infants	125,300
Other[a]	100,240
Long-term:	
Severe physical handicap[b]	68,020
Physical and mental handicap[c]	19,900
Care of mentally retarded (I.Q.'s under 70)	46,540
Care of infants who may require special educational service (I.Q.'s 70 to 79)	114,560
Total	474,560

[a]For example, strabismus, inguinal hernia, talipes.
[b]For example, congenital heart disease, cerebral palsy.
[c]For example, multiple handicap, developmental defect (central nervous system).

From Siegel and Morris, 1970.

TABLE 6–3 FETAL AND PERINATAL DEATHS FROM FOUR WEEKS' GESTATION TO TWO YEARS OF AGE (ESTIMATED AND REPORTED): UNITED STATES, 1967

Stage at Which Death Occurred	*Number of Deaths*
Fetal:	
Between four and 20 weeks' gestation	1,023,880
After 20 weeks' gestation[1]	89,500
After 20 weeks' gestation[2]	54,939
Perinatal:	
Under 28 days	58,127
28 days to one year	20,901
One to two years	5,006

[1]estimated
[2]reported

From Siegel and Morris, 1970.

TABLE 6–4 CAUSES OF DEVELOPMENTAL DEFECTS IN MAN, %

Known genetic transmission	20
Chromosomal aberration	5
Environmental causes:	
Radiations	<1
Infections	2–3
Maternal metabolic imbalance	1–2
Drugs and environmental chemicals	2–3
Combinations and interactions	?
Unknown	65–70

From Wilson, 1972.

always made a great impression upon people. For example, cave paintings from prehistoric times have been found in Australia that show congenital malformations in children. Likewise, small statues made by both Australian aborigines and ancient Egyptians depict children with striking deformities.

BIRTH DEFECTS AND ASTROLOGY

In addition to these artistic sources, written records also exist documenting the observation of birth defects by the ancients, such as the Chaldean tablets in the British Museum in London, which describe in great detail children with birth defects. The ancient Babylonians who prepared these cuneiform writings were especially interested in having such written descriptions because they used the occurrence of the birth of a deformed infant as a portent for the future. These founders of astrology considered that abnormalities of newborn children were a reflection of stellar constellations and could therefore be used to foretell the future just as could the stars themselves. Thus, the old scientific term "monster," a term used to describe a defective child, originated from the Latin word "monstrum" from "monstrare," which means "to show."

The Babylonian idea that the birth of deformed children was a portent of the future and that predictions could be made from it persisted for hundreds of years. An example of this persistence can be seen in a report of the year 1569, when strife between Protestants and Catholics was strong. Twins were born who were conjoined at the chest (Siamese twins), and only one of the twins was baptized before they died. The physician who performed the autopsy somehow interpreted this event as predicting that the Catholic faith would survive that of the Protestants.

POSSIBLE RELATION TO MYTHOLOGY

The descriptions of congenital defects in the Babylonian tablets are so objectively and carefully reported that, in fact, many of the anomalies can be recognized today. However, not all ancient reporting of the birth of deformed infants was objective and careful. The various exaggerated stories that remain suggest that as these reports were transmitted from one generation to the next, tales and legends developed which may have led to the origins of many of the figures of mythology. For example, Cyclops resembles a malformation of the face in which there is only one eye. Likewise, mermaids look somewhat like a child with a certain birth defect in which there is abnormal development of the legs.

INTERSPECIES CROSS-FERTILIZATION

The derivation of other mythological creatures such as centaurs, minotaurs, the sphinx, and so forth that were believed to exist might, however, have been related to the idea that humans and animals could cross-fertilize and produce offspring. In the time of the ancient Greeks and Egyptians, such actions were not considered evil or sinful. However, when these ideas spread into Europe with its Judeo-Christian tradition, the idea of humans and animals copulating became abhorrent. When children were born that resembled animals, it was thought that they resulted from this kind of crossbreeding. During the Middle Ages in Europe, women who gave birth to deformed infants that in some way resembled an animal were sometimes burned at the stake.

Even much later, during the period 1638–1648, a similar event occurred in Connecticut. As summarized by Warkany,

> Three years after the founding of the colony, a monstrous pig was born (in 1641) that had "butt one eye in the midle of the face" and over the eye "a thing of flesh grew forth and hung downe, itt was hollow, and like a mans instrum' of gen'ation." This was obviously a cyclopic pig with a proboscis, a malformation not rare in that species. However, to the good people of New Haven, cyclopia was not known as a spontaneous defect in pigs, and they attributed the birth of this monster to the "unnatureall spell and abominable filthynes" of a servant, George Spencer, who had "but one eye for use, the other hath (as itt is called) a pearle in itt" and closely resembled the eye of the miraculous pig. The court procedures, the confessions, and retractions, as well as the testimonies are recorded in great detail. This trial continued from 1641 to 1642, but finally the prisoner was executed on April 8, 1642, after the cyclopic sow had been "slaine in his sight, being run through with a sworde." On reading this trial one realizes that the hybridity theory of India and Egypt was, with modifications, imported to this country—but also, the proceedings demonstrate that "brain washing" was not invented in recent times.

MATERNAL IMPRESSIONS

Another idea to explain the causation of congenital malformations was the theory of maternal impressions. It was thought that the development of the infant could be influenced by what the mother saw during her pregnancy. This theory was prevalent for hundreds of years and was accepted by outstanding scientists of the time. Even as late as the end of the nineteenth century, a reference book on diseases of children contained a chapter on "maternal impressions." Cases were cited of defects in children together with "the cause or nature of the impression."

In one case presented in this book, the milkman whom the mother saw every day had one finger amputated and the child born subsequently had only four fingers on one hand. In another case, the mother lived next door to a man with a cleft lip and her infant also had a cleft lip. On the basis of the theory of maternal impressions, pregnant women were encouraged to look only at beautiful things in order to be sure that their children would be beautiful.

Although all the causes of congenital malformations are still not known, it is now clear that they are the result of an alteration in the developmental sequences that must occur normally in order to produce a normal infant at term. The role of nutrition in this course of events is still far from being fully understood. By considering the ideas of the past we may gain insight into possible blind spots in our own thinking about cause-and-effect relationships.

GENETIC CAUSES

After the older ideas described above began to fade, and after 1900 when the Mendelian theory of inheritance came to be accepted, it was recognized that some congenital malformations are caused by genetic factors. By this time, the effect of environmental factors on the development of avian and amphibian embryos was well accepted, but the influence of such nongenetic factors on mammalian embryos was not being considered. It was thought that since the mammalian embryo developed inside the mother, it was completely protected from the external environment. Until very recently this idea was especially prevalent in regard to nutrition. The mammalian embryo was thought of as a parasite that would draw from its mother's body the nutrients it needed for its own growth and development.

The first indication in the scientific literature that nutrition could affect the mammalian embryo was from work done at the University of Wisconsin on the effects of various rations on cows. Hart and his coworkers reported in 1911 that cows fed wheat alone produced stillborn or immature, weak calves that did not live. When the ration was supplemented with bone meal, the calves were normal.

The first demonstration that a nutritional factor could produce congenital malformations in a mammal came in 1933 when Hale was studying vitamin A deficiency in pigs. Some of the pigs born to vitamin A-deficient sows were abnormal, exhibiting cleft palate, small or missing eyes, and hernias. This was a chance observation, but Hale later (1937) proved conclusively that the abnormalities were not of genetic origin but were actually caused by the vitamin deficiency. This observation is of special importance in the history of teratology because it was also the first report that an environmental (as opposed to genetic) factor could bring about a disturbance in the prenatal development of a mammal sufficient to produce a congenital malformation.

Warkany was the first person to produce congenital malformations deliberately in experimental animals for the purpose of studying their development and their causation. He is called the father of experimental teratology.

References and Supplementary Readings

Apgar, V., and G. Stickle. "Birth defects: their significance as a public health problem." *J.A.M.A.* **204**: 371–374 (1968). Copyright 1968, American Medical Association.

Hale, F. "Pigs born without eyeballs." *J. Heredity* **24**: 105 (1933).

Hale, F. "The relation of maternal vitamin A deficiency to microphthalmia in pigs." *Texas State J. Med.* **33**: 37 (1937).

Hart, E. B., E. V. McCollum, H. Steenbock, and G. C. Humphrey. "Physiological effect on growth and reproduction of rations balanced from restricted sources." *Wis. Agric. Exp. Sta. Res. Bulletin*, No. 17 (1911).

Hart, E. B., H. Steenbock, G. C. Humphrey, and R. S. Hulce. "New observations and a reinterpretation of old observations on the nutritive value of the wheat plant." *J. Biol. Chem.* **62**: 315–322 (1924).

Kretchmer, N. "Whither birth defects?" *Perspectives in Biol. Med.* **8**: No. 1 (1964).

Siegel, E., and N. Morris. "The epidemiology of human reproductive casualties, with emphasis on the role of nutrition." In: *Maternal Nutrition and the Course of Pregnancy*. Washington, D.C.: Food and Nutrition Board, NRC, NAS, 1970, pp. 5–40.

Warkany, J. *Pediatrics* **5**: 708–725 (1950). Copyright American Academy of Pediatrics, 1950.

Warkany, J. "Congenital malformations and pediatrics." In: *Conference on Teratology*, J. Warkany, ed., *Pediatrics* **19**: 725 (1957).

Warkany, J. "Congenital malformations in the past." *J. Chronic Dis.* **10**: 83 (1959).

Wilson, J. G. *Environment and Birth Defects*. New York: Academic Press, 1973.

Wilson, J. G. "Environmental effects on development-teratology." In *Pathophysiology of Gestation*, N. S. Assali, ed., Vol. 2. New York: Academic Press, 1972, pp. 269–320.

7

General malnutrition and prenatal development

GENERAL MALNUTRITION IN HUMANS

The influence of nutritional factors on prenatal development is difficult to study in human populations, especially when conditions of malnutrition are mild or when conditions of nutrition are suboptimal, because of the numerous factors that usually occur in combination with nutritional inadequacy. However, severe malnutrition can be studied in human populations in famines such as have occurred during wars.

It should be remembered that the term *general malnutrition* usually means *undernutrition*: the intake or availability of insufficient or suboptimal quantities of food or nutrients. Thus, general malnutrition is partly, probably primarily, a deficiency of calories. However, it is most likely that under conditions of general malnutrition or undernutrition, deficiencies of specific nutrients may also occur (see the section on protein deficiency in Chapter 9).

WAR AND FAMINE

Although statistical evidence is not complete concerning the outcome of pregnancies during famines associated with wars, some information is available.

Germany. Hytten and Leitch have reviewed reports of pregnancy outcomes during World War I in Germany. In the winter of 1916–1917 during the blockade of Germany there was acute privation and starvation. There was a marked lowering of the birth rate. Hytten and Leitch have summarized the information available and have concluded that under these conditions the young women who were potential mothers did not conceive. The babies that were born were those of women in rural areas or those of women with priority rations (that is, they had more food available than did the general population). Finally, even those children that were born were not of normal vitality and seemed to be of lower birth weight.

In another period, after World War II, while food supplies were limited and other conditions were also still bad, infants born in Germany in the first few years after the war showed a higher-than-usual incidence of malformations, especially those of the central nervous system.

Holland—World War II. During World War II part of the Netherlands was under blockade, and for a period of about eight months food supplies were extremely low. The famine became progressively worse from October to December of 1944, and availability of food stayed at a very low level until the country was liberated by the Allied Forces in May of 1945. In the attempt to evaluate the effects of this deprivation of food on pregnancy, timing was a complicating factor, since the period of malnutrition lasted for eight months. In each pregnancy there were thus some distinct overlapping factors to be considered.

Shortly after the war, Smith made a study of some of the statistics available at that time on outcome of pregnancy. One very obvious result of the malnutrition in Holland was that the fertility of the women was greatly decreased. Only one-third of the normally expected number of births occurred during this time. About 50% of the female population stopped menstruating, and only about 30% had normal menstrual cycles. This condition, called "war amenorrhea," is a common finding in all instances where famine conditions prevail. (This observation is comparable to those of Keys in his study of young men under near starvation conditions; all sexual desire and interest in women was lost.)

Thus, the most obvious finding in the Rotterdam study was a marked reduction in the birth rate. Because the number of samples was therefore so small, all birth data from this period in Rotterdam were considered statistically questionable. However, when prewar births were compared to those that were the result of conception during famine, it was seen that miscarriages and abortions, stillbirths, neonatal deaths, and malformations were all increased in infants conceived during famine (see Table 7–1). In infants alive at birth, birth weights and lengths were lower at a statistically significant level.

The effects of the Dutch famine of the winter of 1944–1945 have recently been studied in depth. Both the outcome of pregnancy—that is, the condition of the newborn and infant—and the long-range consequences of severe maternal undernutrition were investigated for all Dutch males conceived or born during this period. The study is based on systematic and comprehensive data compiled by various agencies of the Netherlands government on food rationing during the war, birth and death statistics, military

TABLE 7–1 PREGNANCY OUTCOME IN ROTTERDAM IN WORLD WAR II

Condition	*Incidence (Percent of Births)* Prewar	Conceived in Hunger
Abortion and miscarriage	1.67	8.3
Prematurity	5.27	8.4
Stillbirth	3.5	4.0
Neonatal death	1.55	5.1
Malformed	1.36	2.4

Adapted from Smith, 1947.

induction records, and maternity hospital records. The infants who were born during the period under study, both in the famine areas and in comparable communities of Holland that were not subjected to famine, remained almost fully accounted for in government health statistics from birth until examination for military induction.

Figure 7–1 Fertility and caloric ration (number of births and official average daily caloric ration at estimated time of conception for the period June 1944 to December 1946 inclusive). *From Stein et al., 1975.*

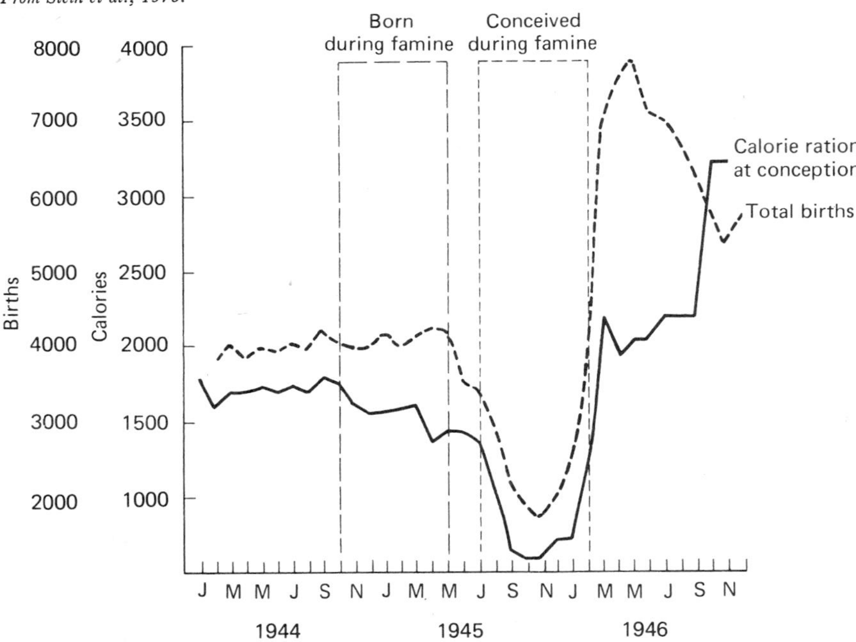

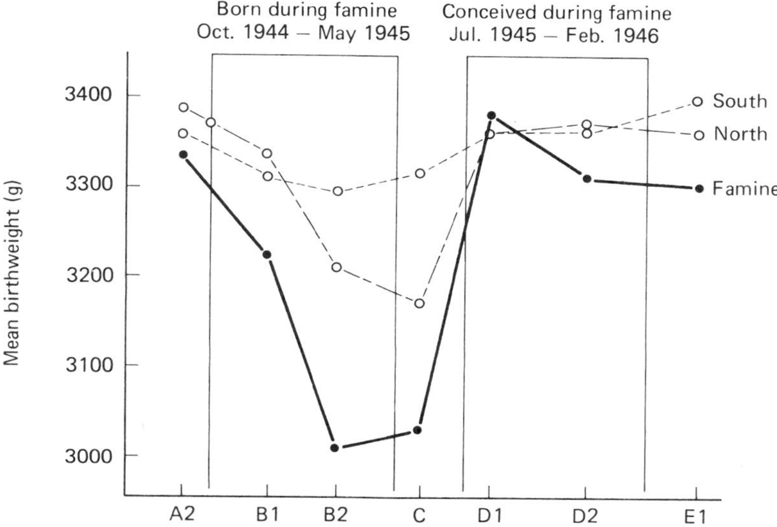

From Stein et al., 1975.

Figure 7–2 Birth weight by time and place (mean birthweight in grams for births in maternity hospitals for seven birth cohorts: famine, Northern control, and Southern control areas compared for the period August 1944 to March 1946 inclusive).

This extremely extensive as well as detailed analysis confirmed some of the findings made by Smith on far more limited data. In addition, important relationships between nutrition and the outcome of pregnancy are apparent from this study.

The number of births was markedly reduced by severe nutritional deprivation at conception (see Figure 7–1), and famine during the first trimester caused increased premature births. On the other hand, undernutrition during late gestation retarded fetal growth, resulting in low birth weight (Figure 7–2). Prenatal exposure to famine in early gestation also appeared to be related to perinatal mortality. There was an increase in stillbirths (Figure 7–3) and first-week deaths in infants conceived at the height of the famine and exposed to famine only during the first trimester of gestation. In addition, this group also showed a rise in the incidence of congenital anomalies of the central nervous system, namely spina bifida and hydrocephalus (Figure 7–4), and an increased death rate from meningitis in later life.

This remarkable study clearly demonstrates the effects of severe caloric restriction during early or late gestation on the postnatal as well as prenatal development of the infant. It is especially significant as an indication of the effect of nutritional deprivation *during gestation alone*, since both before the war and immediately after the famine period, Dutch women were in general well fed. The conditions here were therefore quite similar to those of animal

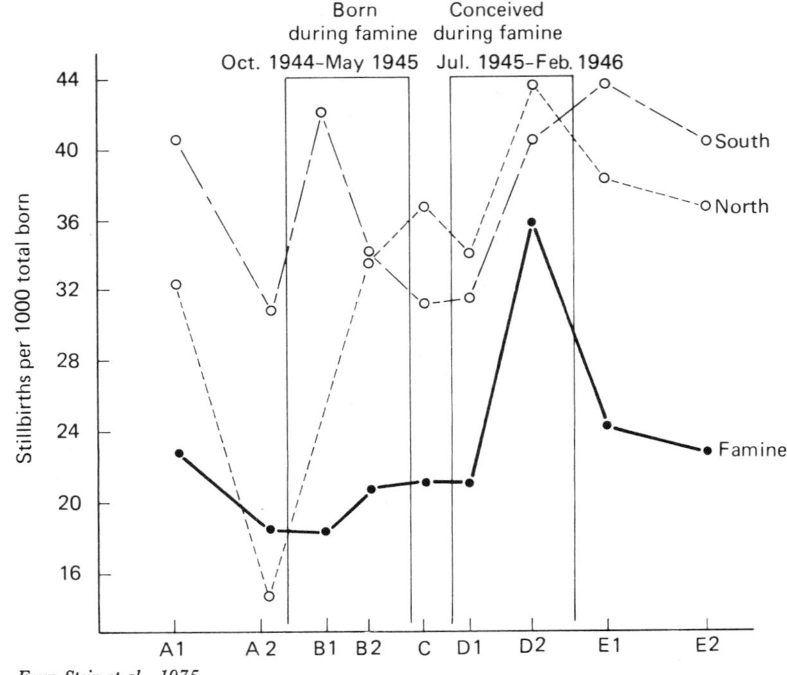

From Stein et al., 1975.

Figure 7–3 Stillbirths by time and place (stillbirths per 1000 total births: famine, Northern control, and Southern control areas by cohort for births January 1944 to December 1946).

Figure 7–4 Incidence of malformations of the central nervous system in groups of male infants born between October 1944 and February 1946 in Holland. Solid line = famine area; dotted line = control area.

From Stein et al., 1975.

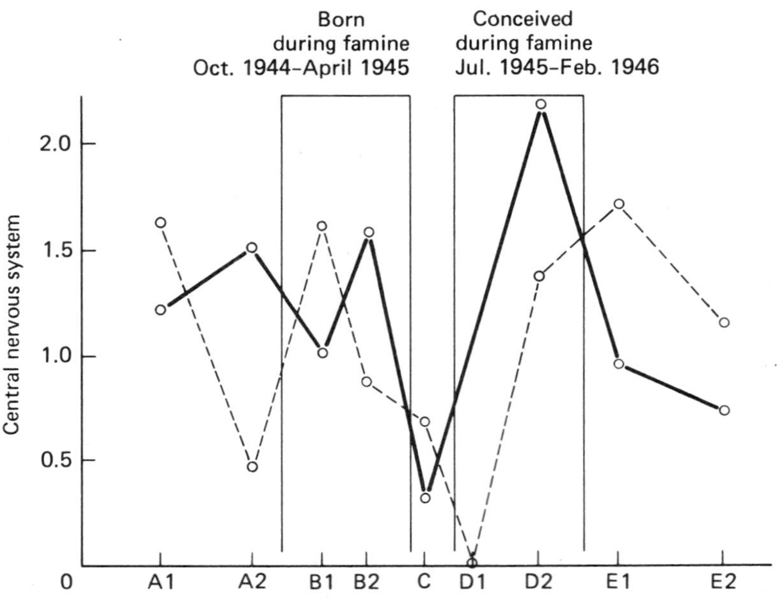

experiments in which the period of malnutrition is limited to pregnancy. In human studies such demarcation is usually not possible.

It is possible that because these women were so well nourished prior to pregnancy, they were less affected by malnutrition during pregnancy than would otherwise have been the case. Through studies on animals, and some information from humans, it is thought that nutrition *prior* to pregnancy also influences its outcome.

Leningrad. Another well-known study concerning the influence of nutrition during human pregnancy was made on the effect of starvation during the seige of Leningrad. During World War II, Leningrad was besieged by the Germans from August 1941 to January 1943. In September of 1941 the city was encircled, and from this date no supplies came into the city and conditions were extremely bad until the pressure was eased in February of 1942. At the same time, bombings were occurring, air raids were constant, and long-range shells were falling. Food supplies were low in quality and quantity, mortality was high, and alimentary dystrophy increased greatly. Bread was rationed in February 1942 at a rate of 500 g per day for manual workers and 400 g for mental workers. This was the principal ration, and its nutritional value was low as it consisted of 50% poor quality rye flour, with the other 50% made up of cellulose, bran, and malt.

Again, as in Holland, the lack of menstruation was evident; the number of infants born was much lower than normal, and the incidence of stillbirths was doubled during the first half of 1942 (Table 7–2). In the second half of 1942 only 79 infants were born, and these pregnancies were all of women who did not suffer from acute food shortage, either because food was available through their jobs or because of priority rations. In these 79 pregnancies the incidence of stillbirths as well as the birth weights were significantly better than in the pregnancies of the first half of 1942.

The effect of starvation was also evident in the birth weights of infants born during the period (Table 7–3). In the latter half of 1941 some depression of birth weight was already apparent and can be correlated with the food shortages during this time. However, the effect was most striking in January to June of 1942, when birth weights were over 500 g lower than those of the previous year. Premature births were also very high in 1942, with an incidence of 35.5%, as compared with the normal rate of about 6.5%.

In addition, the condition of the infants at birth was much poorer than normal, and the most noticeable characteristic was their low vitality. Most were inert, did not maintain their body temperature satisfactorily, and became chilled easily. Their sucking action was weak. They had little resistance to all outside influences and for this reason were susceptible to various diseases that resulted in death. The conditions in the hospitals were appalling. There was no heat, buildings suffered from bomb damage, water supply was poor, and many newborns died of pneumonia. Thus, many other

TABLE 7–2 BIRTHS IN A LENINGRAD CLINIC, 1941–1942

	January to June			*July to December*		
Year	*Livebirths*	*Stillbirths*	*Ratio Stillbirths / All births*	*Livebirths*	*Stillbirths*	*Ratio Stillbirths / All births*
1941	2,007	49	2.44%	1,049	34	3.24%
1942	391	23	5.55%	77	2	2.53%

Adapted from Antonov, 1947.

TABLE 7–3 BIRTH WEIGHT IN A LENINGRAD CLINIC, 1941–1942

	January to June				*July to December*			
	Boys		*Girls*		*Boys*		*Girls*	
	No.	*Wt., g*	*No.*	*Wt., g*	*No.*	*Wt., g*	*No.*	*Wt., g*
1941	933	3444	874	3302	503	3344	447	3222
1942	135	2815	120	2760	39	3199	32	2890

Adapted from Antonov, 1947.

deleterious factors accompanied malnutrition, but neverthless it seems clear that the poor nutrition of pregnant women resulted in abnormal development of their infants.

CLINICAL STUDIES IN HUMANS

Under conditions of malnutrition less severe than those of famine, it is more difficult to see effects on prenatal development, but some information is available. There have been a number of studies on the relationship between the nutrition of pregnant women and the outcome of pregnancy, the condition of the infant. Such studies are difficult to conduct and have yielded conflicting results. Among the many problems involved, it is difficult to evaluate the dietary intake of people, to establish their nutritional intake, and to control all the possible factors that may affect development. However, the consensus now indicates that the diet of pregnant women can affect development of the fetus.

An early, well-controlled (double-blind) clinical study done at Harvard by Burke and her colleagues was published in the 1940s. Dietary records were taken of pregnant women who came to the prenatal clinic, and their nutritional value was evaluated. When the infants were delivered, pediatricians (who were unaware of the nutritional evaluation of the mother) examined the infants. The mothers whose diets were classified as good or excellent gave birth to babies whose condition was superior or good (Figure 7–5). Forty-two percent of the mothers with good or excellent diets had babies that were classified as superior. Over half the mothers with good or excellent diets had babies that were classified as good. Of the mothers with good or excellent diets, only 3% had infants that were classified as fair to poorest. In contrast, of mothers whose diets were fair, only 6% had babies that were considered superior, 44.5% were good or fair, and 5% were poorest. There was thus a definite correlation between the quality of the mother's diet during pregnancy and the condition of the infant at birth.

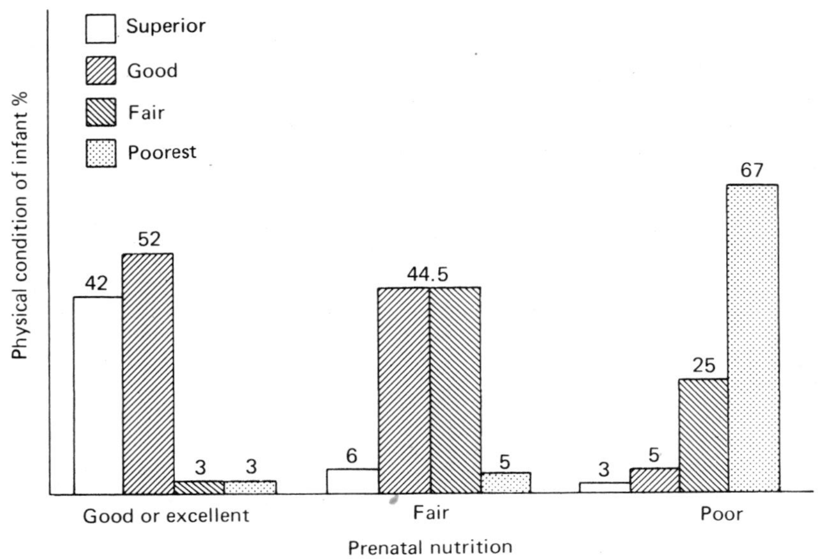

Adapted from Burke, 1943.

Figure 7–5 Correlation of prenatal nutrition of mother with condition of the infant at birth. Numbers over bars indicate percentages of newborns in that category.

When protein was considered, it was found that the birth weights and the birth lengths of the infants correlated with the amount of protein in the maternal diet. When the amount of protein was under 45 g per day, the birth weight averaged 5.8 lb; when the protein was 65 to 74 g, the average weight was 8 lb; and when the protein was 85 g or more, the average birth weight was 9.2 lb.

Similar findings were reported by Jeans and coworkers from the University of Iowa in 1955. In this study, the dietary habits of 400 pregnant rural women of low income were evaluated and were correlated with the condition of their infants at birth. Again, the lowest birth weights, lowest vitality, and largest number of deaths in the newborn period were observed among the infants born to the most poorly nourished mothers. Furthermore, this study found that the incidence of prematurity rose sharply as the nutritional status of the pregnant woman decreased. In the women whose dietary habits were classified as fair to excellent, 4.0% of their infants were delivered prematurely, while in those whose dietary habits were considered poor to very poor, the incidence of prematurity was 9.6%. Even more striking was the condition of the infants at birth (Table 7–4). In the mothers whose dietary habits were classified as fair to excellent, there were no abnormalities —all 11 infants born to them were living and in good condition on leaving

TABLE 7-4 CORRELATION OF CONDITION OF INFANT AND MOTHER'S DIET

	Mothers				*Infants*			
		Delivered Prematurely				*Birth Weight, g*		
Dietary Habits	*No.*	*No.*	*Percent*	*Avg. No. Preg.*	*No.*	*Mean*	*Range*	*Remarks*
Fair to excellent	227	9	4.0	7	11	2344	1970–2490	All infants in good condition on leaving hospital
Poor to very poor	177	17	9.6	3	17	1814	750–2420	1 stillbirth 4 severe congenital anomalies 5 neonatal deaths

Adapted from Jeans et al., 1955.

the hospital. In contrast, the mothers whose dietary habits were classified as poor to very poor gave birth to 17 infants of whom one was stillborn, four had severe congenital anomalies, and five died in the neonatal period.

In more recent clinical investigations, various abnormalities have been reported in infants malnourished before birth, such as cardiovascular anomalies and retarded development of postnatal bone growth. A study of infants with fetal growth retardation indicated that about 10% had postnatal physiological problems resulting from congenital abnormalities.

Primrose and Higgins carried out a different kind of clinical study. This was an intervention study in Montreal in which the dietary history of pregnant women was recorded, and nutrition education was given. If the women were poor, nutritional supplements were also given as well as the nutrition education. The extra food provided was milk, eggs, and oranges. In addition, a commercial vitamin, iron, and mineral dietary supplement was given to mothers. In the group of pregnant women who received supplementary foods as well as nutrition education, the incidence of stillbirths, perinatal mortality, and neonatal mortality was lower than it was in the province of Quebec or in Canada as a whole (Table 7–5).

HUMAN FETAL GROWTH RETARDATION

Fetal malnutrition can arise in two general ways: (1) the nutritional status of the mother's body during pregnancy and her dietary intake can affect the nutrient supply available to the fetus, (2) abnormal or insufficient function of the placenta may deprive the fetus of adequate nutrients through inadequate placental transfer. In addition, the placenta and its function may be affected by other factors such as diseases, drugs, or chromosomal abnormalities.

Fetal malnutrition is studied by examining infants with intrauterine

TABLE 7–5 INFLUENCE OF NUTRITION INTERVENTION ON BIRTHS IN MONTREAL DIET DISPENSARY STUDY

	Rates/1000 Live Births		
	Diet Dispensary Study	*Quebec Province*	*Canada*
Stillbirths	8.7	11.8	11.4
Neonatal mortality in first week	5.7	16.2	14.4
Perinatal mortality	14.4	28.0	25.8

Adapted from Primrose and Higgins, 1971.

growth retardation, which most experts consider to be a sign of fetal malnutrition. Intrauterine growth retardation is defined as small size for the gestational age of the infant. Metcoff and his colleagues have studied human fetal growth retardation as an index of fetal malnutrition. They analyzed isolated leucocytes from blood of the umbilical cord of newborn infants for various biochemical parameters such as protein/DNA ratio (cell size) and various enzyme patterns. These were compared with those from the corresponding maternal leucocytes and with those from mothers whose infants were of normal size for their gestational age. The cell size of leucocytes from infants with fetal malnutrition and their mothers was larger than that of any other group of newborns. Furthermore, enzyme analyses showed an altered pattern of energy metabolism in leucocytes of the infants with intrauterine malnutrition and in their mothers. There was a low content per cell of ATP, of pyruvate kinase, and of adenylate kinase. This pattern was similar to that found in young infants with severe postnatal protein-calorie malnutrition, providing further evidence that fetal growth retardation is an index of prenatal malnutrition.

SIGNIFICANCE OF LOW BIRTH WEIGHT

Why are we concerned with low birth weight in infants? The studies discussed so far on the effects of undernutrition in humans on the outcome of pregnancy are suggestive but do not provide absolute proof that maternal undernutrition produces deleterious effects on the offspring. However, other parameters of fetal development such as birth weight may give us additional information.

Low birth weight is, in general, an important index of the condition of the newborn. There is a very high correlation between low birth weight and perinatal mortality (Figure 7–6). There is also strong evidence from a number of large-scale studies that low birth weight is correlated with congenital abnormalities. Thus, fetal malnutrition as evidenced by low birth weight appears to cause an increase in the incidence of birth defects.

Infants with fetal growth retardation who were followed for eight years after birth continued to show heights and weights below their siblings with normal birth weight. As birth weight increases, neonatal death decreases up to a certain point. However, when the infant's birth weight is higher than normal, as in the case of diabetic mothers, neonatal mortality rises.

Examination of a variety of data in humans suggests that, in general, maternal nutrition in the latter part of gestation affects final growth of the fetus and thus the birth weight, but that maternal nutrition during the earlier part of pregnancy affects fetal mortality and development. The nutrition of the mother during her own development and childhood may also be a crucial factor. For example, women who have had rickets in their early years may

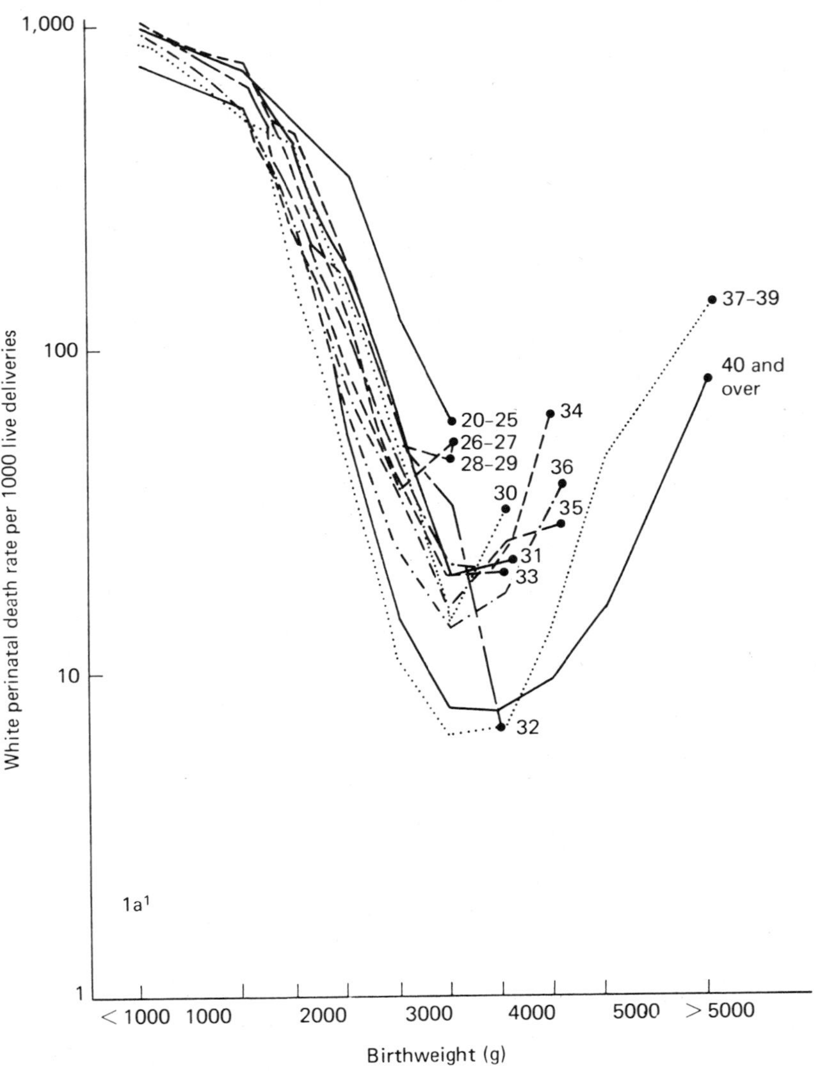

From Bergner and Susser, 1970.

Figure 7–6 Perinatal mortality for specified durations of pregnancy by birth weight, New York City whites, 1958 to 1961.

have deformities of the pelvis that prevent normal childbearing. Similarly, other nutritional factors during pre- and postnatal growth may influence subsequent reproductive performance and mask the influence or the effects of maternal nutrition during the period of the pregnancy itself. Thus, poor nutrition may produce an intergenerational effect, which would be seen in the generation following the one subjected to the nutritional insult. This is a question that needs a great deal of research and for which there is at present very little information available.

As is probably apparent by now, direct proof of the influence of nutrition and of undernutrition in human pregnancy is difficult to obtain because of the many interacting factors that influence the outcome of the pregnancy, the development of the fetus. Socioeconomic factors are also related. Low birth weight is correlated with poverty and race, and race and poverty are themselves correlated with malnutrition, so that these apparently interacting factors form a syndrome. Other complicating factors, for example, include lack of education, less well-integrated family units, poor hygienic conditions, and disease. In human studies it is seldom possible to differentiate these various factors.

ANIMAL STUDIES

We have seen that it is difficult to obtain precise information on the role of maternal malnutrition in fetal development in human studies because of the large number of interacting factors that can influence development and the difficulties in performing rigidly controlled investigations. Animal studies are, therefore, extremely useful, since specific single factors can be isolated and questions can be investigated experimentally. Studies on the effect of maternal malnutrition or of nutritional factors on prenatal development can be divided into two general types: (1) those on the effects of undernutrition in which the quantity of food intake is restricted and (2) those concerned with deficiencies of specific nutrients. Investigations of the effects of undernutrition in pregnant animals can further be divided into two kinds of experiments: (1) short-term total starvation or fasting studies and (2) longer-term experiments in which the animals' food intake is restricted.

FASTING

There are surprisingly few reports in the scientific literature of the effects of fasting during pregnancy in animals. Most of the work reported is in mice. In this species, total fasts of 24 or 30 hours during the period between the seventh and tenth days of gestation (total gestation period is 20 days) produced congenital malformations of the skeleton and the brain. When pregnant mice were fasted as long as 40 hours, no fetuses were carried to term and the pregnancy was interrupted. At the end of the fast, the pregnant females were severely hypoglycemic. Small quantities of glucose or amino acids could counteract the teratogenic effects of fasting. The effects of fasting on embryonic development were influenced by the age and the body weight of the mothers; that is, the fetuses of larger females were less severely affected than those of smaller ones, but teratogenic effects of fasting were more conspicuous in "elderly" than in young females.

In women fasted during the second trimester of pregnancy, plasma levels of glucose and insulin fell to a greater extent and ketone acid in the blood rose more rapidly than in nonpregnant controls. Nitrogen excretion in the urine was increased in the pregnant group. Thus it is possible that continuous glucose utilization by the conceptus may exaggerate and accelerate the metabolic consequences of starvation. Similar observations were made in rats.

RESTRICTION OF FOOD INTAKE

The effects of undernutrition during pregnancy—that is, restriction of total food intake—have been studied extensively in animals. Chow and his colleagues in a long series of studies showed that the offspring of rats whose food intake during pregnancy and lactation was restricted to 75% or 50% of the amount normally eaten were permanently stunted in growth (Figure 7–7). Under these conditions, there was a high mortality of the young during early postnatal life. When the intake during pregnancy alone was reduced to 50% of the normal amount, the young had low birth weights and their growth during the suckling and postweaning periods was persistently lower than normal.

Some investigators have reported that offspring of females subjected to undernutrition during pregnancy or lactation showed metabolic derangements. No gross congenital malformations have been observed in the offspring of experimental animals receiving restricted food intake during pregnancy, but some permanent anatomical aberrations have been found. For example, the skeletons of the young of undernourished female rats were smaller and less mature than those of controls, even after more than three months of ad libitum feeding. In this experiment, undernutrition occurred during both prenatal and postnatal life—that is, during pregnancy and lactation—with ad libitum feeding at weaning. By four months after weaning, the fore and hind limbs and the skull had recovered their normal lengths, but the lengths of the spine and of the pelvis were still abnormal.

Another structure that has been found to be affected by maternal undernutrition during pregnancy and lactation is the perineurium, the outer layer of peripheral nerves. In normal rats this structure provides a barrier to the diffusion of protein that is functionally apparent at the age of four weeks. In the animals subjected to pre- and postnatal undernutrition, no effective barrier was present even after three months of ad libitum food intake. This occurred even when the animals received ad libitum food from the age of

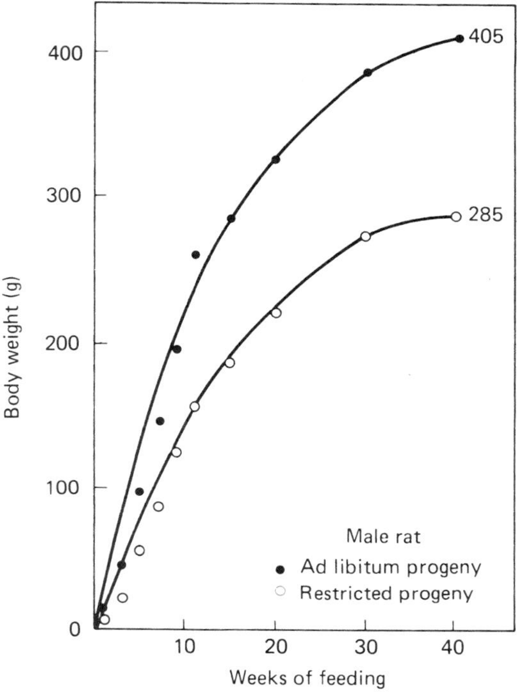

From Chow and Lee, 1964.

Figure 7–7 Growth rates of male rats born to mothers whose dietary intake was unrestricted, or restricted to one-half that of the unrestricted group.

five days. Such irreversibly impaired barriers may be significant in the development of diseases of the nervous system.

Many of the studies of maternal undernutrition are linked with studies of protein deficiency and are discussed in Chapter 9.

CELLULAR GROWTH

The effects of maternal undernutrition on the fetus are often studied in terms of cellular growth (see Chapters 2 and 7). If the maternal diet is restricted during the period of cell replication (hyperplasia) in the embryo or fetus, there is a decreased number of cells in the fetus, and this change appears to be permanent. If, however, the maternal dietary restriction occurs during the period of hypertrophic growth of a tissue or organ (increase in cell size), the effect is to reduce the cell size but not the cell number. Reduction in cell size does not appear to be an irreversible change, and the cell size will return to normal if the animal is refed. Thus, depending in part upon timing during gestation, maternal undernutrition during the prenatal period may lead to a decreased number of cells in various fetal organs and in the placenta in both animals and man.

References and Supplementary Readings

ANTONOV, A. N. "Children born during the siege of Leningrad in 1942." *J. Pediatrics* **30**: 250 (1947).

BERGNER, L., AND M. W. SUSSER. "Low birth weight and prenatal nutrition: an interpretative review." *Pediatrics* **46**: 946–966 (1970). Copyright American Academy of Pediatrics, 1970.

BRASEL, J. A., AND M. WINICK. "Maternal nutrition and prenatal growth." *Arch. Dis. Childhood* **47**: 479–485 (1972).

BURKE, B. S., V. A. BEAL, S. B. KIRKWOOD, AND H. C. STUART. "The influence of nutrition during pregnancy upon the condition of the infant at birth." *J. Nutrition* **26**: 569 (1943).

CHOW, B. F., AND C.-J. LEE. "Effect of dietary restriction of pregnant rats on body weight gain of the offspring." *J. Nutrition* **82**: 10–18 (1964).

DICKERSON, J. W. T., AND P. C. R. HUGHES. "Growth of the rat skeleton after severe nutritional intrauterine and post-natal retardation." *Resuscitation* **1**: 163–170 (1972).

FELIG, P., AND V. LYNCH. "Starvation in human pregnancy: Hypoglycemia, hypoinsulinemia, and hyperketonemia." *Science* **170**: 990–992 (1970).

FITZHARDINGE, P. M., AND E. M. STEVEN. "The small-for-date infant. I. Later growth patterns." *Pediatrics* **49**: 671–681 (1972).

HYTTEN, F. E., AND I. LEITCH. *The Physiology of Human Pregnancy*, pp. 440–450. Oxford: Blackwell Scientific Publications, 1971.

JEANS, P. C., M. B. SMITH, AND G. STEARNS. "Incidence of prematurity in relation to maternal nutrition." *J. Amer. Diet. Assn.* **31**: 576–581 (1955).

METCOFF, J. "Maternal leukocyte metabolism in fetal malnutrition." *Adv. Exp. Biol. Med.* **49**: 73–118 (1973).

MILLER, J. R. "A strain difference in response to the teratogenic effect of maternal fasting in the house mouse." *Can. J. Genet. Cytol.* **4**: 69–78 (1962).

NAEYE, R. L. "Cardiovascular abnormalities in infants malnourished before birth." *Biol. Neonat.* **8**: 104–113 (1965).

NAEYE, R. L., M. M. DIENER, H. T. HARCKE, JR., AND W. A. BLANC. "Relation of poverty and race to birth weight and organ and cell structure in the newborn." *Pediat. Res.* **5**: 17–22 (1971).

NAEYE, R. L., W. BLANC, AND C. PAUL. "Effects of maternal nutrition on the human fetus." *Pediatrics* **52**: 494–503 (1973).

PRIMROSE, T., AND A. HIGGINS. "A study in human antepartum nutrition." *J. Reprod. Med.* **7**: 257–264 (1971).

ROEDER, L. M., AND B. F. CHOW. "Maternal nutrition and its long-term effects on the offspring." *Amer. J. Clin. Nutrition* **25**: 812–821 (1972).

RUNNER, M. N., AND J. R. MILLER. "Congenital deformity in the mouse as a consequence of fasting." *Anat. Rec.* **124**: 437–438 (1956).

SCOW, R. O., S. S. CHERNIK, AND M. S. BRINLEY. "Hyperlipemia and ketosis in the pregnant rat." *Am. J. Physiol.* **206**: 796–804 (1964).

SIMA, A., AND P. SOURANDER. "The effect of perinatal undernutrition on perineurial diffusion barrier to exogenous protein." *Acta Neuropath.* (*Berl.*) **24**: 263–272 (1973).

SMITH, C. "The effect of wartime starvation in Holland upon pregnancy and its product." *Am. J. Obstet. Gynecol.* **53**: 599 (1947).

SMITH, C. "Effects of maternal undernutrition upon the newborn infant in Holland (1944–1945)." *J. Pediatrics* **30**: 229 (1947).

STEIN, Z., M. SUSSER, G. SAENGER, AND F. MAROLLA. *Famine and Human Development. The Dutch Hunger Winter of 1944/45.* New York: Oxford University Press, 1975. Copyright © 1975 by Oxford University Press, Inc. Reprinted by permission.

TUNCER, M. "Bone development, incidence of hypoglycemia and effect of maternal and fetal factors in low birth weight infants." *Turk. J. Pediatrics* **12**: 59–71 (1970).

WILSON, M. G., H. I. MEYERS, AND A. H. PETERS. "Postnatal bone growth of infants with fetal growth retardation." *Pediatrics* **40**: 213–223 (1967).

YASUDA, M., H. NANJO, AND M. SUZUKI. "The effect of fasting upon the development of embryos in elderly pregnant mice." *Kaibogaku Zasshi* **41**: 43–48 (1966).

8

Malnutrition, brain growth, and learning

The subject of malnutrition and learning may be resolved into three main questions.

1. Does early malnutrition have a *permanent* effect on brain size or on other physical parameters? Whether or not malnutrition affects the size or some other physical parameter of the brain at the time that malnutrition is taking place is of interest, but it is not in itself of very great consequence if these effects can be overcome. The important question is thus whether or not there are *permanent* effects on physical parameters of the brain.
2. If malnutrition does have a permanent effect on some physical aspect of the brain, what is the *functional* significance of this effect? Does a brain that is smaller than normal or otherwise different in some physical or chemical parameter necessarily mean that there is a deficit of function as well as of physical characteristics?
3. What do such changes mean in terms of the human condition? What do they mean in terms of a functioning individual, or an individual in a group, or a group of individuals in a society? In other words, if there are deficits of function, are these meaningful in terms of human ability in both short-term and long-run considerations?

MALNUTRITION AND BRAIN GROWTH

NORMAL BRAIN GROWTH

In Chapter 2, the changes during growth in DNA content of various organs were described. Figure 2–5 shows that the number of cells in various organs increases at different rates. Also, the number of cells in each organ stops increasing at different times during the development of the animal. The brain stops its cell replication earlier than does the body as a whole or than do liver, spleen, thymus, kidney, and lung. Furthermore, the time scales at which these various growth patterns change are different in different animals.

The increase in growth of the brain can be plotted as a percentage of its adult weight. Although the general pattern of brain development is similar in various mammalian species, there are species differences in the timing with respect to birth of the growth spurt of the brain. The growth spurt is the period in which increase in brain weight occurs at the highest rate. Other important developmental processes also take place at high velocity during this period.

Figure 8–1 shows the curves of growth rate of the brain in relation to developmental age in various species. The growth spurt of the brain of a rat occurs after birth, during the suckling period. For the dog, it comes much earlier in the neonatal period, almost immediately after birth. In the pig, the curve of growth rate plateaus before and after the birth period. In man, the growth spurt occurs just about the time of birth, while in the guinea pig the maximum rate of growth of the brain is before birth. This latter observation is consistent with the fact that the guinea pig is more developed at birth than is the rat or man.

Achievement of the total adult brain weight in terms of time is also different among the guinea pig, the rat, and man. For the human, much of the

Figure 8–1 Rate curves of brain growth in relation to birth in different species. Values are calculated at different time intervals for each species.

From Dobbing, 1972.

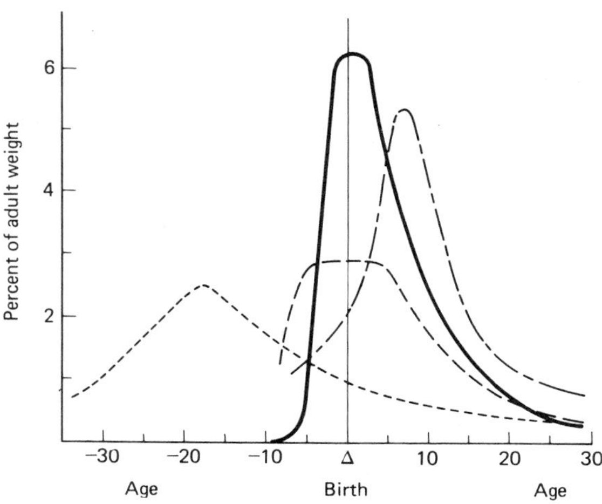

final growth of the brain takes place after birth, up to about two years, as is seen in Figure 8–2. In the rat, even more growth takes place after birth than in the human, while in the guinea pig relatively little brain growth occurs after birth.

The differences among these three species in brain growth are seen even more clearly in the relative increases in number of brain cells (DNA) during development. Figure 8–3 shows that in the guinea pig all brain cells are present at birth, about 75% of the adult number are present in the newborn human, and only 17% of the final number of brain cells are found in the newborn rat.

CHANGES IN BRAIN COMPOSITION

At the time of the growth spurt of the brain, other changes in physical and chemical parameters are also occurring. There is an increase in myelin

Figure 8–2 Relative increases in total brain weight during development of the human, guinea pig, and rat brains. Growth characteristics of the rat brain have been made comparable to those of the human by taking into account the thirtyfold difference in life span. All adult values have been adjusted for valid comparisons. Human ———; guinea pig --------; rat ············.

From Chase, 1971.

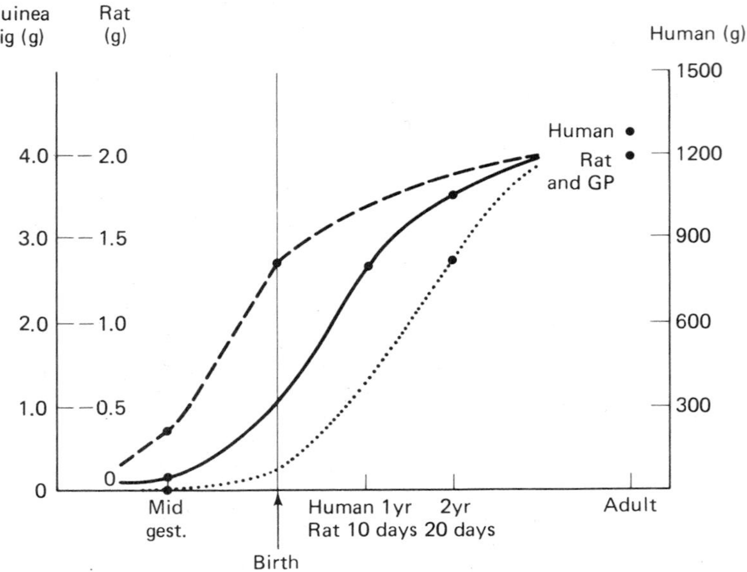

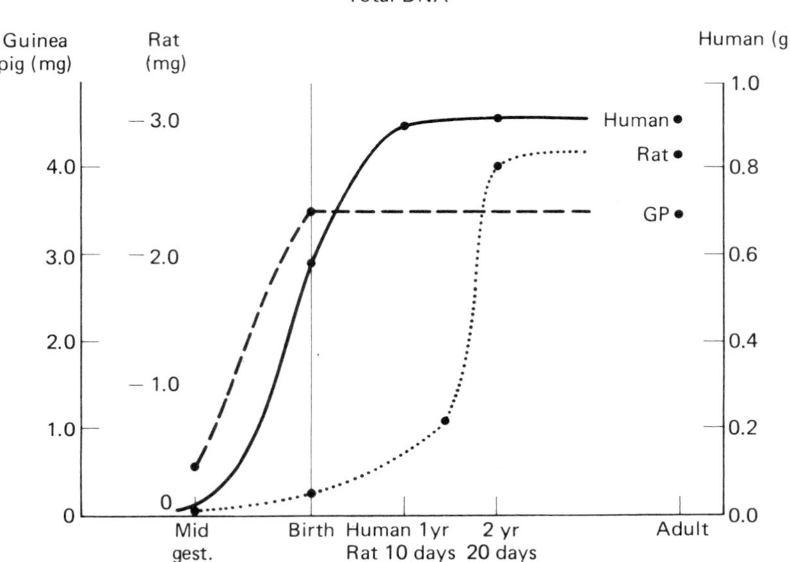

From Chase, 1971.

Figure 8–3 Relative increases in cellularity (DNA) during development of the human, guinea pig, and rat brains. Growth characteristics of the rat brain have been made comparable to those of the human by taking into account the thirtyfold difference in life span. All adult values have been adjusted for valid comparisons. Human ———; guinea pig - - - - - - - -; rat ············.

lipid; this is a period when there is rapid myelination of the brain. As seen in Figure 8–4, myelination in the human and in the rat occurs almost entirely after birth, while in the guinea pig only about half the myelin is laid down after birth and into the first year.

Along with myelination, other changes occur at this time. There is multiplication of glial cells, and many enzyme systems that are important for brain function are developing. There are also changes in the metabolism of the brain, especially its carbohydrate metabolism, development of certain reflex patterns, and changes in water and cation content. Figure 8–5 shows the changes in cholesterol, DNA, and water concentration in the developing guinea pig brain. The water decreases during development, and the concentration of cholesterol and other substances increases. Since cholesterol is a component of myelin, its concentration is used as an indicator of myelination. In Figure 8–6, the same data are shown as weight increments at two-day intervals, and again it is seen that DNA and cholesterol increase at about the same time.

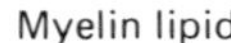

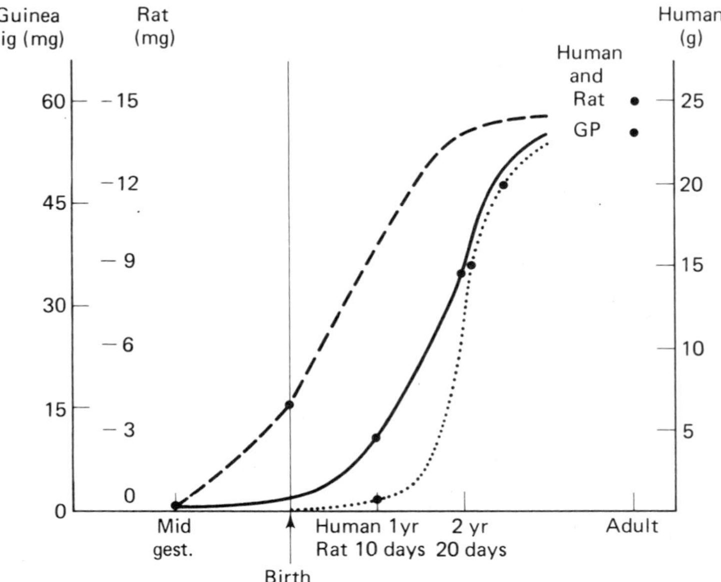

From Chase, 1971.

Figure 8–4 Relative increases in myelin lipids (cerebroside and sulfatide) during development of the human, guinea pig, and rat brains. Growth characteristics of the rat brain have been made comparable to those of the human by taking into account the thirtyfold difference in life span. All adult values have been adjusted for valid comparisons. Human ———; guinea pig - - - - - - -; rat ············.

Figure 8–5 Composition of the developing brain in the guinea pig.

From Dobbing and Sands, 1970.

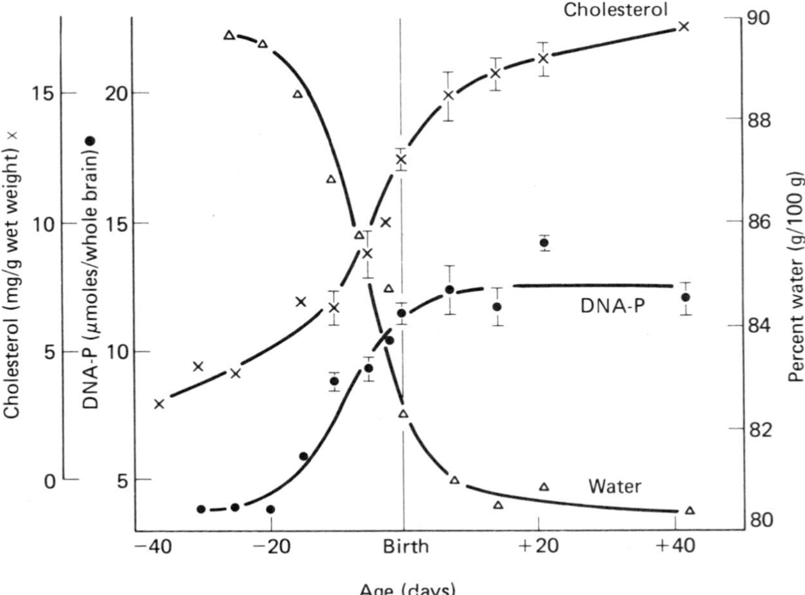

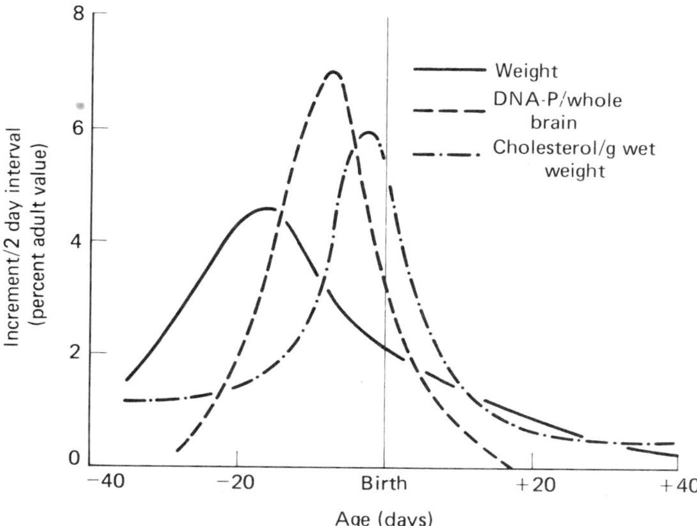

From Dobbing and Sands, 1970.

Figure 8–6 Velocity curves showing increments of wet weight, whole brain DNA-P, and cholesterol concentration per unit wet weight, expressed as percentage of the adult value.

EFFECT OF MALNUTRITION

Growth. What happens if malnutrition occurs? According to Dobbing, the brain is especially vulnerable to malnutrition during its period of growth spurt, so that relatively mild restriction of food intake during this period leads to permanent effects on growth of the brain and the body as a whole in experimental animals. Whether such effects are caused by prenatal or by postnatal nutrition thus depends on the timing of brain growth and development with respect to birth for each species. These growth deficits may be expressed in terms of cell size and number.

The work of Winick and Noble in relation to cell number and cell size was discussed in Chapter 2. The most important contribution of these investigators was to show the effect of malnutrition on these parameters. They showed that if animals were restricted in their nutritional intake, the effect on the brain (or other organs) was related to the period at which the restriction took place. If the restriction was early, during the period of cell replication, or hyperplasia, it interfered with cell division, and even after a period of refeeding the total cell number was lower than normal. If the malnutrition was late, during the period of hypertrophy, then there was a decreased ratio of protein to DNA, which means there was a decreased cell size. After refeeding, however, the ratio became normal; there was recovery. This principle was established in experiments in which groups of rats were restricted in their food intake: some were restricted for a period beginning at birth, some at weaning, and some for a period beginning at 65 days of age. All were refed at a later period.

The easiest way to restrict the feeding of a rat at birth is to increase the number of rats in the litter so that the mother has to suckle a large litter. Each individual rat pup in this case gets a smaller amount of food. Restricting the food intake at weaning or thereafter is done by decreasing the amount of food given to the animal. In the rats that were malnourished from weaning to 42 days of age, which would be the period in human beings comparable to childhood, all of the organs were reduced in total weight and protein concentration, but the brain and the lungs had normal DNA content. The other organs had a reduced DNA content. Thus, in the brain and the lungs the cell size was reduced but the cell number was normal. In the other organs the cell number was reduced but the cell size was normal. In these animals, only the brain and the lung recovered upon refeeding. As seen in Figure 2–5, this period from day 21 to day 42 in the rat is past the time when cell division is taking place in the brain and the lung, and when increased numbers of cells are accumulating. Malnutrition during this period did not affect the total cell number, but malnutrition during the period of active cell division reduced the number of cells.

These experiments suggest that any interference with cell division will produce a permanent effect on the number of cells. If malnutrition occurred at the time when the organ was normally in its period of hyperplasia, then even if the animal was later fed as much as it would eat, it could not make up for its reduced number of cells because the period of cell division was over. If, however, malnutrition took place during the time of the increase in cell size, then refeeding at a later time could make up the deficit.

Another aspect of the effect of malnutrition on the brain involves the nature of brain cells. The brain is not composed of a single cell type as is the liver, for example; the brain is really a composite of different structures, different parts, and different cell types. Each region of the brain has its own pattern of cellular growth and can accordingly be affected in different ways. It is oversimplification to say that growth or DNA content of the brain is affected or is not affected by a certain treatment. Thus, as shown in Figure 8–7, in rats malnourished for the first ten days of life only glial cell division was inhibited in the cerebral cortex, but in the cerebellum and lateral and third ventricles cell division of many different types of cells was decreased (Winick, 1976).

Overfeeding during the critical period of brain growth has also been shown to affect its total cell number. In some experiments, suckling rats were overfed by altering the number of rats in the litter. In this case, the animals were nursed in litters of three to six (instead of the usual eight to

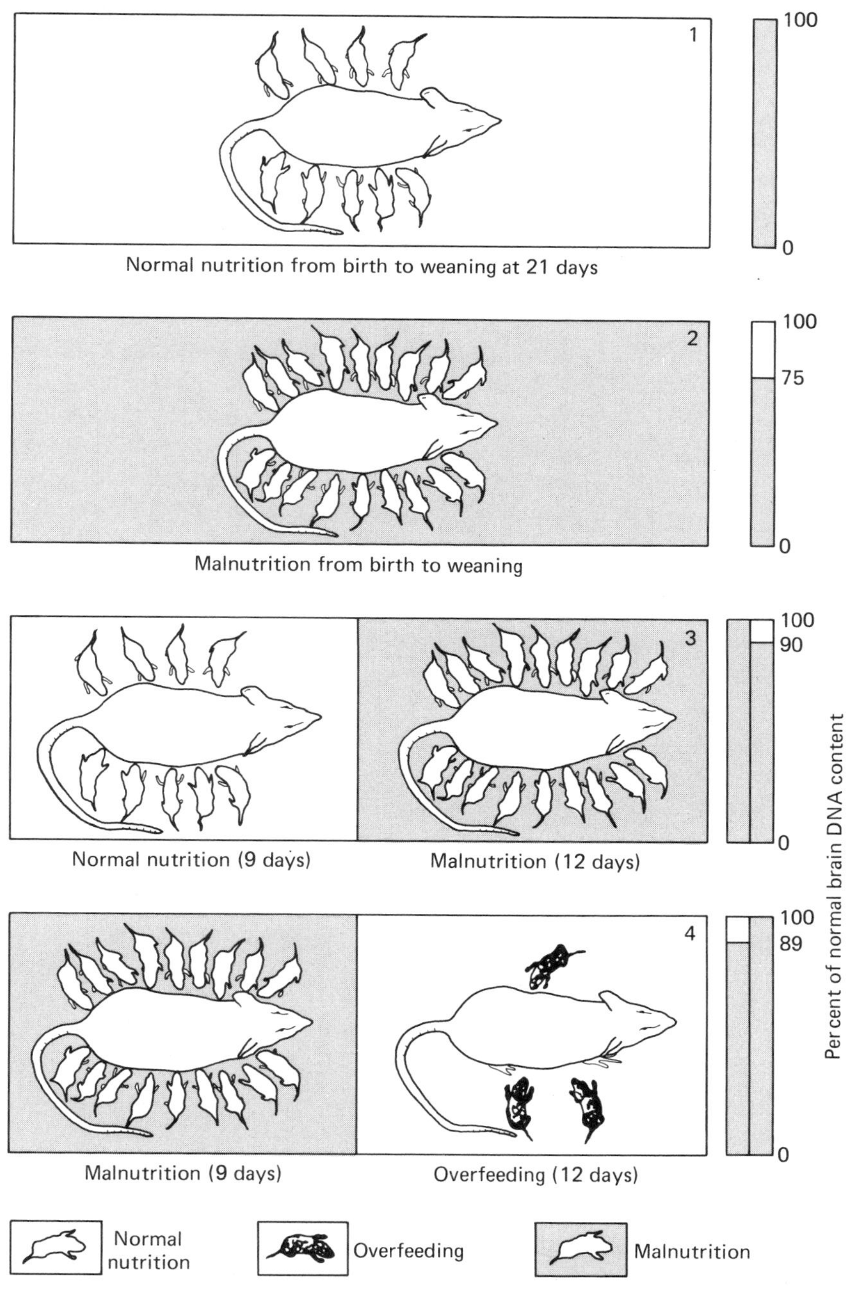

From Winick, 1976.

Figure 8–7 Effect of malnutrition on individual cell types in rat brain.

twelve) and they grew to a very large body size. In such animals, the organs contained more cells than normal, but the individual cell size was normal. There was apparently an increased rate of cell division. Later experiments showed that the deficit in brain cell number produced by undernutrition during the first nine days of life could be entirely overcome by overnutrition during the next 12 days (see Figure 8–8). These results suggest that changes caused by malnutrition in infants could also be reversed by extra feeding as long as it occurred during the period of cell replication.

Chemical composition. Malnutrition during the vulnerable period has an effect on the chemical composition of the brain as well as on its growth. Myelination occurs at a rapid rate at the same time as the growth spurt of the brain. If malnutrition is imposed during the period of most rapid myelination, decreased cholesterol content and decreased cholesterol concentration result. Cholesterol is one of the components of myelin, along with cerebrosides, phosphatidylethanolamine, and sphingomyelin. All of these components are reduced under conditions of malnutrition in the vulnerable period, which leads to a reduced rate of myelination and a reduction in the ultimate amount of myelin in the brain.

Figure 8–8 Methods of altering nutritional status during the suckling period.

From Winick, 1976.

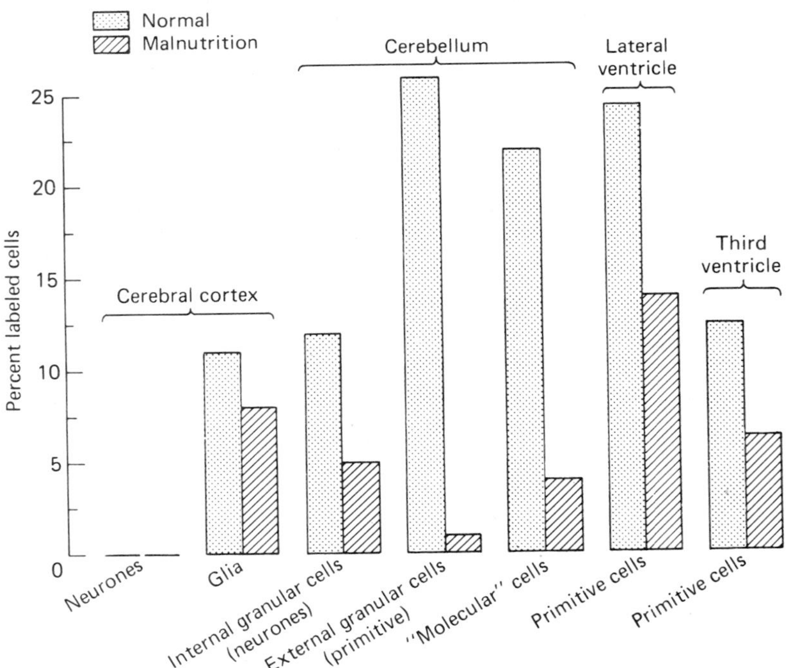

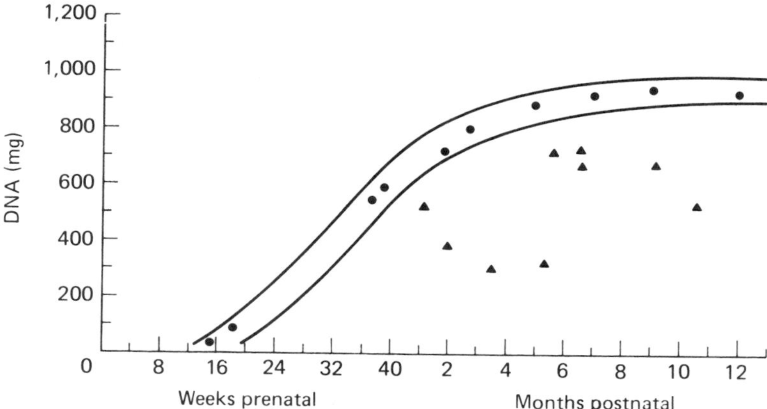

From Winick, 1969.

Figure 8–9 Reduction in cell number in nine children who died of malnutrition in Santiago, Chile. Lines indicate United States norms. ○ = brains of normal Chileans; △ = brains of Chilean children who died of marasmus.

Human studies. Similar findings have been observed in infants who were exposed to severe malnutrition during early life. In Chile, where there is a serious problem of infant malnutrition, studies were carried out on the brains of children who died. Normal children who had not been malnourished and who died suddenly in accidents had brain weights that fell within the normal range for U.S. children. In contrast, the brain weights of children in Chile who died of marasmus or malnutrition were all below the normal range (Figure 8–9). The concentrations of RNA, of protein, and of DNA were also lower in children suffering from malnutrition or marasmus than in normal children. These effects of malnutrition on the number of cells in the brain could be overcome if refeeding took place during the time when cell division was still going on. The exact timing of this critical period in the human is still uncertain, but evidence suggests that it lasts into the second year after birth.

Chase, studying a 12-month old infant who died of malnutrition (Figure 8–10), found that in comparison with two control children of similar age, the weight of body and brain were reduced, as were also content of brain cholesterol, gangliosides, and cerebrosides-sulfatides.

INFLUENCE ON BRAIN FUNCTION

Malnutrition in early life can thus have permanent effects on brain size, composition, and number of cells. This has been shown to occur in human infants as well as in animals. What does this mean in terms of brain function?

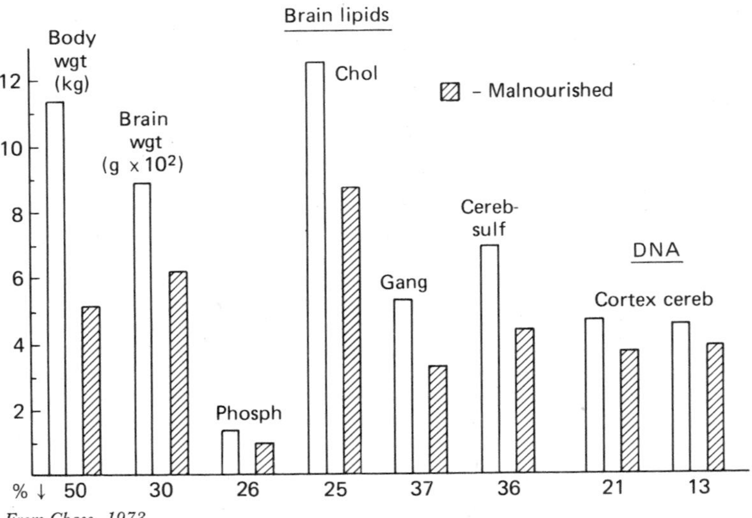

From Chase, 1973.

Figure 8–10 Comparison of body and brain weight, grams of brain lipid (phosph = lipid phosphorous, chol = cholesterol, gang = ganglioside, and cereb-sulf = cerebroside sulfatide) and brain DNA (cortex = cortex plus brain stem; cereb = cerebellum) from a 12-month-old malnourished child from Guatemala ▨, and two control children ▨ of similar age. Numbers on the abscissa represent the percent decrease of the undernourished subject compared to the two controls. It can be seen that the body weight is affected more than brain weight and that the alterations occurring in the brain are multiple.

Many studies have been carried out on experimental animals and human beings. It is extremely difficult to separate the various factors that can influence behavior in human beings, so for this reason behavioral studies on animals are most useful and can yield a great deal of information.

There is now a good deal of evidence that malnutrition at critical periods can produce alterations in behavior in experimental animals. A number of techniques have been used, such as learning tests, behavioral tests, and tests for emotionality. There are still many questions regarding the relevance of the tests themselves to human behavior. Nevertheless, it is well established that malnutrition during these critical periods does change the behavior of animals.

It is also clear from these studies that learning, however it is defined, seems to result from an interaction of response and stimulus. When an animal is put into a new environment, it responds to the environment by exploratory behavior, by investigating the new environment. This in turn elicits new stimuli to which the animal reacts. There is thus a constant feedback, and the animal learns as it is responding to the stimulus. From this interaction between stimulus and response, learning occurs. Malnutrition can alter this feedback response drastically by producing a decrease in the interaction between response and stimulus. When the malnourished animal is put into the new environment, it is apathetic. One of the outstanding features of malnutrition in infants is also apathy. They are not responsive to stimuli, therefore there is no reaction that can in turn call forth a new stimulus—the interaction of which forms the process of learning.

Another kind of situation, which does not start out as malnutrition but which can produce the same kind of result, is sensory deprivation. It can be seen in infants and in adults as well. An example of this effect is from an experiment that was published in 1930 on children in an orphanage. The orphanage was overcrowded and understaffed, so that the attendants had no time to do anything but feed the children in a very mechanical way and take care of their bodily needs. There was almost no socialization or personal interaction of any kind. The children were mentally retarded. The experiment consisted of removing some of the children into a home for mentally retarded children. It was a pleasant place, and the children were taken care of by attendants and by some of the older children in the home in an intensive one-to-one relationship. Twenty-one years later they were reinvestigated and they were all found to be self-supporting; the median school grade passed was the twelfth grade, which fits well within the U.S. norms for the time. The controls, who remained in the orphanage, all had low I.Q.'s; they were all still institutionalized, and the median grade passed was the third. Apparently, the sensory deprivation experienced in the orphanage had affected the learning ability of the children.

Sensory deprivation is also known to produce failure to thrive in children. They do not eat, do not grow, and are very apathetic. Such sensory deprivation can in itself produce mental defects.

Malnutrition helps to increase sensory deprivation, and this in turn has a negative effect on mental development, so that there is a synergistic effect of malnutrition and sensory deprivation. Work by Levitsky and Barnes with rats indicates that some of the effects of malnutrition can be overcome by increased sensory stimulation. In this experiment, rats were either well nourished or malnourished for seven weeks and then subjected to one of three environments—normal, isolated, or "enriched," that is, providing additional stimulation. After refeeding, behavioral testing revealed a highly significant interaction between early malnutrition and isolation. Environmental stimulation seemed to compensate for early malnutrition. Under similar conditions, activity of choline-acetyltransferase was depressed in brains of malnourished rats unless they were provided additional stimulation in the environment. Malnutrition and isolation thus appear to exert synergistic effects that are evident at the biochemical as well as behavioral level and that can be overcome at least in part by additional stimulation by the environment (Figure 8–11).

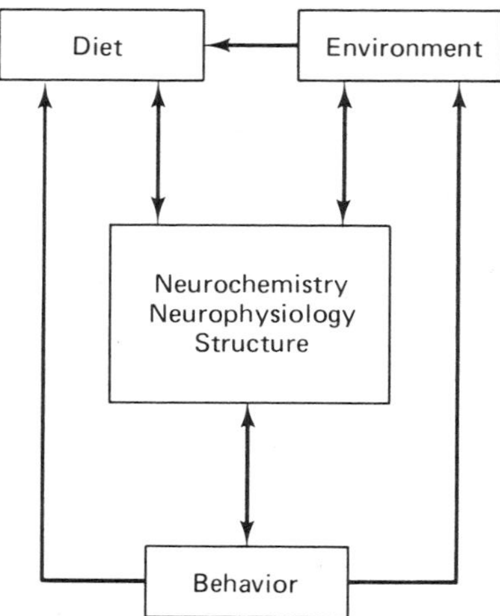

From Food and Nutrition Board, NRC, 1973.

Figure 8–11 Interrelationship of diet, environment, and behavior.

EARLY MALNUTRITION AND LEARNING CAPACITY

The important question in terms of human society is the following: does early malnutrition have any effect on learning capacity? The difficulty in trying to answer this question is in isolating the factor of malnutrition from all the other factors that can influence learning capacity and I.Q. under the conditions where malnutrition is found. Malnutrition is rarely found as a single factor. It is found in combination with poverty, low socioeconomic level, poor home environment, lack of intellectual incentive, and other factors that are related to development of low learning capacity.

A study was recently made in which children who had suffered from malnutrition during their first two years of life were compared with siblings who had not suffered malnutrition. The children were studied at school age, and it was found that those who had been malnourished had lower I.Q.'s than their own siblings. However, even in this carefully done study, the factor of hospitalization could not be eliminated, since the children had been hospitalized because of their malnutrition and their siblings had not.

The multifactorial nature of the interrelationships between malnutrition and intellectual ability is schematized in Figure 8–12. It is seen that in developing countries lack of education, technologic backwardness, problems of sanitation, infection, large families, inadequate child care, and malnutrition form a vicious cycle. Some of these factors can also be found in developed

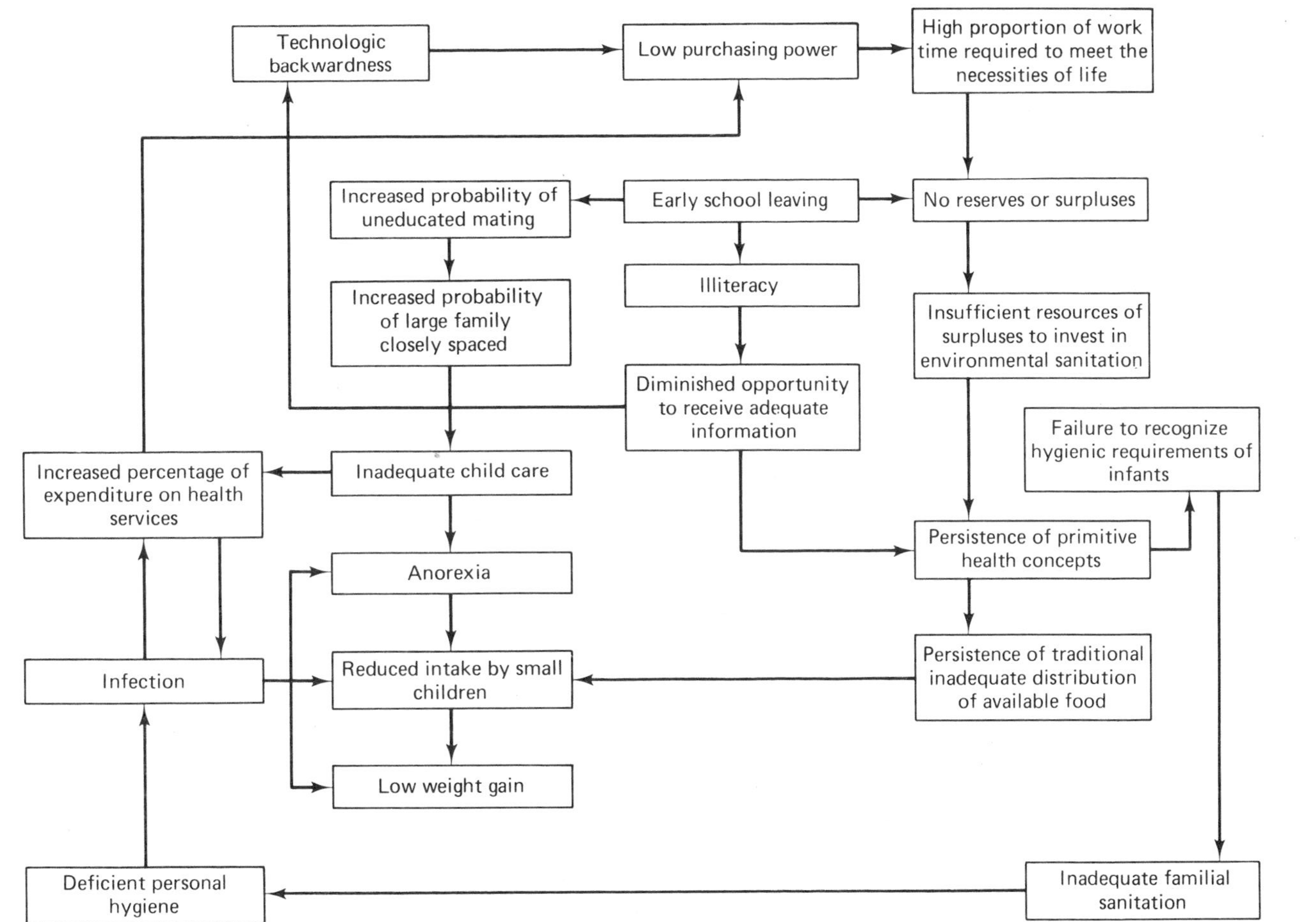

From Cravioto, 1970.

Figure 8–12 Interrelation among biosocial factors and malnutrition.

countries among people living at the poverty level. The recent finding that prenatal exposure to the Dutch famine of 1944–1945 (see Chapter 7) did not seem to be related to the mental performance of young men at age 19 may thus be related to environmental factors other than nutrition that influence development of mental performance.

A recent retrospective study of Korean orphans suggests a similar conclusion. In this group, all of whom were adopted by American families before the age of two, some of the children were severely malnourished during the first year of life. Tests of intelligence and achievement were tabulated between the ages of seven and 16. The mean I.Q. and achievement of the previously well-nourished children were significantly higher than that of the previously malnourished children, although the latter reached a level of I.Q. and school achievement that was perfectly normal for American children of their age and grade.

In conclusion, early nutritional deprivation appears to result in permanent anatomical or biochemical changes, but its direct causal relationship to permanent and irreversible alteration in intellectual capacity in humans is not clear.

References and Supplementary Readings

BARNES, R. H. "Nutrition and man's intellect and behavior." *Fed. Proc.* **30**: 1429–1433 (1971).

CHASE, H. P. "The effects of intrauterine and postnatal undernutrition on normal brain development." *Ann. N.Y. Acad. Sci.* **205**: 231–244 (1973).

CHASE, H. P., C. S. DABIERE, N. N. WELCH, AND D. O'BRIEN. "Intrauterine undernutrition and brain development." *Pediatrics* **47**: 491–500 (1971). Copyright American Academy of Pediatrics, 1968 and 1971.

CRAVIOTO, J. "Complexity of factors involved in protein-calorie malnutrition." In: P. GYORGY AND O. L. KLINE, eds., *Malnutrition is a Problem of Ecology*, Nutritio et Dieta, No. 14. Basel: S. Karger, 1970.

DOBBING, J. "Vulnerable periods of brain development." In: A. VON MURALT, ed., *Lipids, Malnutrition and the Developing Brain*, pp. 9–29. Amsterdam: Associated Scientific Publishers, 1972. Ciba Found. Symp., Ud. 3. Copyright © Ciba Found.

DOBBING, J., AND J. SANDS. "Growth and development of the brain and spinal cord of the guinea pig." *Brain Res.* **17**: 115–123 (1970).

DOBBING, J., AND J. SANDS. "Quantitative growth and development of human brain." *Arch. Dis. Childhood* **48**: 757–767 (1973).

ECKHERT, C. D., D. A. LEVITSKY, AND R. H. BARNES. "Postnatal stimulation: the effects on cholinergic enzyme activity in undernourished rats." *Proc. Soc. Exp. Biol. Med.* **149**: 860–863 (1975).

FOOD AND NUTRITION BOARD, NRC, NAS. *The Relationship of Nutrition to Brain Development and Behavior.* Washington, D.C., 1973.

HERTZIG, M. E., H. G. BIRCH, S. A. RICHARDSON, AND J. TIZARD. "Intellectual levels of school children severely malnourished during the first two years of life." *Pediatrics* **49**: 814–824 (1972).

LEVITSKY, D. A., AND R. H. BARNES. "Nutritional and environmental interactions in the behavioral development of the rat: Long-term effects." *Science* **176**: 68–71 (1972).

STEIN, Z., M. SUSSER, G. SAENGER, AND F. MAROLLA. *Famine and Human Development. The Dutch Hunger Winter of 1944–1945.* New York: Oxford University Press, 1975.

WINICK, M., AND A. NOBLE. "Cellular response in rats during malnutrition at various ages." *J. Nutrition* **89**: 300–306 (1966).

WINICK, M., AND A. NOBLE. "Cellular response with increased feeding in neonatal rats." *J. Nutrition* **91**: 179 (1967).

WINICK, M. "Malnutrition and brain development." *J. Pediatrics* **74**: 667–669 (1969).

WINICK, M. *Malnutrition and Brain Development.* New York: Oxford University Press, 1976.

ZAMENHOF, S., AND E. VAN MARTHENS. "Study of factors influencing prenatal brain development." *Molecular Cellular Biochem.* **4**: 157–168 (1974).

9

Protein and amino acids

When general malnutrition or undernutrition occurs during pregnancy, a crucial nutritional factor that is limited by total food restriction is protein. Thus many of the same effects that occur with starvation or low food intake are also seen with protein deficiency. In fact, few studies have attempted to differentiate among caloric deprivation, protein deficiency, and protein-calorie malnutrition. This section will be concerned with studies of dietary protein deficiency in which caloric restriction was not a factor, so that the effects of protein deprivation alone could be investigated.

PROTEIN DEFICIENCY

The relation of protein intake to reproduction in rats was first studied with purified diets by Nelson and Evans. Various levels of from zero to 25% protein were used in the diet. With diets containing very low amounts of protein (0, 2.5, or 5% protein), there was a high incidence of resorptions, but no congenital malformations were seen (Table 9–1). Furthermore, the young at birth were very small. The birth weight of young born to mothers fed a diet containing 25% protein was 6.5 g, while young born to mothers given 2.5% protein weighed only 3.8 g. The gain in body weight of the mothers was also correlated with the protein content of the diet. Control mothers (with 25% protein in the diet) gained 120 g during the pregnancy, while those receiving only 5% protein in the diet gained only 24 g. Without any protein in the diet at all, the pregnant females lost body weight—41 g.

In a later experiment (see Table 9–1) embryonic death could be prevented by giving the mother injections of estrogen and progesterone or of progesterone alone. When no protein at all was given in the diet, but progesterone was injected, the body weight of the mothers again decreased during pregnancy, but their litters were maintained until birth. These findings suggest that the absence of protein in the diet affected gonadotrophic

TABLE 9-1 RELATION OF DIETARY LEVELS TO REPRODUCTION IN THE RAT

Dietary Protein Level, %	*No. of Rats Bred*	*Weight Change During Gestation, g*	*Resorptions, %*	*Birth Weight, g*
25	10	+120	0	6.5
20	10	+116	0	6.0
15	10	+ 95	0	6.0
10	10	+ 82	0	5.5
5	10	+ 24	0	4.7
2.5	10	− 22	70	3.8
0	10	− 41	89	2.9
0 + progesterone and estrogen	10	− 22	0	—[a]

[a]Not measured

Adapted from Nelson and Evans, 1953, 1954.

hormone production by the pituitary gland, and the resulting absence of the hormones estrogen and progesterone caused the pregnancy to be terminated. The offspring were thus not maintained *in utero* because of an *indirect* effect of the protein deficiency. That is, protein deficiency affected the mother's metabolism, and this indirectly affected the embryo by causing inadequate hormonal support. However, the effect of protein deficiency on the birth weight of the fetuses is not explained entirely by the hormonal imbalance.

These studies also show that in the case of protein deficiency, the fetus was to a significant extent acting as a parasite, because the mother was able to use her body tissue for protein to synthesize fetal tissue. However, under conditions of protein deficiency, if the fetuses survive to term and postnatal growth is studied, it can be seen that these offspring are not normal (see below). Their neonatal survival is poor, growth and development are abnormal, cell number is reduced, and kidney and intestinal function are impaired. The low birth weight indicates that their prenatal development and postnatal prognosis are not optimal.

Pregnancy could also be maintained in protein-deficient rats by injections of adrenal cortical steroids or ACTH, apparently through mobilization of maternal tissue protein. However, body weights of the fetuses were much lower than in protein-fed controls. In pigs, protein deficiency was less deleterious to the embryo than in rats. Embryonic mortality was not significantly reduced by lack of protein, although the newborn pigs were only about 80% of normal birth weight.

An extensive and well-controlled series of studies on the effect of prenatal protein deficiency in rats has been carried out by Zeman and her colleagues. In these experiments, the effects of prenatal deficiency were differentiated from those of postnatal (lactational) deprivation by cross-fostering studies during the suckling period. In cross-fostering studies, the offspring of females protein deficient during gestation were given at birth to normally fed females; conversely, the offspring of control females that had received the same purified diet but with a normal amount of protein were given to females who had received the protein-deficient diet during pregnancy. During the lactation period all groups received the normal diet. These studies showed that under conditions of prenatal protein deficiency there is decreased birth weight, birth length, and liver and kidney weights. However, heart, brain, and thymus weights in relation to body weight were higher in young protein-deficient dams than in controls. A decreased number of cells was found in the fetus at term, and this depression of cell number appeared to be irreversible even after long-term supplementation of food intake. When litters of rats whose mothers were protein deficient during pregnancy were reduced to four sucklings in order to increase their food intake, the liver, kidney, and heart increased in weight and their cells increased in size, but there were no increases in the number of cells in these organs. In the thymus, the number of cells increased and cell size decreased, but in the brain, the weight, number, and size of cells were unaffected. Thus, the effect of prenatal protein deficiency in reducing the number of cells in these organs was irreversible even with increased feeding after birth.

The postnatal effects of prenatal protein deficiency are thus a combination of the damage to the developing fetus in the prenatal period and the consequences of its inability to suckle adequately in the postnatal period. Furthermore, in females with inadequate protein during pregnancy, there was failure or inadequacy of lactation.

In addition to decreased cell number and cell size, the kidneys of newborn young from protein deficient rats had fewer glomeruli, proportionately more connective tissue, and fewer collecting tubules than normal controls. Glomeruli were also less well differentiated. The changes in the kidney were not only morphological but functional as well, and tests showed reduced kidney function in these animals. Both the morphological and functional differences were irreversible after birth, even with increased feeding. Other tissues also showed morphological abnormalities, especially intestine and skeleton. In the intestine of pups from protein-deficient dams there was delayed morphological development (see Figure 9–1) and reduced absorptive activity. Such reduced intestinal absorption is probably an important factor in the poor postnatal development of such young. Skeletal growth and development in these animals was significantly retarded and was not cor-

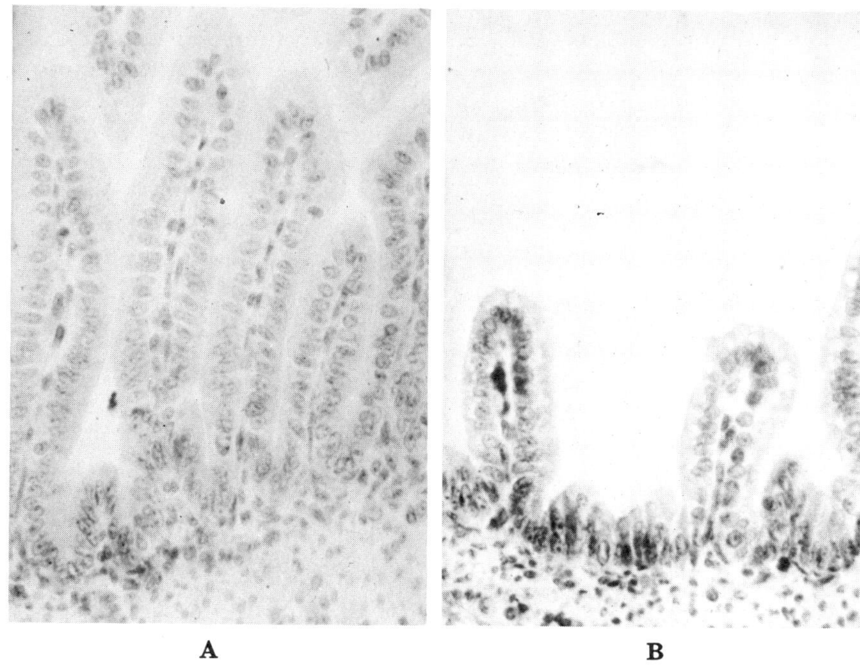

From Loh et al., 1971.

Figure 9–1 (a) Jejunal villi of newborn control rat pup. Microvilli (m) are present on the luminal surface of enterocytes. Intervillus crypt (c) cells contain mitotic figures. H&E. × 240. (b) Jejunal villi of newborn young of protein-deficient dam. Villi are widely separated. Crypts are not distinguishable. Cells appear vacuolated and lack brush borders. H&E × 240.

rected by increased postnatal food intake. The observations on skeletal growth and development appeared to be related to depressed synthesis of growth hormone.

AMINO ACIDS

DEFICIENCY

It is a principle of nutrition that deficiencies of single amino acids have, in general, effects similar to those of deficiency of protein as a whole, since for maximum utilization of dietary protein or amino acids for efficient protein synthesis all of the essential amino acids must be available to the body at approximately the same time. Thus it can be said in general terms that omission of single essential amino acids from the diet of pregnant animals produces effects similar to those of protein deficiency. However, there have been relatively few studies of effects of deficiencies of specific amino acids on prenatal development in mammalian species.

Pike, using an experimental diet with acid-hydrolyzed casein providing the amino acid mixture, found that tryptophan deficiency caused congenital cataracts in the offspring of rats. However, these congenital cataracts could not be prevented by addition of tryptophan alone but required additional niacin as well. The cataracts thus appeared to result from an inadequate supply of either tryptophan or niacin.

In other experiments in which diets containing mixtures of amino acids rather than hydrolyzed casein were used, the omission of one essential amino acid (except for lysine) resulted in a higher number of resorptions in rats. Growth of the uterus, placenta, and fetuses was also decreased. In a systematic study of the effect of amino acid deficiencies on the developing rat fetus, Zamenhof and his colleagues found that omission of trytophan, lysine, or methionine produced decreases in birth weight and in the cerebral weight, cerebral cell number, and protein content of the brain. These effects were similar to those produced by total protein deprivation. Thus, omission of single amino acids during pregnancy may be as harmful as total absence of dietary protein.

Another means of producing an amino acid deficiency was used by Persaud and Kaplan, who gave an analogue of leucine to pregnant rats. This compound, hypoglycin-A, was injected intraperitioneally during the first six days of gestation. Most fetuses at term had malformations including gastroschisis, encephalocele, syndactyly, and abdominal herniation. Malformations occurred in 92% of the young. Hypoglycin-A is of interest because it occurs naturally in certain fruit growing in the West Indies. This fruit is an important constituent of the Jamaican diet and has been incriminated as the causative factor of "vomiting sickness," which apparently results from ingestion of the unripe fruit. Clinical evidence suggests that hypoglycin-A might be teratogenic in humans. This experiment suggests the importance of leucine for fetal development, but it is difficult to interpret the results with respect to the teratogenesis of the compound for humans, since it was injected in the rats rather than being given by mouth. Also there was no control group that received both the leucine analogue and additional leucine as well.

EXCESS

Excessive amounts of single amino acids are also detrimental, since they result in amino acid imbalances or antagonisms. Large amounts of lysine or leucine in the diet of pregnant rats resulted in fetal mortality and retarded fetal growth. When injected, leucine also caused resorption and malformation.

Phenylalanine in excessive amounts is extremely deleterious to the developing embryo and fetus. This has been shown in rats, mice, monkeys, and humans. In rhesus monkeys, marked elevation of phenylalanine and tyrosine was produced in the blood of pregnant animals by feeding excess phenylalanine in the diet. The plasma of umbilical-cord blood under these conditions was also high in these amino acids, so that the embryo and fetus were subjected to excessive amounts of these compounds (see Figure 9–2). Infant monkeys born to hyperphenylalaninemic mothers were normally proportioned without gross congenital abnormalities. However, infants of mothers who had received the excessive phenylalanine throughout their pregnancies and who had shown the highest elevation of the amino acid in their serum had very low birth weights. Measurement of the free amino acid pattern in umbilical-cord serum showed that the concentrations of phenylalanine and tyrosine were extremely elevated in these fetuses, and in all cases free amino acids were higher in the fetus than in the mother. Tests of learning behavior

Figure 9–2 Free amino acids of umbilical cord venous serum at full-term gestation of *M. mulatta*. Blocks indicate mean value, ±1 standard deviation, from eight control pregnancies. Solid circles indicate values from the infant born to a pregnant female receiving excess dietary L-phenylalanine (pregnancy 3). Value for 3-CH_3-histidine could not be accurately determined.

From Kerr et al., 1968.

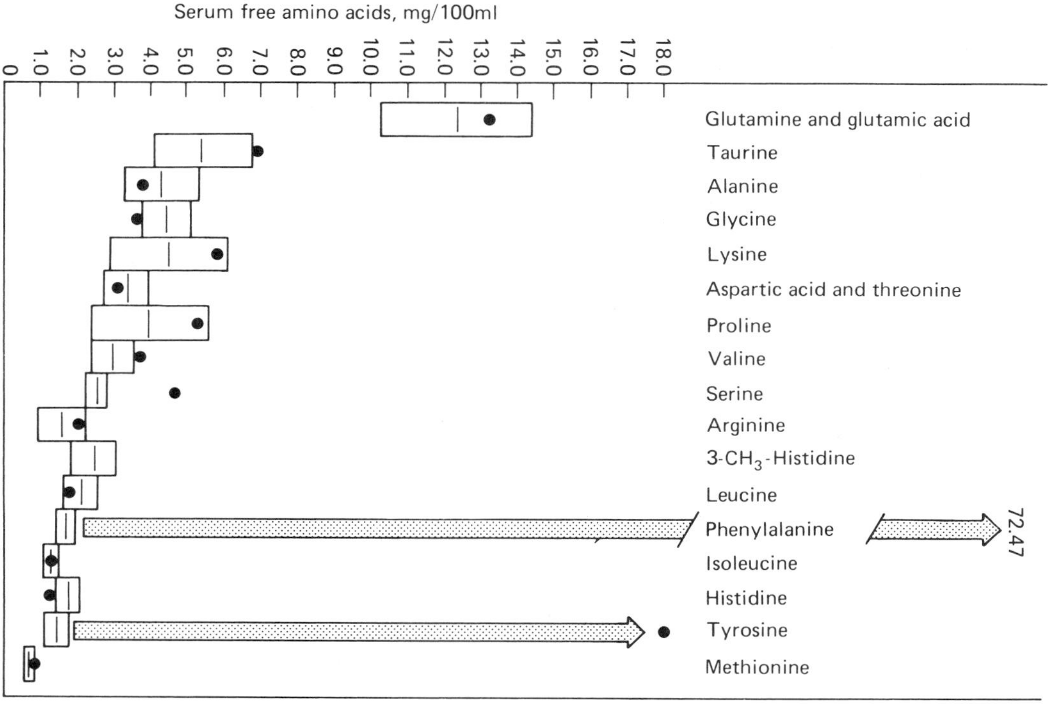

in these infant monkeys showed that those born to mothers with hyperphenylalaninemia had a significant reduction in learning behavior.

In rats, a high level of dietary phenylalanine plus daily injection of the amino acid led to fetal death, resorption, and congenital malformation in the offspring.

In humans, children born to women with phenylketonuria are often mentally retarded, even though the women themselves do not have the genetic disease. Maternal phenylketonuria may also result in intrauterine growth retardation, microcephaly, and other congenital malformations. Skeletal anomalies, cardiac defects, abnormal development of esophagus and spleen, and lung abnormalities have been observed. Spontaneous abortions have also occurred. Retardation of postnatal growth is also seen, and an inverse relationship was found between the level of phenylalanine in the mother's blood and the intelligence of the offspring. Thus it appears that if the maternal plasma phenylalanine level is high, fetal brain damage occurs, but at lower levels of maternal plasma phenylalanine there may be no damage to the fetal brain.

In one case a mother with phenylketonuria had three retarded children while on an unrestricted diet. In a subsequent pregnancy she was given a low-phenylalanine diet and gave birth to a normal infant. There are thus good prospects for the prevention of such abnormalities in the future.

References and Supplementary Readings

ALLAN, J. D., AND J. K. BROWN. "Maternal phenylketonuria and foetal brain damage. An attempt at prevention by dietary control." In: K. S. Holt and V. P. Coffee, eds., *Some Recent Advances in Inborn Errors of Metabolism*, pp. 14–38. Edinburgh: E. & S. Livingstone Ltd., 1968.

BERG, B. N., E. B. SIGG, AND P. GREENGARD. "Maintenance of pregnancy in protein-deficient rats by adrenocortical steroid or ACTH administration." *Endocrinology* **80**: 820–834 (1967).

KERR, G. R., A. S. CHAMOVE, H. F. HARLOW, AND H. A. WAISMAN. "Fetal PKU: The effect of maternal hyperphenylalaninemia during pregnancy in the rhesus monkey (*Macaca mulatta*)." *Pediatrics* **42**: 27–36 (1968).

LOH, K.-R. W., R. E. SHRADER, AND F. J. ZEMAN. "Effect of maternal protein deprivation on neonatal intestinal absorption in rats." *J. Nutrition* **101**: 1663–1672 (1971).

NELSON, M. M., AND H. M. EVANS. "Relation of dietary protein levels to reproduction in the rat." *J. Nutrition* **51**: 71–84 (1953).

NELSON, M. M., AND H. M. EVANS. "Maintenance of pregnancy in the absence of dietary protein with estrone and progesterone." *Endocrinology* **55**: 543–549 (1954).

NELSON, M. M., AND H. M. EVANS. "Maintenance of pregnancy in absence of dietary protein with progesterone." *Proc. Soc. Exp. Biol. Med.* **88**: 444–446 (1955).

PERSAUD, T. V. N., AND S. KAPLAN. "The effects of hypoglycin-A, a leucine analogue, on the development of rat and chick embryos." *Life Sci.* **9**: 1305–1313 (1970).

PIKE, R. L. "Congenital cataract in albino rats fed different amounts of tryptophan and niacin." *J. Nutrition* **44**: 191–204 (1951).

ZAMENHOF, S., S. M. HALL, L. GRAUEL, E. VAN MARTHENS, AND M. J. DONAHUE. "Deprivation of amino acids and prenatal brain development in rats." *J. Nutrition* **104**: 1002–1007 (1974).

ZEMAN, F. J. "Effect of protein deficiency during gestation on postnatal cellular development in the young rat." *J. Nutrition* **100**: 530–538 (1970).

ZEMAN, F. J., R. E. SHRADER, AND L. H. ALLEN. "Persistent effects of maternal protein deficiency in postnatal rats." *Nutrition Rep. Intl.* **7**: 421–436 (1973).

10

Carbohydrates and lipids

CARBOHYDRATES

Neither the requirement of the embryo and fetus for carbohydrates nor the effect of low-carbohydrate diets in the pregnant female on embryonic development is well understood. From experiments with early chick embryos *in vitro* it appears that carbohydrates are the primary source of energy in the early embryonic period and that glucose and fructose are utilized better than other carbohydrates at this time. It also seems that specific organs have various requirements for glucose, since different concentrations of the sugar were needed in order for the organ to be maintained in culture.

In the preimplantation blastocyst of the rabbit, glucose was found to occur, but its concentration was low relative to that in the maternal tissue. Glucose is transferred very readily by the placenta, and the rate of transfer is especially high near term. However, fetal blood contains a lower concentration of glucose than does maternal blood. During the first month of pregnancy in the human, glycogen is formed from glucose in the placenta, but later, near term, glycogen is synthesized in the fetal liver itself, and its concentration in this organ rises (see Chapter 3). Thus it appears that glucose, glycogen, and possibly other carbohydrates are important in embryonic and fetal metabolism.

A dietary practice that is poorly understood in regard to both its etiology and its consequences is that of amylophagia, or starch eating. The starch referred to in this condition is laundry starch. Amylophagia is a form of pica or perversion of the appetite. In one study of a group of pregnant women with this condition, very large amounts of starch were eaten, as much as one pound per day. There was a distinct correlation between starch eating and the incidence of severe anemia. The anemia results from iron deficiency, because the calories supplied by the starch replace those that would otherwise be obtained from food containing iron. There also seem to be relationships between starch eating in pregnancy and perinatal mortality.

Thus, excessive intake of carbohydrate will have bad nutritional repercussions if the carbohydrate is obtained from pure sources such as starch, because foods containing other essential nutrients are not eaten.

Large amounts of a simple sugar, galactose, have also been shown to be extremely deleterious to the developing embryo and fetus. When pregnant rats were fed diets containing 25% galactose, there were abnormalities of limb development in the fetuses. With dietary levels of 40% galactose in pregnant rats, a high incidence of cataracts was seen in the newborn young. Under such conditions there was also retardation of body growth and brain growth and reduced numbers of brain cells in the offspring.

In humans, congenital galactosemia is a disease that leads to mental retardation and opaque lenses of the eye. Galactosemia is a hereditary defect characterized by a block in the metabolism of galactose, so that galactose or galactose-containing sugars such as lactose in milk cannot be metabolized (Figure 10–1). Cataracts and mental retardation are clinical features of the condition (Table 10–1). Infants with this condition usually appear normal at birth, but after a short period of milk feeding gastrointestinal symptoms occur, followed by cataract formation and mental retardation. The development of the clinical syndrome of galactosemia depends on exposure to galactose, and therefore it is possible that the syndrome may be initiated

Figure 10–1 The effect of an oral galactose tolerance test on the blood glucose and galactose levels in an eight-year-old patient with galactosemia.

From Isselbacher, 1959.

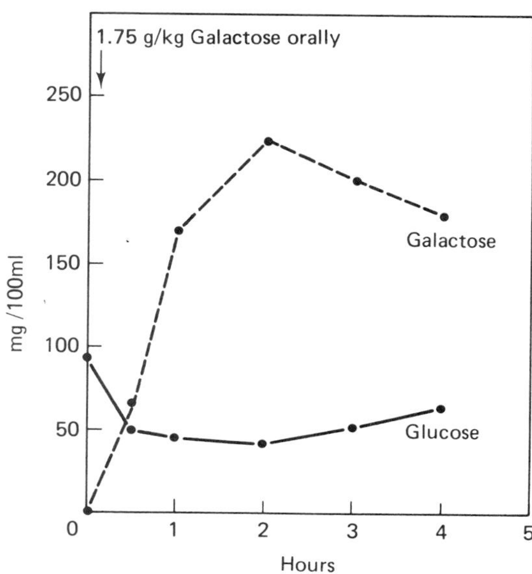

TABLE 10-1 CLINICAL AND LABORATORY FINDINGS IN GALACTOSEMIA

Clinical Features	*Laboratory Findings*
Nutritional failure Hepatosplenomegaly, jaundice, cirrhosis Cataracts Mental retardation	Elevated blood galactose Reduced galactose tolerance Deficient erythrocyte galactose-1-phosphate uridyl transferase Urine: galactose, amino acids, albumin

From Isselbacher, 1959.

in utero by passage of galactose through the placenta from the mother. In experimental studies in which high-galactose diets were fed to pregnant rats, cataracts were found in the newborns (see Figures 10–2 and 10–3). These

Figure 10–2 Normal series: (A) eye of a 16-day embryo, hybrid strain; (B) eye of an 18-day fetus, Wellesley College strain; (C) eye of an 18-day fetus, Wellesley College strain; (D) eye of a full term rat, Wellesley College strain.

From Bannon et al., 1945.

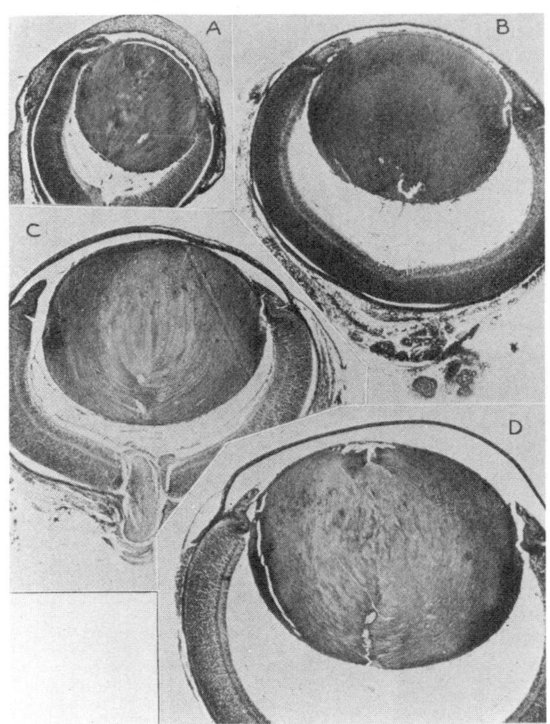

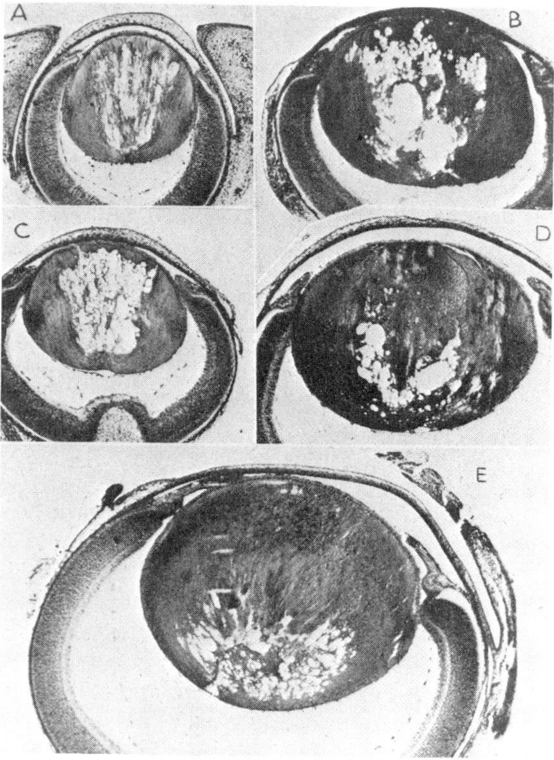

From Bannon et al., 1945.

Figure 10–3 Cataract series (A) eye of a 16-day embryo, hybrid strain; (B) eye of an 18-day fetus, Battle Creek strain; (C) eye of a 17-day fetus, hybrid strain; (D) eye of a 19-day fetus, Wellesley College strain; (E) eye of 19-day fetus, Battle Creek strain.

findings suggest that women known to be heterozygous for the galactosemia gene should take a diet low in lactose during pregnancy in order to decrease the possibility of harming the fetus by placental transfer of galactose.

LIPIDS

During development of the fetus its proportion of body lipids increases greatly (see Chapter 3). In the human, for example, lipid concentration of the whole body goes from 0.5% at 12 weeks to 9.0% at 42 weeks of fetal age. Differentiation of tissues and morphological development of new structures and organs requires synthesis of new cells containing phospholipids and sterols. Finally, toward the end of gestation, the large accumulation of fat during the last six weeks in the human requires an important quantity of lipids as well as lipid metabolism.

Despite the importance of these components, however, detailed information concerning the influence on embryonic development of lipid concentration in the maternal diet is limited in experimental animals as well as in man. Alterations in the composition of fat in the maternal diet do seem to produce some modifications of fetal fat composition. For example, the iodine number of fat could be varied in fetuses by changing the degree of saturation of the fatty acid in the maternal diet. However, the extent of alteration in the mother's tissue was much greater than in that of the fetus. In the guinea pig, chronic feeding of cholesterol to pregnant animals influenced the uptake of cholesterol by the fetus. Some alteration in fatty acid composition of fetal tissues was also noted in humans. Thus it appears that alterations in lipids of maternal diets can influence the composition of fetal lipids, but these changes are small compared to those of the mother's tissues and to the changes in the diet.

DEFICIENCY

A requirement of fat, actually essential fatty acids, for normal reproduction has been recognized since the early work on the discovery of essential fatty acids by Burr and Burr in 1930. In a systematic study of the effect of various levels of fat in the diet of rats from the time of weaning, Deuel and his colleagues found that rats fed a fat-free diet produced a small number of young per litter and that these offspring died within a few days after birth. Thus, normal pregnancy could not be maintained without essential fatty acids. Likewise, lactation and neonatal survival also required these essential nutrients (Table 10-2). A low level of essential fatty acids for two generations in rats resulted in young with low birth weight and a lower concentration of cerebrosides in their brains than in normal animals.

EXCESS

The influence of high-cholesterol diets on fetal development has been studied in experimental animals. In rabbits, high-cholesterol feeding produced fetuses of low body weight and caused high fetal mortality. In rats, on the other hand, these effects were not seen. However, drugs that alter the cholesterol level of the blood have been studied in experimental animals; a drug that increases the cholesterol level of the blood as well as a drug that decreases this constituent in maternal plasma have both been shown to be

TABLE 10–2 THE EFFECT OF DIFFERENT LEVELS OF COTTONSEED OIL ON PREGNANCY, SURVIVAL, AND GROWTH OF YOUNG FROM FEMALES ON A FAT-FREE DIET

Category	Group No.						
	1	2	3	4	5	6	7
Cottonseed oil fed daily, mg	0	10	40	100	200	400	1000
Females bred	23	24	25	25	25	25	25
Litters cast, percent	83	96	92	100	96	92	100
Litter (at birth):							
Total number of rats	122	196	192	228	210	227	232
Average number per litter	6.4	8.5	8.3	9.1	8.8	9.9	9.3
Litter (at 3 days):							
Total number of rats	0	46	117	162	162	196	175
Total litters represented		9	18	22	21	23	21
Average weight per rat, g		4.7	6.1	6.3	6.8	6.4	6.6
Litter (at 21 days):							
Total number of rats	0	9	88	124	114	122	126
Total litters represented		3	16	21	18	20	21
Average weight per rat, g		24.6	26.9	29.4	33.4	32.0	29.4
Mortality (0–3 days):							
Total	122	150	75	66	48	31	57
Percent	100	76	39	29	23	14	25
Mortality (3–21 days):[a]							
Total		32	9	11	18	22	14
Percent		77	9	8	14	15	11

[a]Litters were cut to seven at three days.

From Deuel et al., 1954.

teratogenic in experimental animals. The mechanism by which congenital malformations can be caused by these apparently contradictory treatments is unknown.

References and Supplementary Readings

ALLING, C., A. BRUCE, I. KARLSSON, O. SAPIA, AND L. SVENNERHOLM. "Effect of maternal essential fatty acid supply on fatty acid composition of brain, liver, muscle and serum in 21-day-old rats." *J. Nutrition* **102**: 773–782 (1972).

BANNON, S. L., R. M. HIGGINBOTTOM, J. M. MCCONNELL, AND H. W. KAAN. "Development of galactose cataract in the albino rat embryo." *Arch. Ophthal.* **33**: 224–228 (1945).

DEUEL, H. J., Jr., C. R. MARTIN, AND R. B. ALFIN-SLATER. "The effect of fat level of the diet on general nutrition. XII. The requirement of essential fatty acids for pregnancy and lactation." *J. Nutrition* **54**: 193–199 (1954).

FORD, R. C., AND J. L. BERMAN, "Phenylalanine metabolism and intellectual functioning among carriers of phenylketonuria and hyperphenyl-alaninaemia." *Lancet* **1**: 767–771 (1977).

HAWORTH, J. C., J. D. FORD, AND M. K. YOUNOSZAI. "Effect of galactose toxicity on growth of the rat fetus and brain." *Pediat. Res.* **3**: 441–447 (1969).

ISSELBACHER, K. J. "Galactose metabolism and galactosemia." *Am. J. Med.* **26**: 715–723 (1959).

KEITH, L., H. EVENHOUSE, AND A. WEBSTER. "Amylophagia during pregnancy." *Obstet. Gynec.* **32**: 415–418 (1968).

ROUX, C., AND M. AUBRY. "Action tératogène chez le rat d'un inhibiteur de la synthese du cholesterol, le AY 9944." *C. R. Soc. Biol.* **160**: 1353–1357 (1966).

ROUX, J. F., AND T. YOSHIOKA. "Lipid metabolism in the fetus during development." *Clin. Obstet. Gynec.* **13**: 595–620 (1970).

SEGAL, S., AND H. BERNSTEIN. "Observations on cataract formation in the newborn offspring of rats fed a high-galactose diet." *J. Pediatrics* **62**: 363–369 (1963).

SHELLEY, H. J., AND G. A. NELIGAN. "Neonatal hypoglycaemia." *Br. Med. Bull.* **22**: 34–39 (1966).

11

Fat-soluble vitamins

VITAMIN A

DEFICIENCY

Vitamin A deficiency has special significance in the history of teratology and developmental nutrition. The importance of this vitamin for normal prenatal development has been known since 1933, when Hale reported on experiments with vitamin A deficiency in pigs (see Chapter 6). A sow given a vitamin A-deficient ration for five months before breeding and for the first 40 days of pregnancy gave birth to a litter of 11 piglets, all of which were born without eyes (Figure 11–1). Similar treatment of additional sows also caused abnormalities of the eyes. This was the first report that congenital malformations in a mammal could result from environmental manipulation, and it led to the development of experimental teratology (see Chapter 6). In addition to various ocular defects, other anomalies such as accessory ears, subcutaneous cysts, cleft lip, and misplaced kidneys were found in the offspring of vitamin A-deficient sows. Experiments showed that these abnormalities were not due to genetic problems but were actually caused by the nutritional deficiency.

Major advances in the study of teratogenic effects of vitamin A deficiency were made by Warkany and his colleagues in a series of comprehensive studies in rats. In addition to eye defects, which they described in detail, these investigators also found histological abnormalities of the genitourinary tract, including fused kidneys, absence of male accessory sex glands, and lack of vaginal development. Diaphragmatic hernia was also observed in these animals, and there were pronounced cardiovascular abnormalities consisting of defects in the septa between ventricles and various anomalies of the aortic arch (Figure 11–2). In fetuses from vitamin A-deficient rats epithelial keratinization, a cardinal sign of vitamin A deficiency, was observed in the genitourinary tract.

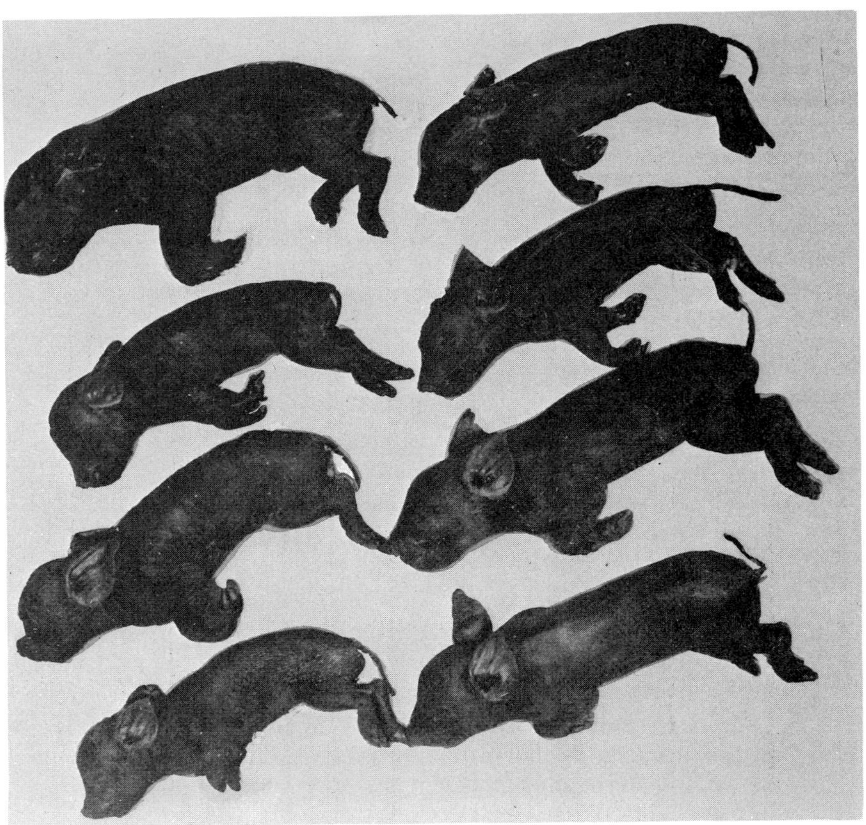

From Hale, 1933.

Figure 11–1 A Litter of Eyeless Pigs. Progeny of normal Duroc-Jersey sow all showing complete absence of eyeballs.

Even relatively mild deficiency of vitamin A caused abnormal development. Urogenital and eye anomalies were found in offspring of pregnant rats, even when the deficiency was so mild that the mother herself appeared to be normal. In pregnant rabbits, vitamin A deficiency produced premature degeneration of ova and reduced the number of fertilized eggs before implantation. If such pregnancies were allowed to continue, resorption and abortion occurred during late gestation, so that the final number of living fetuses was greatly reduced. Fetal size was small, and ocular abnormalities were present. Postnatally, hydrocephalus was also seen in the newborn and postnatal young.

Wilson and his colleagues analyzed the syndrome of malformations produced by vitamin A deficiency by giving single large doses of the vitamin to deficient pregnant rats on various days of gestation (Table 11–1). Administration of the vitamin at progressively earlier times during pregnancy resulted in a progressive reduction in the number of malformed young. Associated with this reduction in the malformation rate was an alteration in the types of defects. The congenital malformations resulting from the maternal vitamin

Figure 11–2 Aortic-arch anomalies in rat fetuses resulting from maternal dietary deficiency of vitamin A. Upper left: Hypothetic embryonic pattern of aortic arches. All arches are not present simultaneously in mammals but are shown here in cumulative arrangement to emphasize their positional relationships. Upper right: Definitive pattern of arteries. Parts of embryonic system that undergo regression are indicated by broken lines. Lower left: Anomaly of right aortic arch. Lower right: Anomaly of right subclavian artery.

Adapted from Wilson and Warkany, 1950, from Hurley, 1978.

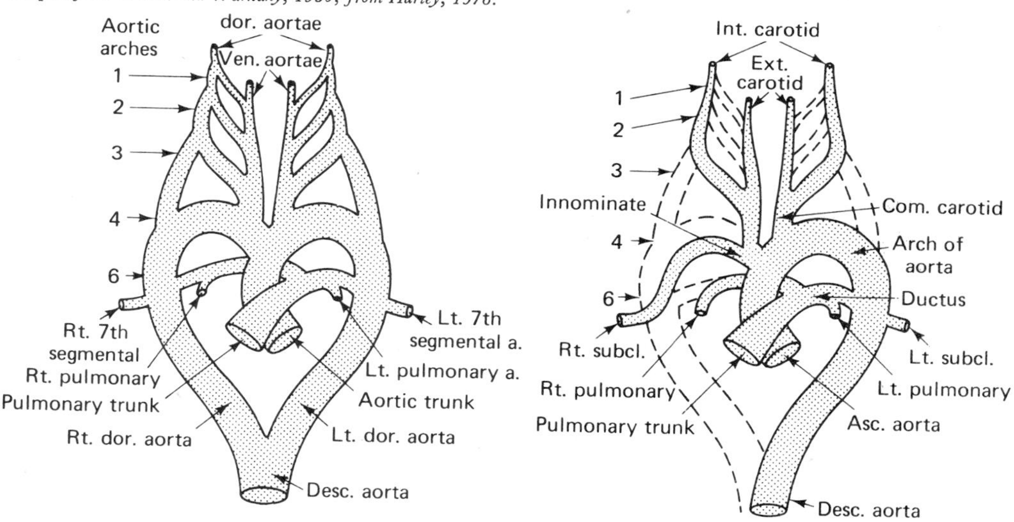

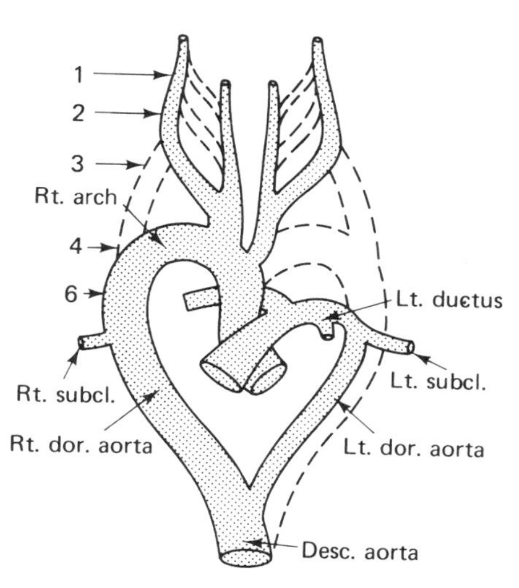

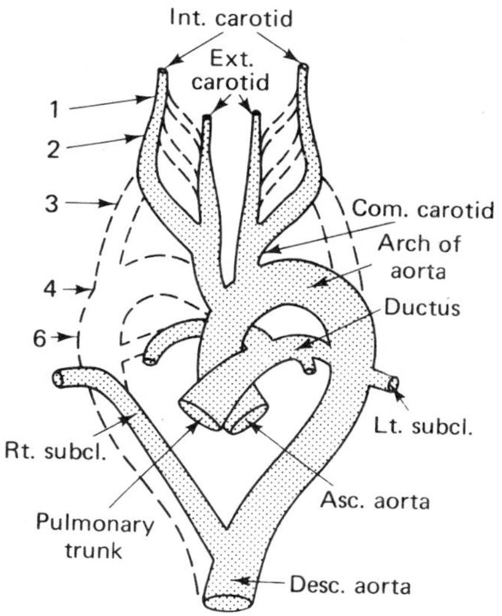

TABLE 11–1 SUMMARY OF DEVELOPMENTAL ANOMALIES IN VARIOUS ORGANS AND SYSTEMS

	Percentage of Offspring Affected						
	After Treatment of Mothers with Vitamin A on Specific Days of Pregnancy						*Without Therapy*
	10th	*11th*	*12th*	*13th*	*14th*	*15th*	
Offspring with typical defects	5	6	19	25	42	33	53
Organs affected:							
Eyes	0	0	0	4	17	28	49
Aortic arch	0	0	15	14	17	17	9
Heart	5	6	8	18	25	13	4
Lungs	0	0	4	8	6	7	4
Diaphragm	0	0	8	16	23	24	31
Kidneys	0	0	0	2	13	20	38
Ureters	0	0	0	2	11	24	36
Genital ducts	0	0	8	10	10	13	42
Lower genitourinary tract	0	0	0	2	0	2	20

From Wilson et al., 1953.

A deficiency appeared to be determined during the period of active morphogenesis of the organ involved.

Thus an important principle was established. The time period of the deficiency (or other teratogenic influence) affects the type of defect produced. Timing of the prenatal insult is important, because it relates to the various developmental stages during which different organs develop. If a part of the body is in the process of structural formation, its development can be adversely affected by a nutritional deficiency or other teratogenic influence, and it will develop in an abnormal way. If, however, the critical period for development of the structure is over, its normality will not be impaired. Thus, when vitamin A was given to the vitamin A-deficient rat at specific times during pregnancy, malformations of certain organs could be prevented. For example, a malformation of the aortic arch was prevented if vitamin A was fed before the 11th day of pregnancy. After that time, the heart would already have formed with the malformation in process, and additional vitamin A would not reverse the sequence. Once an organ has developed beyond a certain point, the developmental process is irreversible.

Although its effects on the developing embryo have been described extensively in many species, the mechanism of action of vitamin A deficiency remains unknown.

EXCESS

An excessive amount of vitamin A during pregnancy is also detrimental to the developing young. When pregnant rats were given by mouth 35,000 IU of vitamin A from the second, third, or fourth through the 16th day of gestation, gross anomalies of the skull and brain occurred in 54% of the offspring. The major developmental defect was an extrusion of the brain (exencephaly). Other malformations were cleft lip, cleft palate, and eye defects. There was also a marked reduction in the number of litters carried to term.

Excess vitamin A in pregnant animals produces many types of birth defects, depending on the amount as well as on the gestational stage at which it is administered. Anencephaly (lack of cerebral cortex) and cleft palate appear to be the most common malformations, but anophthalmia (missing eyes) and other eye anomalies, as well as spina bifida (open spinal column), syndactyly (fused or missing digits), and face malformations also occur (Figures 11–3 and 11–4). Dental malformations have also been found in rats subjected to hypervitaminosis A in the prenatal period.

Excessive amounts of vitamin A have also produced congenital defects in a number of species besides rats. The mouse, for example, responds to relatively small doses of excess vitamin A with abnormal development. Congenital malformations have also been produced with hypervitaminosis A in the guinea pig, the rabbit, the pig, the hamster, and the monkey. In all these animals cleft lip and palate and malformations of the brain, spinal cord, and eyes were common findings.

Figure 11–3 Twenty-day fetuses. Left, control. Others, mother given vitamin A on day 8. Left to right: meningocoele, open eye, microstomia; meningo-encephalocoele, microstomia; exencephaly. All show absence of pinna, protruding squamosal, and exaggerated cephalic flexure.

From Morriss, 1972.

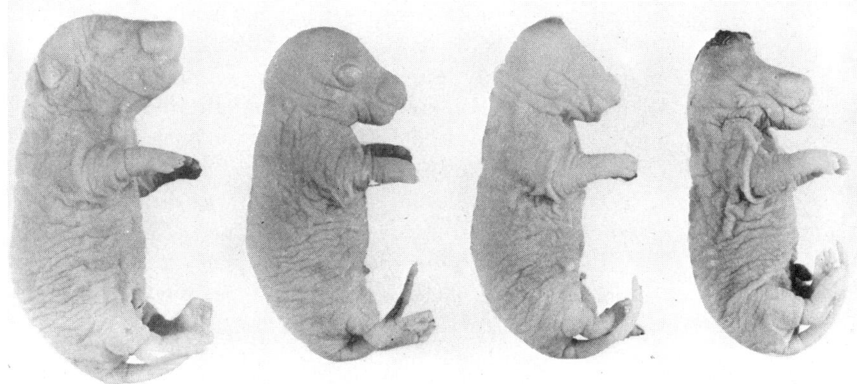

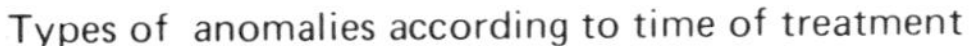

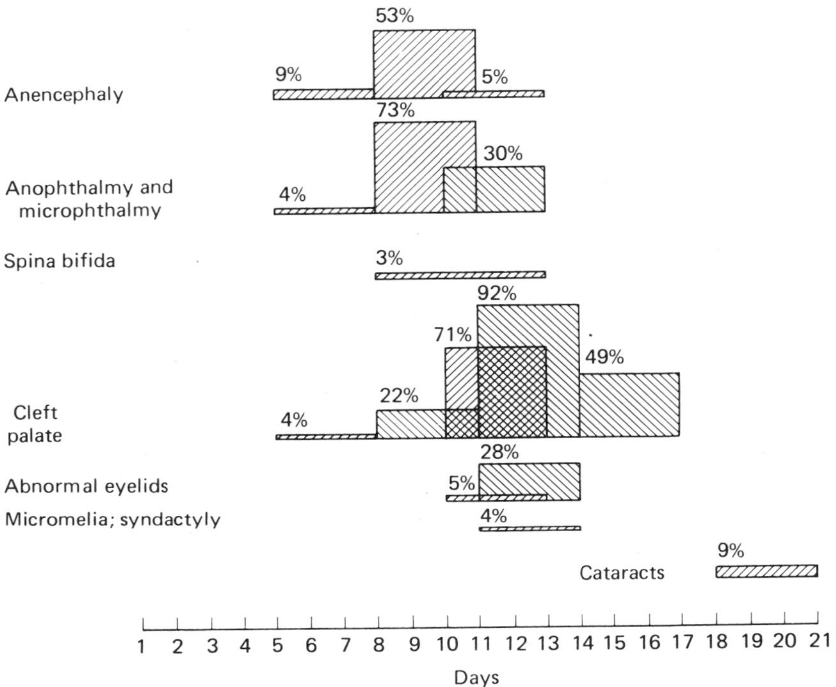

From Giroud and Martinet, 1956.

Figure 11–4 Distribution of malformations as related to dates of vitamin A administration.

Mechanism of action. As in the case of vitamin A deficiency, the mechanism by which hypervitaminosis A produces abnormal development of embryos and fetuses is not understood. The morphogenesis of the brain malformations produced by excessive amounts of vitamin A has been subjected to detailed microscopic study, following the development of the brain from its earliest stages. At the cellular level, tritiated thymidine has been used. Both the morphological and the cellular approach seem to indicate that the abnormal development results from changes in differential growth rates among various tissues. For example, large doses of vitamin A prevented the neural groove from closing, possibly by interfering with the mitotic activity of the neuroepithelial cells. Thus there was a loss of normal synchrony in the differential growth rates necessary to produce normal development. The studies with tritiated thymidine suggest that this loss of synchrony may occur through interference with DNA synthesis in neuroepithelial cells. Thus a lengthening of the cell cycle would occur, and this in turn could lead to a decreased rate of cell proliferation.

Findings of studies on the development of cleft palate using tritiated thymidine are consistent with those of brain development. They suggest that vitamin A excess retards the growth of the palatal processes so that they do not come in contact with each other at the required time, thus producing cleft palate.

Another hypothesis suggests that the role of vitamin A in metabolism of sulfated mucopolysaccharides is the basis for its teratogenic action. Thus it is possible that abnormal biosynthesis of mucopolysaccharides may be a basic defect in developing tissues subjected to this teratogenic agent. The role of vitamin A in mucopolysaccharide biosynthesis might also be related to the general effect of the vitamin on membranes of cells and of intracellular organelles.

Most of the experiments with hypervitaminosis A have used the ester form of the vitamin, retinyl acetate. However, retinoic acid is also teratogenic and is in fact even more active than the ester form. The incidence of defects produced with the ester can be achieved with only one-fortieth as much retinoic acid. With retinoic acid as a teratogen, it is possible to influence very specific embryonic stages, because this compound, unlike the ester or alcohol form, is rapidly eliminated from the body. These studies also suggested that retinoic acid had a disruptive effect on the spatial organization of the cartilage models of the limbs—again, possibly through effects on mucopolysaccharides.

Postnatal effects of prenatal hypervitaminosis A. The postnatal behavioral effect of relatively mild hypervitaminosis A was examined by giving pregnant rats excess vitamin A on the eighth, ninth, and tenth days of gestation. Only a small percentage of the newborn offspring showed minor malformations. However, when they were tested for maze learning, the offspring of dams who had received vitamin A performed significantly poorer than did controls. This shows that the vitamin A, although not producing visible malformations of the central nervous system, did cause defects that were apparent at the functional level. When rats were given a teratogenic dose of vitamin A later in gestation (on days 14 and 15 or on days 17 and 18), their young also showed behavioral abnormalities but of different types, depending upon the timing of the treatment.

VITAMIN A IN HUMAN PREGNANCY

There is now considerable knowledge concerning the teratogenic effects of both vitamin A deficiency and vitamin A excess in experimental animals. Every species tested has shown congenital malformations with both too little and too much vitamin A. It is thus somewhat surprising that little research has been carried out on the possible teratogenic effects of vitamin A in humans, especially since vitamin A deficiency is a serious problem in many human populations. However, there is no good information on the incidence of congenital abnormalities in these areas, or the relationship of congenital malformations in humans to vitamin A deficiency.

One case report from India concerns a woman who was severely deficient in vitamin A and was blind as a result. She gave birth to a premature baby with microcephaly and anophthalmia. Other observations also suggest that prenatal vitamin A deficiency may be partially responsible for eye abnormalities and impaired vision in children. Several cases have been reported of women who took excessive amounts of vitamin A during pregnancy with apparent teratogenic consequences. Their infants were born with congenital anomalies of the urogenital system. Although such cases do not prove that vitamin A was responsible for the abnormal development, they are certainly suggestive, since the malformations produced were very similar to those caused by the same treatment in experimental animals.

In an attempt to assess the correlation between congenital malformations in infants with vitamin A intake of the mother, maternal serum vitamin A was measured after delivery. The level of vitamin A was significantly higher in mothers of infants with central nervous system malformations than in those with normal babies. Measurements of vitamin A in the livers of fetuses that were aborted, or of premature infants that died shortly after birth, were also higher in those with malformations. This study, with a rather small number of subjects, should be repeated on a larger scale.

More information is obviously needed on vitamin A in human pregnancy and its possible relationship to congenital abnormalities or postnatal functional problems. The placental transfer of vitamin A to the fetus, the correlation of maternal, fetal, and neonatal serum levels of the vitamin, and the effect of either low or high maternal intake of the vitamin on neonatal and postnatal development in the infant are all subjects demanding further investigation.

VITAMIN D

DEFICIENCY

Vitamin D functions in the absorption and utilization of calcium. In the absence of this vitamin, normal calcification of the skeleton cannot occur. Thus, deficiency of vitamin D in the maternal diet during pregnancy results in abnormal development of the fetal skeleton.

Animal studies. In rats, a diet deficient in vitamin D during pregnancy produced offspring with skeletal abnormalities resembling those of rickets. When cows were given a vitamin D-deficient diet, plasma calcium declined to one-half and blood phosphorus to one-fifth of normal values. The animals were shown to be in negative balance for both elements. The calves produced under these conditions showed gross evidence of rickets (Figure 11–5).

Humans. In humans, vitamin D deficiency combined with low calcium intake during pregnancy results in the birth of infants with fetal rickets. Recent studies suggest that nutritional vitamin D deficiency may occur more frequently than was thought. Plasma concentration of 25-hydroxycholecalciferol(25-OH-D), the active form of vitamin D, was measured in both premature infants with neonatal hypocalcemia and their mothers. Most of the infants with this condition, as well as their mothers, had very low levels of 25-OH-D, suggesting that the low blood calcium may be due to vitamin D deficiency in the infants and their mothers. Further examination of the women showed that they, too, had low calcium, and low albumin in their blood, together with low vitamin D intake. The group also experienced inadequate prenatal care (see Table 11–2).

Enamel hypoplasia of the teeth has been observed in connection with neonatal tetany in maternal vitamin D deficiency. Further evidence that

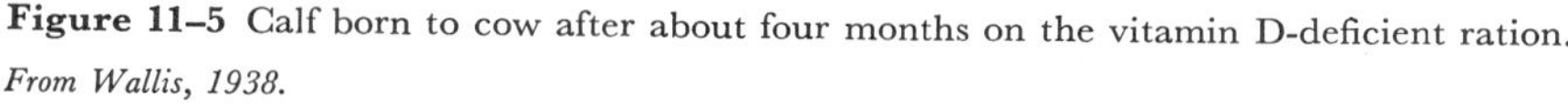

Figure 11–5 Calf born to cow after about four months on the vitamin D-deficient ration. *From Wallis, 1938.*

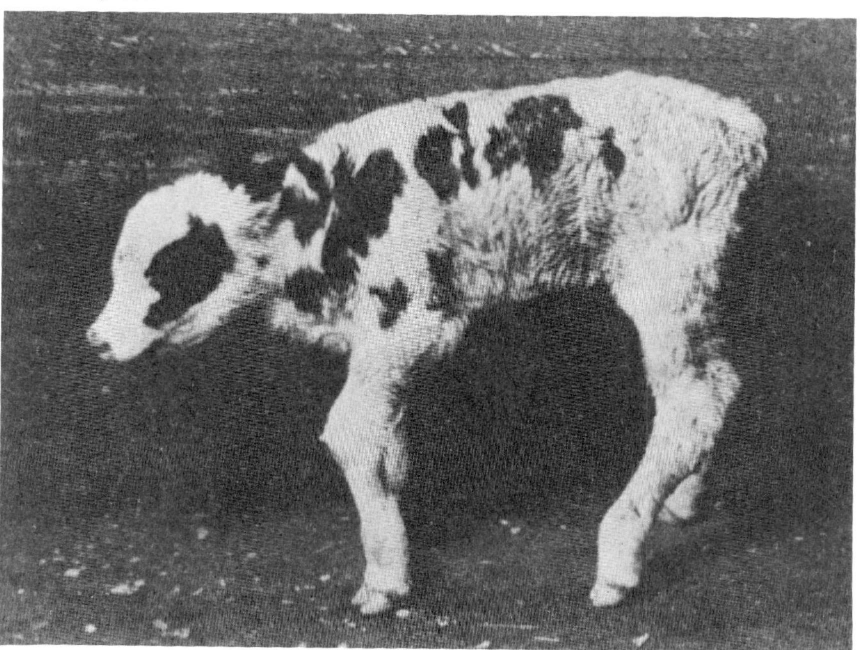

TABLE 11–2 SERUM OR PLASMA VALUES OF 25-HYDROXYVITAMIN D(25-OHD), CALCIUM, AND PHOSPHORUS IN ALL SUBJECT GROUPS

	No. of Subjects	*Plasma 25-OHD, Mean ± SE, ng/ml*	*Serum Calcium, Mean±SE, mg/100 ml*	*Serum Phosphorus, Mean±SE, mg/100 ml*	*Range of Weight, g*
Group 1					
Premature infants with neonatal hypocalcemia[a]	11	7.0 ± 1.0 (5–9)[d]	6.1 ± .17	8.1 ± .24	794–2,166
Mothers of premature infants with neonatal hypocalcemia[a]	11	11 ± 1.0 (.98)[c] (8–13)[d]	8.5 ± .18	3.8 ± .1	
Estimated maternal intake of vitamin D, 100–200 units/day					
Group 2					
Premature infants with neonatal hypocalcemia[b]	4	24 ± 3	6.1 ± .2	7.5 ± .27	837–1,361
Mothers of premature infants with neonatal hypocalcemia[b]	4	31 ± 3 (.96)[c]	9.52 ± .23	3.8 ± .1	
Estimated maternal intake of vitamin D, 600–1000 units/day					
Group 3, controls					
Full-term infants	15	23 ± 2	10.12 ± .25	5.4 ± .09	> 2,500
Mothers of full-term infants	15	28 ± 2 (.97)[c]	9.40 ± .14	3.8 ± .09	
Estimated maternal intake of vitamin D, 600–1000 units/day					

[a]Group of mothers and premature infants with significantly low plasma levels of 25-OHD.
[b]Group of mothers and premature infants with normal plasma levels (compared to controls) of 25-OHD.
[c]Numbers in parentheses indicate linear correlation coefficients (r) between maternal-infant levels.
[d]Numbers in parentheses indicate range of values.

From Rosen et al., 1974.

vitamin D deficiency during prenatal life may influence development of the teeth comes from large comparative dental surveys of London school children in 1929 and 1943. The findings suggest that nutritional improvement, especially of vitamin D, had increased the quality of the teeth so that poor dentition and high susceptibility to caries were greatly reduced.

A number of genetic diseases involve vitamin D metabolism. These have been called vitamin D-resistant or vitamin D-dependent rickets (Table 11–3). Manifestations include growth failure, convulsions, severe rickets, and, in some types of vitamin D dependency, hypophosphatemia. The recent elucidation of the biochemical role of vitamin D and its metabolism has led to new treatment for these genetic disorders. The genetic diseases whose victims formerly required massive doses of vitamin D can now be treated with very small quantities of the active metabolite of the vitamin (see Table 11–4).

EXCESS

Animal studies. Like vitamin A, excessive as well as inadequate amounts of vitamin D are detrimental to the developing fetus. Excess vitamin D in the diet of pregnant rats resulted in young with low birth weights and low calcium and phosphorus content in fetal bones and whole body. The long bones of the fetuses showed impairment of osteogenesis and of skeletal development. The abnormal bone development of such offspring persisted during the postnatal period even though their intake of vitamin D was normal after birth. Because of the abnormal bone development, multiple fractures occurred as early as the fifth day of life, and healing of the fractures was impaired. The growth retardation also persisted throughout life; in fact, it became more marked with time (Figure 11–6). The abnormal bone formation

Figure 11–6 Postnatal weight curve of experimental and control rats. C = control; E = experimental (prenatal vitamin D treatment).

From Ornoy et al., 1972.

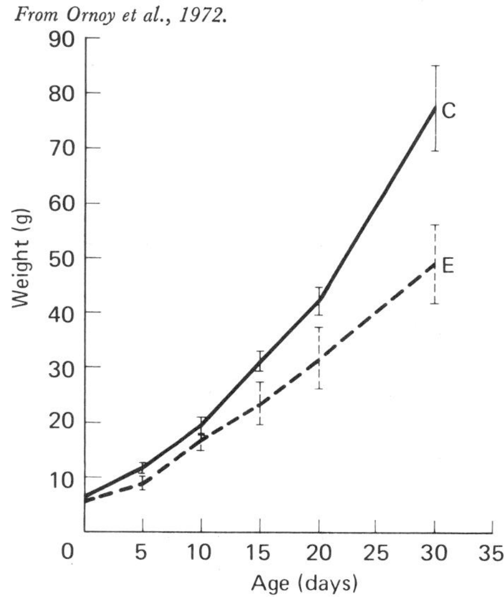

TABLE 11–3 FAMILIAL FORMS OF VITAMIN D-RESISTANT RICKETS

	Causes of Rickets "Refractory" to Vitamin D[a]	
	Calciopenic Causes	*Phosphopenic Causes*
Nutritional	Calcium deprivation	Phosphate deprivation (in antacid therapy with magnesium-aluminum hydroxides)
Transport	Defective absorption; bile salt depletion (effect on vitamin D absorption)	X-linked hypophosphatemia
	Sprue, celiac disease, etc. (effect on calcium and vitamin D absorption)	Tubulopathies involving phosphate and other solutes; includes the Fanconi syndrome
Metabolic	(1) Defective synthesis of 25-OH-D; —Hepatocellular disease; —Drug-induced increase of microsomal oxidation (2) Defective synthesis of 1α,25-$(OH)_2D$; —Renal parenchymal (cortex) disease; —Hereditary vitamin D dependency (pseudodeficiency rickets)	Secondary forms (secondary to hyperparathyroidism with calciopenia)

[a]Refractory to physiological doses of vitamin D (prohormone), can be responsive to pharmacological doses of vitamin D or "physiological" doses of vitamin D metabolites (25-OH-D or 1α-OH-vitamin D analogues).

From Fraser and Scriver, 1976.

TABLE 11–4 VITAMIN D METABOLIC REQUIREMENT

	Normal, μg/day	*Vitamin D Dependent, μg/day*
Vitamin D_2 or D_3	10	1000
25-OH-D_3	3	300
1,25-$(OH)_2$-D_3	1	1

and abnormal fracture repair in these animals was thought to result from fundamental damage to fetal tissues induced by the teratogenic effects of vitamin D. However, these studies did not distinguish between the prenatal effects of hypervitaminosis D and the possible effects of this treatment on the development of the mammary gland and lactation. Thus, impaired milk production with reduced food intake during the suckling period might have been a factor.

The pregnant female rat subjected to hypervitaminosis D, although unable to produce a fully normal offspring, is herself less susceptible to the toxic effects of the vitamin than is the nonpregnant animal. Nonpregnant rats given large amounts of vitamin D displayed hyperlipidemia and structural damage involving degeneration and calcification in the cardiovascular, respiratory, and excretory organs. In pregnant rats given the same amount of the vitamin, however, organ injury of this kind was rarely seen and then only to a mild degree. However, serum lipid concentration was higher in pregnant females with hypervitaminosis D than in nonpregnant animals. Furthermore, pregnant rats treated with vitamin D showed fatty degeneration of the liver and elevated levels of esterified fatty acids.

Hypervitaminosis D did not produce hypercalcemia in pregnant rats, although it did in nonpregnant rats. In fetuses, the magnesium content of bone was increased and the placenta showed reduced size, wet weight, and ash content.

In rabbits, the teratogenic effects of hypervitaminosis D resemble those of a disorder in infants called supravalvular aortic stenosis syndrome (SASS). In both conditions there are aortic lesions and anomalies of the cranial, facial, and dental development. Newborn rabbits subjected to hypervitaminosis D during prenatal development showed hypoplasia of the lower jaw and of the tooth enamel, a congenital absence of teeth, or malocclusion. In addition, they showed premature closure of the cranial bones, strabismus (cross-eyedness), odd-shaped ears, and low birth weight. The blood level of the vitamin was much higher in these pregnant rabbits and their fetuses than in controls, showing that placental transfer had occurred. Serum calcium levels were also higher than normal in both fetuses and mothers treated with vitamin D.

Humans. Although many pregnant women take vitamin D supplements, we have little information on the possible effect of an excessive intake of this vitamin during gestation. In women treated for hypoparathyroidism with high doses of vitamin D during pregnancy, there was no evidence of cardiovascular or craniofacial abnormalities in their children. These 27 children born to the 15 women appeared to be perfectly normal when examined at ages ranging from six weeks to 16 years. However, the patients with hypoparathyroidism did not show the usual hypercalcemic effect of vitamin D, and in this respect they differed from some of the animal models in which fetal anomalies have been produced.

A genetic disorder in children, idiopathic infantile hypercalcemia, seems to be similar in many respects to the effect of hypervitaminosis D on the offspring of pregnant rabbits. In the severe form of the disease there is impairment of kidney function, dwarfism, mental retardation, persistent hypercalcemia, and osteosclerosis. Serum vitamin D activity was 20 to 30 times higher in these children than in normal infants, suggesting that a defect in the metabolism of vitamin D or related substances is the primary etiologic factor in this genetic syndrome. Serum cholesterol levels are also significantly raised in patients with this disease.

In the mild form of hypercalcemia, however, mental and growth retardation and osteosclerosis do not occur. This condition can be reversed by removal of vitamin D from the diet or by a reduction of calcium intake. It has been postulated that excessive intake of vitamin D or unusual sensitivity to the vitamin may be related to this mild form of idiopathic hypercalcemia, but the evidence is conflicting.

VITAMIN K

Vitamin K functions in blood clotting. Thus, in the absence of vitamin K hemorrhages occur, and finally death ensues from internal bleeding.

ANIMAL STUDIES

The first report of vitamin K deficiency in prenatal animals appeared in 1929 in the description of sweet clover disease in cattle, later recognized to be vitamin K deficiency. This disease is caused by ingestion of dicoumarol, a vitamin K analogue, which produces a deficiency of the vitamin. Cattle that were eating white clover gave birth to calves that died of hemorrhage shortly after birth.

In pregnant rats given a diet low in fat and deficient in vitamin K, the young had a high incidence of brain hemorrhages at birth. They were either born dead or died within 24 hours. In vitamin K-deficient pregnant rabbits, hypoprothrombinemia was demonstrated and embryos were aborted at the end of the first trimester of gestation.

Dicoumarol was also used to produce vitamin K deficiency in rabbits. However, the dose given was monitored by measuring the prothrombin level of the mother. When given in doses that produced a prothrombin level below 10% of normal even for only two days, the fetuses died *in utero*. When prothrombin levels considered "safe" (that is, more than 10% of normal) were maintained in the mother, the prothrombin level of the offspring was extremely low at birth, and they had a tendency to hemorrhage. Pups born to a pregnant dog given dicoumarol at low levels during the last week of pregnancy had reduced prothrombin levels despite the normal prothrombin concentration of the mother. Half of the litter was given vitamin K at birth, and these animals survived, but the rest died of hemorrhage in the neonatal period.

HUMANS

Dicoumarol is used in clinical medicine for the treatment and prevention of clotting diseases (thromboembolic diseases) in humans. Patients with thromboembolism or with artificial heart valves are subject to long-continued treatment with dicoumarin anticoagulants. There has therefore been considerable concern regarding the effects of this drug in pregnant women and their infants. The overwhelming evidence appears to favor the conclusion that fetal mortality and morbidity and fetal malformation may result from the use of this compound in pregnant women.

Numerous cases have been reported in which fetal abnormalities were found in infants of women treated with these anticoagulants. In one report, fetal or neonatal death occurred in high incidence, with multiple hemorrhages visible on autopsy. In another case, the infant was blind and mentally retarded. It is now accepted that prenatal vitamin K deficiency caused by dicoumarol drugs produces a particular group of characteristics called the coumadin syndrome. The outstanding feature of this syndrome is hypoplastic nasal structures (Figure 11–7). Mental retardation and bone abnormalities are other aspects. Conflicting findings, however, suggest that anticoagulant therapy is not deleterious to the fetus if the dosage is properly managed.

VITAMIN E

DEFICIENCY

It was the role of vitamin E in reproduction that first led to its discovery as an essential nutrient by Evans and Bishop in 1922. Rats given a diet deficient in what was later shown to be vitamin E were sterile. With a milder deficiency of vitamin E, mating and pregnancy were initiated but fetuses were not carried to term unless vitamin E was administered. If the vitamin was given at the beginning of gestation, normal young were produced, but when it was given later in gestation there was a high incidence of multiple congenital abnormalities, including exencephaly, anencephaly, umbilical hernia, scoliosis (curvature of the spine), club feet, cleft lip, syndactyly, and

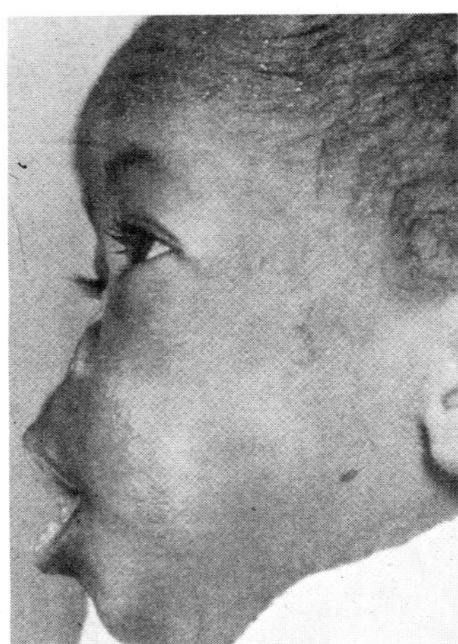

From Kerber et al., 1968.

Figure 11–7 Profile view of infant (two months old) with coumadin syndrome. Note hypoplastic development of nose.

kinked tail. The incidence of malformation varied with the composition of the ration and the amount of vitamin E. The tocopherol content of the fetuses was not correlated with the degree of malformation.

In another study, rats depleted of vitamin E showed complete resorption of their fetuses and lowered concentration of serum tocopherol. Oral supplements of tocopherol on the eighth and ninth days of gestation permitted fetal development to continue, but the offspring were not normal. Gestation was prolonged and most of the young were stillborn. Maternal mortality at parturition was high, with death following lethargy, pallor, dyspnea, and vaginal hemorrhage. These effects were considered to be similar to those of women with toxemia of pregnancy. Fetal death and stillbirth also occur in the mouse as a result of vitamin E deficiency.

An association between low tryptophan and vitamin E deficiency has been found in rats. Pregnant rats given diets low in both of these nutrients gave birth to offspring of which a high proportion had opaque regions in the lens of the eye—varying degrees of cataracts.

EXCESS

Excessive intake of vitamin E (as high as 500 mg/day) during gestation and lactation in rats produced no teratogenic effects on their newborn young. The survival, birth weight, and litter size were also unaffected. Some eye abnormalities were seen in older pups of rats given extremely high amounts of the vitamin. Offspring of mothers who had received 500 mg/day of vitamin E (2252 mg/kg/day) during gestation and lactation had a higher concentration of liver and plasma vitamin E than did controls. Vitamin E transfer across the placenta was negligible, and mammary transfer was quite efficient. This study suggests that supplemental vitamin E during pregnancy is relatively harmless to the fetus.

References and Supplementary Readings

Bernhardt, I. B., and D. J. Dorsey. "Hypervitaminosis A and congenital renal anomalies in a human infant." *Obstet. Gynec.* **43**: 750–755 (1974).

Bouillon, R., H. Van Baelen, and P. De Moor. "25-Hydroxyvitamin D and its binding protein in maternal and cord serum." *J. Clin. Endocrin. Metab.* **4**: 679–684 (1977).

Bunce, G. E., and J. L. Hess. "Lenticular opacities in young rats as a consequence of maternal diets low in tryptophan and/or vitamin E." *J. Nutr.* **106**: 222–229 (1976).

Butcher, R. E., R. L. Brunner, T. Roth, and C. A. Kimmel. "A learning impairment associated with maternal hypervitaminosis-A in rats." *Life Sciences* **11**: 141–145 (1972).

Cohlan, S. Q. "Excessive intake of vitamin A as a cause of congenital anomalies in the rat." *Science* **117**: 535–536 (1953).

Fraser, D., and C. R. Scriver. "Familial forms of vitamin D-resistant rickets revisited. X-linked hypophosphatemia and autosomal recessive vitamin D dependency." *Am. J. Clin. Nutr.* **29**: 1315–1329 (1976).

Giroud, A., and M. Martinet. "Tératogénèse par hautes doses de vitamine A en fonction des stades du développement." *Archives D'Anatomie Microscopique* **45**: 7–98 (1956).

Hale, F. "Pigs born without eye balls." *J. Heredity* **24**: 105–106 (1933).

Hurley, L. S. "Nutritional deficiencies and excesses." In: J. G. Wilson and F. C. Fraser, eds., *Handbook of Teratology*, Vol. 1, pp. 261–308. New York: Plenum Publishing Corp., 1977.

Hurley, L. S. "Developing organisms as model systems for the study of degradative processes." In: R. D. Berlin, H. Herrmann, I. H. Lepow, and J. M. Tanzer, eds., *Molecular Basis of Biological Degradative Processes.* New York: Academic Press, 1978.

Hutchings, D. E., J. Gibbon, and M. A. Kaufman. "Maternal vitamin A excess during the early fetal period: effects on learning and development in the offspring." *Developmental Psychobiol.* **6**: 445–457 (1973).

Kerber, I. J., O. S. Warr, III, and C. Richardson. "Pregnancy in a patient with a prosthetic mitral valve." *J.A.M.A.* **203**: 223–225 (1968).

Langman, J., and G. W. Welch. "Effect of vitamin A on development of the central nervous system." *J. Comp. Neur.* **128**: 1–16 (1966).

Martin, M., and L. S. Hurley. "Effect of large amounts of vitamin E during pregnancy and lactation." *Am. J. Clin. Nutr.* **30**: 1629–1637 (1977).

Morriss, G. M. "Morphogenesis of the malformations induced in rat embryos by maternal hypervitaminosis A." *J. Anat.* **113**: 241–250 (1972).

ORNOY, A., T. KASPI, AND L. NEBEL. "Persistent defects of bone formation in young rats following maternal hypervitaminosis D_2." *Israel J. Med. Sciences* **8**: 943–949 (1972).

ROSEN, J. F., M. ROGINSKY, G. NATHENSON, AND L. FINBERG. "25-Hydroxyvitamin D. Plasma levels in mothers and their premature infants with neonatal hypocalcemia." *Am. J. Dis. Child.* **127**: 220–333 (1974). Copyright 1974.

WALLIS, G. C. "Some effects of a vitamin D deficiency on mature dairy cows." *J. Dairy Science* **21**: 315–322 (1938).

WILSON, J. G., C. B. ROTH, AND J. WARKANY. "An analysis of the syndrome of malformations induced by maternal vitamin A deficiency. Effects of restoration of vitamin A at various times during gestation." *Am. J. Anatomy* **92**: 189–217 (1953).

WILSON, J. G., AND J. WARKANY. "Cardiac and aortic arch anomalies in the offspring of vitamin A deficient rats correlatd with similar human anomalies." *Pediatrics* **5**: 708–725 (1950).

WARKANY, J. "Warfarin embryopathy." *Teratology* **14**: 205–210 (1976).

12

Water-soluble vitamins

ASCORBIC ACID

DEFICIENCY

Ascorbic acid, unlike the other vitamins, is a required constituent of the diet for only a few species—man and other primates, the guinea pig, and some tropical birds. Experimental studies of the effects of vitamin C deficiency during pregnancy are limited to a few investigations using guinea pigs. In early work, pregnant guinea pigs given an ascorbic acid-deficient diet had a high incidence of spontaneous abortions, especially between the 26th and 30th days of gestation (about halfway through the pregnancy).

In guinea pigs fed a chronically low level of ascorbic acid, viability of offspring and growth during the nursing period were adequate. However, postweaning growth was depressed.

More recently a biochemical and histological study was made of fetal and uterine tissue of guinea pigs given an ascorbic acid-deficient diet during pregnancy. Because of the role of ascorbic acid in maintenance and synthesis of connective tissue (especially collagen), the proline, hydroxyproline, and ascorbic acid concentrations were measured. Collagen synthesis was impaired in both fetal and uterine tissues from deficient animals. Histologically, the deficient fetal and uterine tissues showed abnormalities in mucopolysaccharides, collagen, and elastin. The pregnant females themselves showed no outward signs of ascorbic acid deficiency.

In humans, ascorbic acid deficiency causes scurvy, a disease that has been recognized for hundred of years. It has existed in high incidence at certain periods of history and has been extensively studied. It is therefore surprising that so little information, either historical or modern, is available on the effects of vitamin C deficiency in pregnant women. In a large study of maternal and infant nutrition carried out at Vanderbilt University, the dietary intake, serum vitamin C levels, and pregnancy outcomes were

TABLE 12–1 ASCORBIC ACID CONTENT OF PLASMA OF MATERNAL AND CORD BLOOD TAKEN AT THE TIME OF DELIVERY

Vitamin C Content of Maternal Diet					
Normal or Above Plasma Ascorbic Acid, mg per 100 cc		*Suboptimal Plasma Ascorbic Acid, mg per 100 cc*		*Deficient Plasma Ascorbic Acid, mg per 100 cc*	
Maternal Blood	*Cord Blood*	*Maternal Blood*	*Cord Blood*	*Maternal Blood*	*Cord Blood*
1.0	1.9	0.5	1.8	0.1	0.5
0.8	1.5	0.1	0.5	0.2	0.6
0.6	1.4	0.4	1.5	0.1	1.0
1.0	1.9	0.5	1.0	0.1	0.8
0.9	1.7	0.5	1.0	0.2	1.0
0.9	2.4	0.6	1.3	0.5	1.2
0.8	1.7	0.5	1.4	0.5	1.1
1.0	1.7	0.4	1.0	...	...
1.0	1.8	...	...	...	...
Average Values in mg per 100 cc					
0.88	1.77	0.44	1.19	0.24	0.89

From Teel et al., 1938.

recorded for over 2000 women. In general, serum levels of ascorbic acid decreased during pregnancy except in the women with a high level of vitamin C intake. The frequency of congenital malformations was no higher in the women with the lowest serum level of vitamin C than it was in those with the highest level. However, increased frequency of premature births occurred in the women with the lowest intake of the vitamin; these women also had the lowest serum concentrations of vitamin C of the group. Other studies have also shown that the dietary intake of the pregnant woman is correlated with her plasma level of the vitamin. At the same time, the plasma of the fetus at delivery (cord blood) also seems to be lower in women whose plasma ascorbic acid level is low (see Table 12–1).

EXCESS

Excessive amounts of vitamin C during pregnancy appear to be detrimental to the offspring. Guinea pigs given high doses of vitamin C displayed infertility, fetal mortality, and spontaneous abortions, although the pregnant females themselves did not show toxic symptoms. Stillbirths and abortions have also been reported in rats and mice given large amounts of ascorbic acid during pregnancy. These observations remain to be confirmed, however.

In women who took large doses of ascorbic acid, termination of early pregnancy was reported. In this study, 20 women were selected who showed a 10- to 15-day delay of their menstrual periods. They were given 6 g of ascorbic acid per day for three days for the purpose of terminating the pregnancy. In 16 of the 20 women, menstrual bleeding appeared in one to three days after the ascorbic acid treatment. Excretion of estrogen in the urine was increased in 12 out of the 16 women. These results were interpreted as indicating that the large doses of ascorbic acid increased the estrogen level of the blood and that this in turn brought about interruption of pregnancy. However, in this clinical report no control group was used, and one cannot be certain that these women were in fact pregnant.

Another problem that may be caused by excessive intake of vitamin C during pregnancy concerns "conditioned" scurvy in the offspring. In a few infants, cases of scurvy have been reported that were interpreted as being due to an excessive intake of ascorbic acid by the mother during pregnancy. It is possible that a high rate of ascorbate catabolism resulted which caused deficiency of the vitamin after birth.

Experimental work with guinea pigs supports this idea. Offspring of mothers who received high levels of ascorbic acid during pregnancy developed scurvy sooner than did those of controls. The higher excretion of CO_2 found in the experimental young suggested that an increased rate of catabolism of ascorbic acid was responsible for their higher vitamin C requirement.

B-COMPLEX VITAMINS: RIBOFLAVIN

DEFICIENCY

Riboflavin was the second nutrient whose deficiency during pregnancy was shown to produce congenital malformations in mammals (see Chapter 6). Warkany and his colleagues reported in the early 1940s that rats given a diet deficient in riboflavin for a short period before and throughout pregnancy gave birth to young that had severe congenital malformations, including shortness of the mandible, tibia, fibula, radius, and ulna, fusion of ribs, syndactyly (fused or missing digits), and cleft palate. Further work showed there were also malformations of dental and other oral and facial structures. Hydrocephaly and eye defects as well as conjoined (Siamese) twins were also found. When the riboflavin-deficient diet was given to female rats for 60 days before mating, no young were produced at all; with 40 days of dietary deficiency before pregnancy, fetuses were carried to term, but about 50% had congenital malformations.

Even very mild deficiencies of riboflavin in the mother produced teratogenic effects. In females who produced full-term fetuses of which 68% were dead or malformed, the level of riboflavin in maternal liver was decreased by only 20% of the normal value on the 14th day of gestation and by 32% of the normal value at term. The mildness of the deficiency in the mother was also evident in that she had no signs of deficiency.

The riboflavin antimetabolite galactoflavin has been used to study the effects of an acute transitory deficiency of riboflavin in pregnant rats. When pregnant rats were given during pregnancy a riboflavin-deficient diet without galactoflavin, no abnormal young were found. With increasing amounts of galactoflavin in the diet, however, fetal death and resorption increased, maternal weight gain decreased, and the incidence of malformed young increased. These effects could be prevented by addition of riboflavin to the galactoflavin-containing diet. The malformations observed were primarily skeletal defects such as had been reported previously. However, now soft-tissue defects also occurred. These included subcutaneous edema, cardiovascular and urogenital anomalies, herniation of the umbilicus or diaphragm, hydrocephaly, "open" eyes (abnormal development of eyelids), microphthalmia (small eyes), and epidermal defects. When galacsoflavin was given for only a short period during gestation, malformations also occurred. For example, from days 7 to 11, cardiovascular defects were found, and when the antimetabolite was given from days 7 to 13, both cardiovascular and skeletal defects were found.

In embryos from females given a riboflavin-deficient diet with added galactoflavin during the entire pregnancy, growth retardation of the embryo was seen from an early stage, day 12 of gestation. Embryonic mortality occurred between day 11 and day 15.

Galactoflavin has also been used in combination with a riboflavin-deficient diet in pregnant mice. In this species, too, congenital malformations are produced by this treatment. Using inbred strains, it was found that there are genetic differences in susceptibility to the teratogenic effects of riboflavin deficiency or galactoflavin (Figure 12–1). Offspring of various strains differed greatly in frequency and severity of particular malformations. Further, some strains required a higher dose level of galactoflavin in order to show abnormal development. The pattern of malformations was also different in the various strains and was more or less characteristic of each strain. Overall, however, there was a similarity of the abnormalities produced in rats and in mice.

In pregnant pigs, riboflavin deficiency resulted in young that were dead at birth or died within 48 hours and showed abnormalities of the limbs.

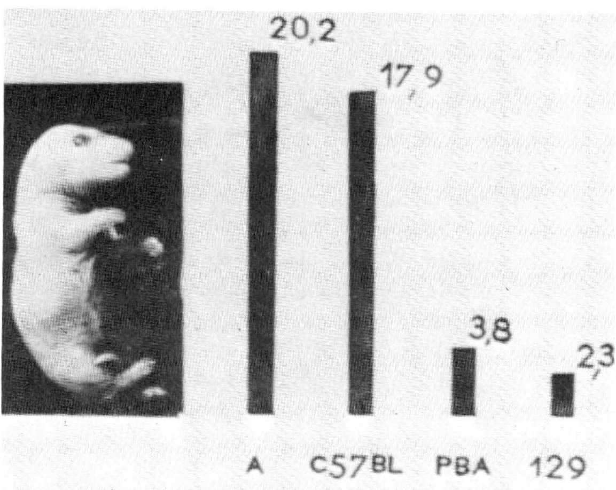

From Giroud, 1970, using data of Kalter and Warkany, 1957, J. Exp. Zool. 136, 531.

Figure 12–1 Variation of the frequency of malformations according to the strains of mice. Open eye in riboflavin-deficient mice induced by an antagonist.

MECHANISM OF ACTION

The basic mechanisms responsible for the teratogenic effects of riboflavin have been the subject of a number of investigations. Concentrations of total riboflavin, FAD (flavin adenine nucleotide), and free riboflavin plus FMN (flavin mononucleotide), as well as those of folate were measured in whole embryos and in fetal and maternal livers after riboflavin deficiency during pregnancy. In embryos from females given the riboflavin-deficient diet containing galactoflavin, there was a 37% decrease in total riboflavin and a 60% decrease in FAD content from the 11th through the 15th days of gestation as compared with controls. When the diet was deficient in riboflavin but did not contain galactoflavin, total riboflavin and FAD content of the embryos were reduced by only 30% (see Figures 12–2 and 12–3).

These results suggested that galactoflavin may inhibit the synthesis of FAD and that the teratogenic effects of galactoflavin-induced riboflavin deficiency might be due to a low level of FAD during the period of embryonic differentiation. Because of the similarity of malformations produced by riboflavin deficiency and by folic acid deficiency (see the section below on folic acid), the folate levels of maternal liver were also measured. After 16 days of the riboflavin-deficient diets, the concentrations of folate and cit-

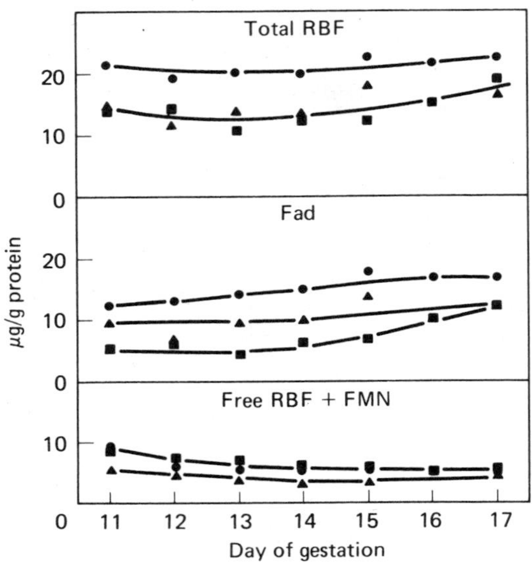

From Miller et al., 1962.

Figure 12–2 Comparison of flavin distribution in embryos and fetuses from diets 1, 2, and 3: ●——●, diet 1, control; ▲——▲, diet 2, riboflavin-deficient; ■——■, diet 3, riboflavin-deficient + galactoflavin (RBF, riboflavin).

rovorum factor in maternal liver were reduced to approximately 50% of the normal values, but there was no correlation between liver folate level and the teratogenicity of riboflavin deficiency.

The effect of riboflavin deficiency on the terminal electron-transport systems in rat embryos was studied by use of a riboflavin-deficient galactoflavin-containing diet in pregnant rats. In such embryos, the succinic and DPNH oxidase systems were markedly reduced from control values (Figure 12-4). However, placenta and maternal heart were unaffected. It was therefore proposed that the mechanism of action of riboflavin deficiency in teratogenesis is through reduced activity of electron-transport systems. However, experiments on limb bud development in organ culture suggested that basic mechanisms for limb defects occurred at the local cellular level and not from a generalized physiological impairment of the embryo.

An extensive study of biochemical effects of riboflavin deficiency during pregnancy on maternal and fetal tissues showed that glycogen, protein, DNA, and RNA levels were reduced in the placenta and the fetus, as well as the number of cells and alkaline phosphatase activity. The concentration of calcium was normal in 13-day embryos from riboflavin-deficient females, but was low at term. This was in contrast to concentrations of zinc, sodium,

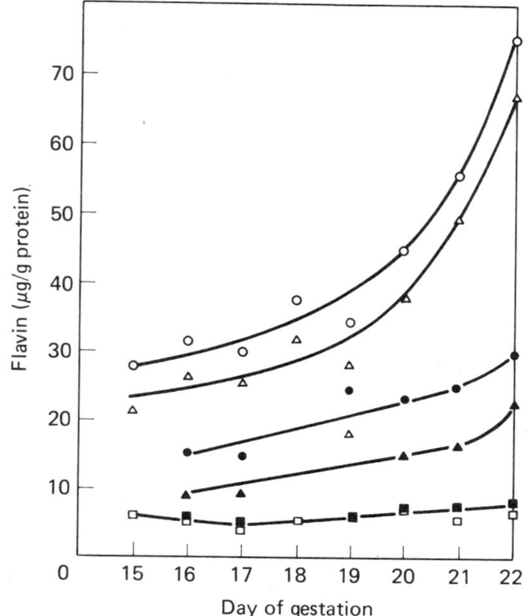

From Miller et al., 1962.

Figure 12–3 Flavin distribution in embryonic and fetal liver. Control: ○, total riboflavin; △, FAD; □, free riboflavin + FMN. Riboflavin-deficient + galactoflavin; ●, total riboflavin; ▲, FAD; ■, free riboflavin + FMN.

Figure 12–4 DPNH oxidase activities of R_2 fractions (ETP) from treated * and control embryos and fetuses at various days of gestation. The mean of the activities of the control series is represented by ●, and the mean of the activities of the treated fractions by ○. The vertical lines show the standard error of the means. * Riboflavin-deficient, galactoflavin fed.

From Aksu et. al., 1968.

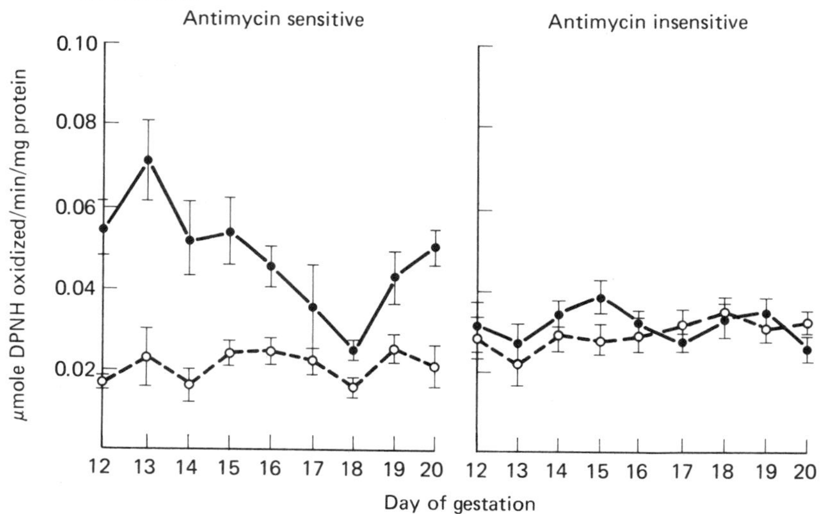

and potassium, which remained at normal levels throughout gestation. There was also a decrease in mitotic activity in the fetal liver, but not in the brain. The brain cells, however, were smaller than normal in size and had reduced metabolic activity. These changes in biochemical composition do not seem to be related to the teratogenic effects of riboflavin deficiency, since similar changes in fetal composition occur in types of malnutrition that are not teratogenic.

RIBOFLAVIN IN HUMAN DEFICIENCY

Relatively little information is available on the role of riboflavin in human pregnancy. In one study of 900 pregnant women, 190 were diagnosed as suffering from riboflavin deficiency. They were studied with respect to the course of pregnancy, labor, condition of the newborn, and neonatal development of their infants. Vomiting during pregnancy and the incidence of prematurity and stillbirths were higher in this group of women than in comparable controls, but no differences were apparent in the incidence of toxemia, infections, or hemmorhagic complications. Likewise, birth weight and incidence of malformations appeared to be normal, but lactation was depressed.

THIAMIN

Thiamin deficiency during pregnancy has deleterious effects on the offspring in both experimental animals and humans. In rats, thiamin deficiency beginning on the day of breeding or one week prior to breeding produced a high rate of stillbirths and living young of low birth weight. There was also marked loss of maternal weight and increase in maternal mortality. Use of pair-fed controls showed that these effects of thiamin deficiency were largely due to the restriction of food intake that is such a striking consequence of lack of this vitamin. Injection of estrogen and progesterone maintained pregnancy in almost all of the animals even though the same reduction of food intake occurred, suggesting that the effect of thiamin deficiency on pregnancy was through endocrine function.

Thiamin deficiency before but not during pregnancy also affected subsequent reproductive performance. Female rats were fed a diet low in thiamin from weaning to mating but were given an adequate supply during pregnancy. The average number of young per litter was reduced by about 30% in animals inadequately fed with thiamin during their growing period. The young were of normal weight, however, and their total serum protein, hemoglobin, and hematocrit levels were similar. Doubling the intake of thiamin and other vitamins during pregnancy was without effect on the reproductive performance. The thiamin content of the young and of the maternal liver was not influenced by low thiamin intake prior to pregnancy but was related to intake during pregnancy. Since the average number of resorptions per litter was the same in both groups, the lower number of young born to animals with inadequate thiamin prior to pregnancy reflected lower fertility, the result of poor nutritional status at the time of conception.

Thiamin deficiency in pregnant sows has also been shown to affect the offspring. In these animals there was a high rate of stillbriths, weak newborn young, and poor maintenance of pregnancy.

The effect of thiamin deficiency on the human fetus is well known. Congenital beriberi, although rare, may occur in the newborn infants of women with thiamin deficiency. In such cases, the mother usually has only mild symptoms but consumes an inadequate diet, frequently consisting mainly of refined carbohydrates.

NIACIN

Rats given a niacin-deficient diet had a marked reduction in the number of young born. A diet that was deficient in tryptophan as well as in niacin (the rat can convert tryptophan to niacin) also produced a high rate of fetal resorption.

Most of the studies on the effects of niacin deficiency in pregnant rats have been carried out with the use of an antimetabolite, 6-aminonicotinamide (6-AN). When this antagonist was fed to pregnant rats, multiple congenital abnormalities resulted. Malformations included defects of the skeleton, central nervous system, eyes, urinary system, trunk, and thyroid and thymus glands. When the antimetabolite was given for only two or three days during pregnancy, there was a high incidence of embryonic death and resorption and a low incidence of malformed young. Single injections of 6-AN during pregnancy in rats also produced congenital malformations. These included hydrocephaly and ocular, urogenital, and vascular defects.

VITAMIN B_6

EXPERIMENTAL ANIMALS

Deficiency. The first reports on the essential nature of pyridoxine in pregnancy came from studies in which a deficiency of the vitamin was produced in rats with the use of an antagonist, desoxypyridoxine. With this diet, both resorptions and stillbirths were high, and birth weight was low. Injections of estrogen and progesterone or gonadotrophic hormones allowed the rats to maintain pregnancy. The influence of pyridoxine deficiency on embryonic death therefore occurred at least partially through its effect on gonadal function in the pregnant animals. With larger amounts of desoxypyridoxine in the diet, congenital malformations resulted, including defects of the digits, cleft palate, omphalocele (failure of the abdominal wall to close), shortness of the lower jaw, and exencephaly (external brain).

When a pyridoxine-deficient diet is given to pregnant rats without the use of a pyridoxine antagonist, no congenital malformations are observed. In fact, in one study the conclusion was reached that the fetus was protected from B_6 deficiency during pregnancy, since no defects were apparent at birth. However, feeding a pyridoxine-deficient diet to pregnant rats during the last two weeks of gestation and during lactation resulted in the birth of young that had convulsions as early as three days of age. Plasma transaminases as well as pyridoxal phosphate were low in the brains of B_6-deficient pups at the time of birth.

The pyridoxine level of the diet prior to pregnancy also affected fetal development. Rats given a diet deficient in vitamin B_6 for seven to 30 days before the beginning of pregnancy, but fed an adequate amount of the vitamin during pregnancy, produced young with low birth weight, as low as or lower than that of young of females given the antagonist during gestation. Thus pyridoxine in the diet *before* mating is apparently as important as pyridoxine during gestation. These findings support the idea that the condition of the mother prior to pregnancy plays a critical role in the course of pregnancy and its outcome.

The influence of B_6 deficiency during gestation, or gestation and lactation, on the biochemical development of the fetal and neonatal brain has also been investigated. Animals deficient in pyridoxine during gestation and lactation showed poor survival, retarded weight gain, reduced activity, and a higher incidence of errors in a maze test. Many of them died with convulsive seizures. Brain tissues showed reduced concentration of γ-aminobutyric acid (GABA) (Figure 12–5) and reduced activity of glutamate decarboxylase, dopa decarboxylase, and GABA transaminase. Brains of pups from B_6-deficient dams also showed decreased concentrations of pyridoxine, cerebrosides, and protein. These findings show that pyridoxine deficiency during prenatal life can have significant effects on biochemical parameters of the offspring that are important in the functional activity of the brain and nervous system, even if there are no grossly visible malformations. In addition, neuromotor development and coordination were also found to be inferior in young of rats fed low levels of B_6 by comparison with those fed larger amounts. Even progeny of rats fed pyridoxine at the level considered to be adequate for this species showed poorer performance than those of females fed four times the requirements.

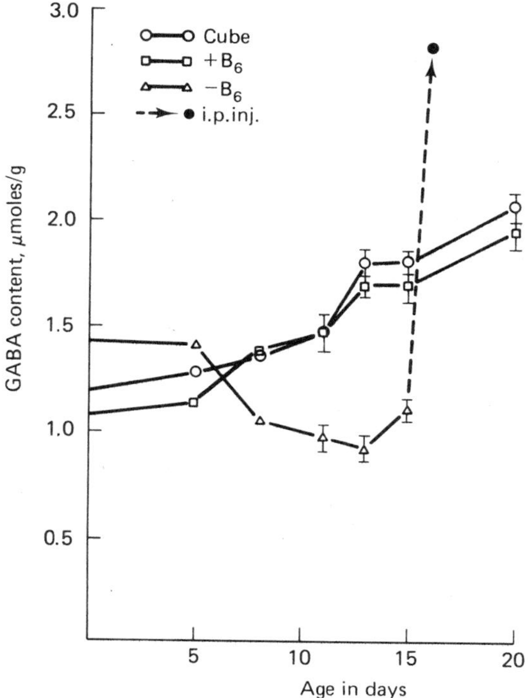

From Bayoumi and Smith, 1972.

Figure 12–5 Whole-brain GABA levels of vitamin B_6-deficient neonates ($-B_6$), vitamin B_6-supplemented neonates ($+B_6$) and normal control neonates (cube) during 0–20 days of age expressed per g wet weight. Points represent the mean value obtained from four to eight animals. Bars indicate ±S.D. On day 16 (24 hours after the intraperitoneal injection of pyridoxine hydrochloride to deficient neonates) the new level of GABA is also shown.

Excess. A high pyridoxine intake during pregnancy in rats produced no abnormalities in the young. Litter size, growth to weaning, and requirement for pyridoxine after weaning were not altered by the high maternal intake during pregnancy.

HUMANS

Pyridoxine nutrition is also a problem in pregnant women. Various indicators of vitamin B_6 status have shown that many pregnant women should have increased intakes of pyridoxine. In a prospective study, for example, maternal and fetal levels of pyridoxal-5-phosphate (PLP) and the degree of coenzyme saturation (activation factor) of aspartate aminotransferase and alanine aminotransferase in maternal erythrocytes were measured. More than 4 mg of B_6 supplementation daily was required to maintain plasma PLP levels in the range found during the first trimester or in nonpregnant women. Plasma PLP in maternal and cord blood were highly correlated, indicating dependence of fetal B_6 nutrition on maternal circulating PLP (Figure 12–6). The findings on activation factor, however, were difficult to interpret.

FOLIC ACID

EXPERIMENTAL ANIMALS

The importance of folic acid during pregnancy in mammals has been studied extensively, primarily with the use of folic acid antagonists. However, even without an antagonist in the diet, folate deficiency causes congenital malformations in rats. With a relatively mild deficiency a variety of

Figure 12–6 The effect of pyridoxine supplementation on the plasma concentrations of pyridoxal phosphate in cord blood at the time of delivery.

From Lumeng et al., 1976.

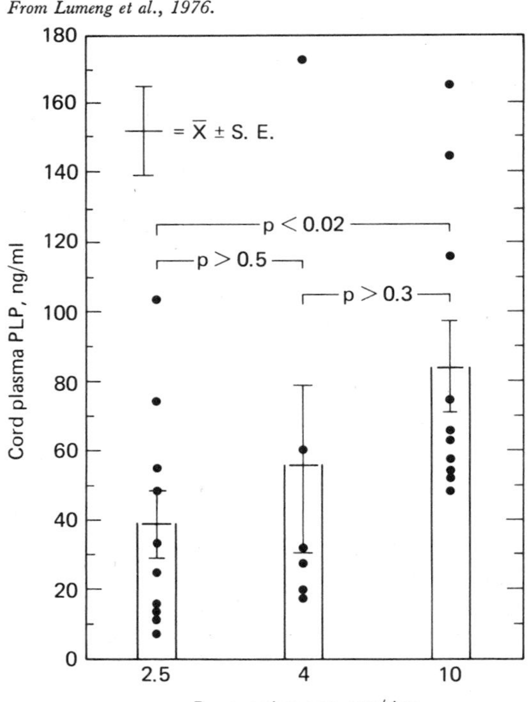

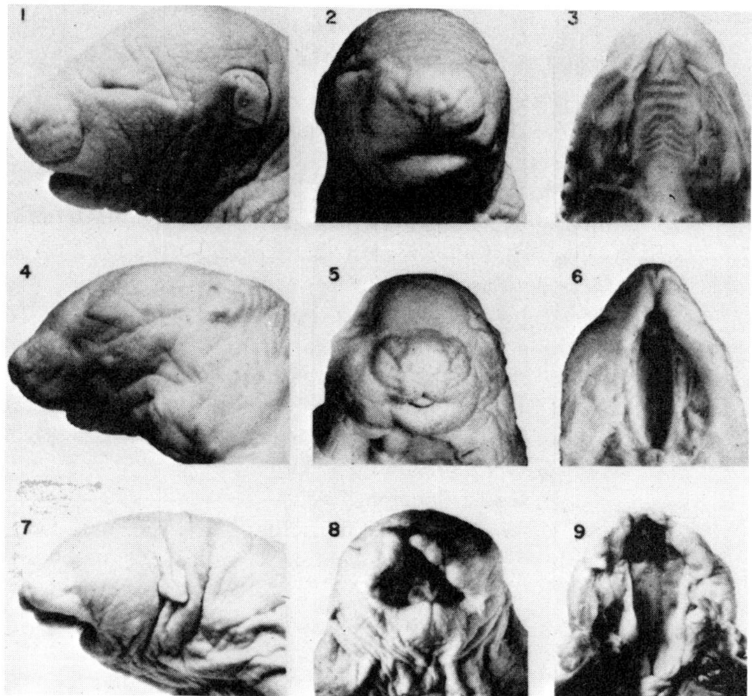

From Nelson et al., 1955.

Figure 12–7 Lateral and frontal views of the head and ventral views of the palate in 21-day-old rat fetuses of mothers maintained on the PGA-control or deficient diet. 1, 2, 3: Control. 4, 5, 6: PGA-deficient, days 10 to 13, showing a wide cleft palate and short mandible. 7, 8, 9: PGA-deficient, days 10 to 13, showing cleft palate, unilateral harelip, and extremely short mandible.

malformations was found, including cleft lip, hydrocephaly, failure of closure of the thoracic and abdominal walls, and eye defects.

Extensive studies of the wide variety of congenital malformations produced by folate deficiency were made in the pregnant rat using an antagonist, X-methyl pteroylglutamic acid (X-methyl PGA), in combination with a folate-deficient diet. There was a high incidence of resorptions as well as multiple congenital defects. The frequency of the various types of defects depended on the timing. The young showed marked edema and anemia, cleft palate, numerous defects of the face, syndactyly, a wide variety of skeletal malformations, and defects of the lungs, eyes, and urogenital and cardiovascular systems (Figure 12–7). Even short-term, transitory deficiency in combination with the folate antagonist caused high incidences of multiple malformations. For example, when this diet was given for only 48 hours between day 7 and day 12, there were gross congenital malformations in 72 to 100% of the young at term. Similar malformations have also been produced in the mouse and the cat with the same antagonist.

Biochemical effects. Although some investigators have attempted to determine the mechanism by which folate deficiency produces teratogenic effects, little progress has been made. Since folate antagonists are known to inhibit nucleic acid synthesis, the influence of maternal treatment with such diets on the nucleic acid synthesis of embryos was studied. In one experiment using aminopterin as a folate antagonist, DNA levels in fetal liver of rats were depressed but RNA was not affected. In another study, however, there were significant decreases in protein, DNA, and RNA of whole body, liver, brain, and placenta of experimental fetuses as compared with controls. These effects could not be altered by administration of DNA, orotic acid (used in DNA synthesis), or ascorbic acid to pregnant rats. The lower content of DNA in the fetuses from treated females seemed to be due to inhibition of DNA synthesis.

In folate deficiency as in riboflavin deficiency, the effects of the teratogenic condition on the mother were minimal. That is, the mother showed neither visible nor biochemical evidence of the vitamin deficiency, although the effect on the developing embryos was very pronounced. As in the case of riboflavin deficiency, the biochemical changes observed in the placenta and the fetuses of folate-deficient females are not specific for folic acid but are also found in other teratogenic vitamin deficiencies. It must therefore be concluded that the specific defect resulting in teratogenic effects of folate deficiency has not yet been discovered.

In another approach to the problem of the biochemical basis of the teratogenicity of folate deficiency, concentrations of adenosine triphosphate (ATP), diphosphate (ADP), and monophosphate (AMP) were measured in developing rat embryos. It was found that the ATP level was markedly reduced and the pool of adenine (as ATP, ADP, and AMP) was decreased in experimental embryos. These findings were thought to be related to the increased oxygen consumption observed in rat embryos from folate-deficient females, suggesting the possibility that cellular energy metabolism is deranged.

The effect on enzymatic differentiation of folate deficiency during prenatal development (using a folate antagonist) was also studied. Alterations in isozyme patterns for a number of enzymes were seen in embryos from folate-deficient rats. Enzymic differentiation of phosphomonoesterases also showed pronounced differences in embryos from folate-deficient females as compared with controls (see Figure 12–8). The specific activity of this enzyme in tissues from experimental fetuses did not parallel that of the controls for any of the fetal ages studied. The changes in enzyme patterns were correlated with abnormal chondrogenesis and osteogenesis.

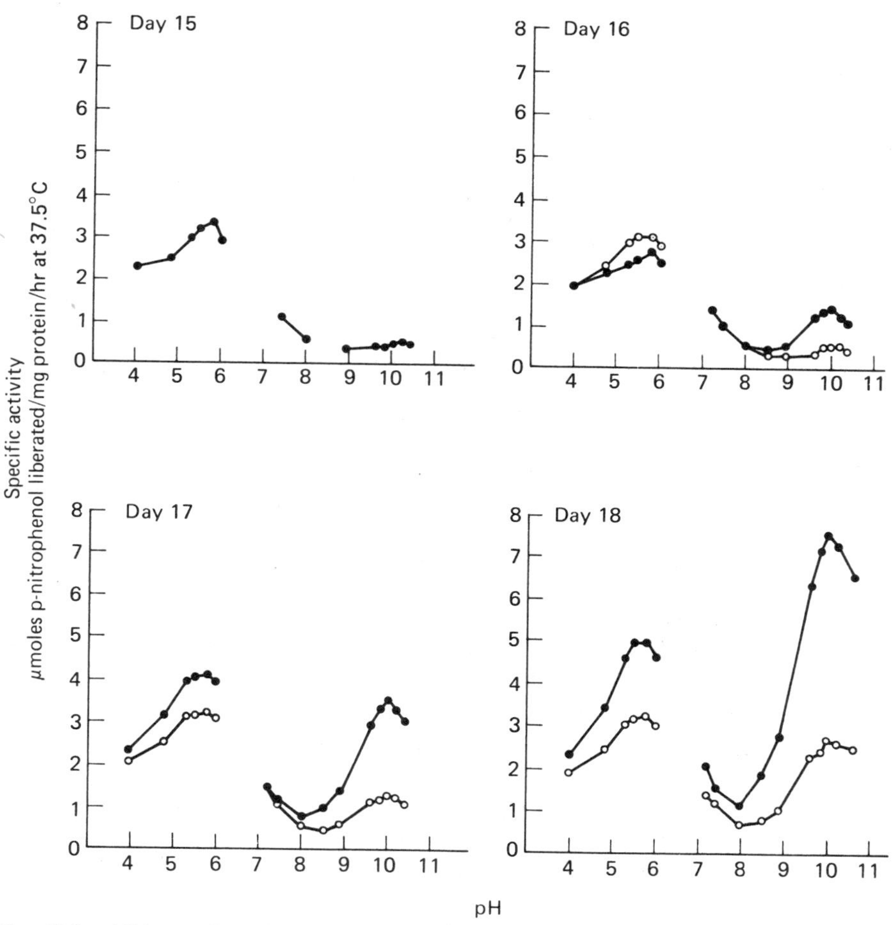

From Jaffe and Johnson, 1973.

Figure 12–8 Specific activity of the *p*H-dependent phosphomonoesterases of limb homogenates from control (●) and experimental (○) fetuses. Each point on the curves represents material from 12 litters.

HUMANS

Folic acid is essential for the developing human embryo, as is clearly evident from clinical reports in which folate antagonists have been used as abortifacient agents. When these compounds were given during the first trimester of pregnancy, fetal deaths followed by spontaneous abortion resulted. However, if the antagonist was given in insufficient quantities, or was given too late during the pregnancy, the result was not abortion but a malformed fetus, usually with brain abnormalities.

In less extreme conditions, however, the possible relationship of folate deficiency during pregnancy to malformation or other abnormalities of pregnancy is not as clear. It is generally agreed that folate deficiency is not rare in pregnant women. The estimate of the incidence of this condition varies from 3 to 22% of pregnant women in this country and as high as 54% of a population of pregnant women in southern India.

In an early retrospective study of 17 pregnant women with megaloblastic anemia (the type of anemia resulting from folate deficiency), five of the women gave birth to infants with congenital malformations. In another retrospective study, the investigators used the histidine load test as a sign of folate deficiency. The urinary excretion of formiminoglutamic acid (FIGLU) is measured after the ingestion of histidine. In the absence of folate, the metabolism of histidine cannot proceed beyond FIGLU, which is then excreted in larger-than-normal amounts in the urine. Of the mothers of malformed infants, 62% had a positive response indicating folate deficiency, as compared with 17% of mothers of normal infants (see Table 12–2). The relationship of positive FIGLU excretion tests with malformations was even more striking when only central nervous system anomalies were considered. There also seemed to be a relationship between folic acid deficiency and the occurrence of placental abruption (premature separation of the placenta) or spontaneous abortions. It is possible that a genetic factor involving folate metabolism may be involved, since in one study many of the women with defective folate metabolism as measured by the FIGLU test developed the same condition in the next pregnancy.

A recent prospective study of over 800 women corroborates these findings. In women with low erythrocyte folate in early pregnancy, the incidence of small-for-dates infants and of malformations was higher than in women with normal folate, and the difference was highly significant (Figure

TABLE 12–2 FIGLU EXCRETION TESTS IN 98 MOTHERS OF MALFORMED INFANTS

Mothers	*FIGLU-Positive, %*
Mothers of all malformed infants	62
Mothers of all infants with CNS malformations	66
Matched pairs:	
Mothers of malformed infants	65
Mothers of normal infants	17
Mothers of infants with CNS malformations	69
Mothers of normal infants	17

Adapted from Hibbard and Smithells, 1965.

12–9). In another large prospective study, significantly lower levels of red-cell folate were found in mothers subsequently giving birth to infants with neural-tube defects than were found in controls.

There is also impressive evidence suggesting that an inadequate level of maternal serum folate brings about a depression of fetal growth rate that may persist into the first year of life. In women who are folate deficient, supplementation with folic acid during pregnancy results in an increase of their infants' birth weight. Table 12–3 summarizes a study in which Bantu women were folate deficient, but white women were not. In the absence of folate deficiency, additional folate did not increase birth weight. Maternal

TABLE 12–3 BIRTH WEIGHT OF INFANTS OF BANTU AND WHITE MOTHERS RECEIVING VARIOUS SUPPLEMENTS

Group	*No.*	*Supplementation*	*Birth Weight, Lb, Mean*	*± S.D.*
Bantu	63	Fe	5.48	1.8
	65	Fe + Folate	6.22	1.1
	55	Fe + Folate + B_{12}	6.38	1.1
White	52	Fe	6.92	1.3
	62	Fe + Folate	7.03	1.3
	58	Fe + Folate + B_{12}	6.91	1.2

From Baumslag et al., 1970.

Figure 12–9 Incidence of subsequent complications in patients with normal and low erythrocyte folate levels in early pregnancy.

From Hibbard, 1975.

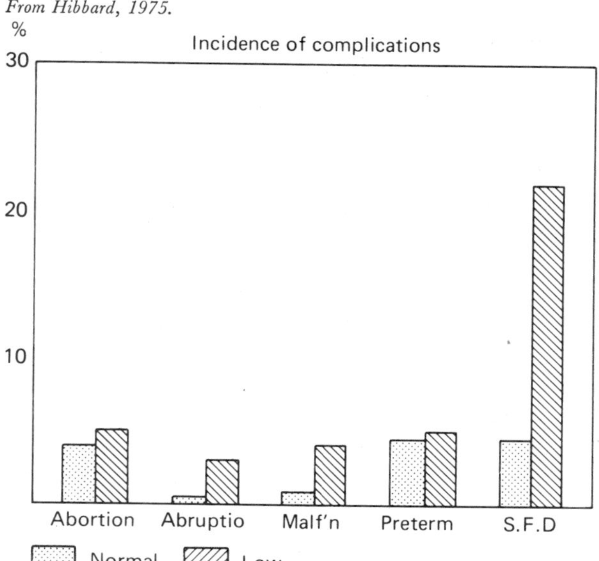

folate deficiency also appears to cause postnatal functional problems. In one study, children whose mothers were severely folate deficient showed abnormal or delayed behavioral development.

Although there is now considerable evidence of a high correlation between folic acid deficiency and various complications of pregnancy, some conflicting findings have been reported. In some studies little correlation was found, for example, between folate status (as measured by plasma folate levels and morphology of red cells) and problems associated with abnormal development.

PANTOTHENIC ACID

Pantothenic acid is an essential nutrient in the diet because it functions in metabolism as part of the molecule of coenzyme A. Experimental studies in several species of animals have shown that it is important for embryonic development. However, there is no information on the role of pantothenic acid in human pregnancy.

Nelson and Evans in 1946 were the first to show that a dietary deficiency of the vitamin in pregnant rats results in deleterious effects on reproduction. When a pantothenic acid-deficient diet was given to female rats during pregnancy beginning 16 to 23 days before mating or as late as the day of mating, failure of implantation and resorption occurred and the young had low birth weights. Later studies by the French workers Giround and Lefebvres-Boisselot reported teratogenic effects as well. Malformations that occurred were edema, hemorrhage, exencephaly, anophthalmia or microphthalmia, limb abnormalities, and malformations of the renal system. Even fetuses that were not malformed at birth showed abnormal intrauterine growth. Dry weights, especially, were markedly lower in fetuses of pantothenic acid-deficient rats from 17 days of gestation to term. Because of their edema, the total body weight was not much different from normal, since the animals contained a higher concentration of water than did the controls.

In some fetuses from pantothenate-deficient rats a peculiar abnormality of the limbs was observed, which resembled partial amputation of the paws. The extremities of the limbs were red and irregularly swollen. Histological examination of the paws on the 16th day of gestation showed an arrest of blood circulation in the marginal veins, apparently resulting in direct contact of the coagulated blood with the tissues. It was concluded that breakdown of the tissues in contact with the blood caused degeneration of the digits.

The teratogenic effects of pantothenate deficiency occurred in the absence of signs or symptoms of deficiency in the mothers. In nonpregnant

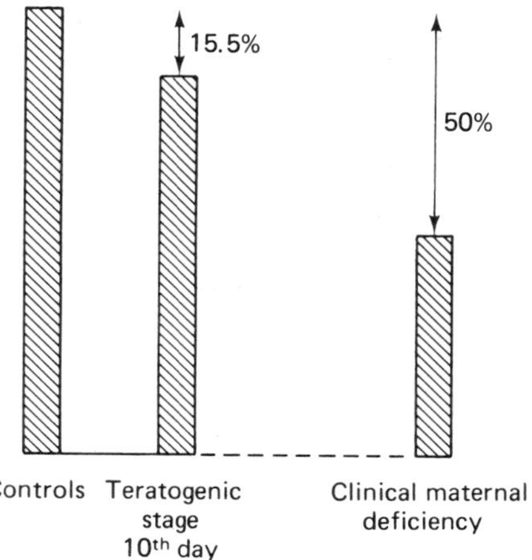

From Giroud, 1970.

Figure 12–10 Slightness of the teratogenic pantothenic acid deficiency. Variations of the pantothenic acid level in the maternal liver (rat). Note that the drop in vitamin is very small at the teratogenic stage, when the malformations are induced. The drop is much more marked when the pathological symptoms appear in the mother.

rats deficient in pantothenic acid, the level of liver pantothenate may fall by 75% of its original value. However, in pregnant rats given a pantothenic acid-deficient diet, when maternal liver pantothenate fell to 40% of the normal value, fetal death occurred. With less severe reduction of pantothenate in maternal liver, however, malformations of the fetus resulted. Indeed, on the tenth day of gestation, a time critical for development of brain and eye malformations in rats, the level of liver pantothenate in pantothenic acid-deficient rats was only 16% lower than normal (see Figure 12–10). This is another example of the principle that deleterious influences on the developing fetus may result from very mild nutritional deficiencies that produce little, if any, pathological effects on the mother herself.

Biochemical studies of fetuses have been made under teratogenic conditions of pantothenate deficiency. In such fetuses at term, the content of protein, DNA, and RNA was low in liver, brain, and total body. The brain, where malformations were of high incidence, showed the least depression of these values. Similar changes were seen in placenta, but the maternal liver was normal with respect to these biochemical parameters.

A pantothenate antagonist, ω-methyl-pantothenic acid, in combination with a deficient diet has also been used to study the effects of pantothenate deficiency during reproduction. With this combination, teratogenic effects were seen in a variety of organ systems. In addition to the defects of the nervous system and limbs previously observed, there were interventricular septal defects, anomalies of the aortic arch pattern, hydronephrosis and hydroureter, club foot, cleft palate, and tail and dermal defects. The tissues of young from pantothenate-deficient females contained at birth only 9% as much pantothenic acid as was present in normal young. Blood concentrations of pantothenic acid were also lower than normal. The injection of ascorbic acid to pregnant females given a pantothenate-deficient diet could compensate partially for the effects of the deficiency. With this treatment the percentages of abnormal young and of resorptions were lower than without the ascorbic acid.

Pantothenic acid deficiency during prenatal life was also found to cause permanent postnatal effects. Pregnant rats were given a pantothenate-deficient diet during the first 14 days of gestation only. The offspring of these females, even though they received a normal diet throughout their lifetime, showed motor incoordination, deficient body-righting reflexes, motor spasms, and poor head orientation. These abnormalities occurred in the absence of other teratogenic effects and persisted into adulthood.

The effects of pantothenic acid deficiency in pregnant guinea pigs has been studied in conjunction with changes in levels of pantothenic acid and coenzyme A in the developing guinea pig liver. (See Chapter 5 for discussion of pantothenic acid and coenzyme A.) Pregnant guinea pigs given a pantothenic acid-deficient diet died within a short time, 9 to 16 days. Liver pantothenic acid and coenzyme A levels in these animals were markedly reduced and liver fat concentration was greatly increased. A transitory dietary deficiency of pantothenic acid during the ninth or tenth (last) weeks of gestation (total period 70 days) resulted in loss of fetuses through abortion or death of the mother. Deficiency during the tenth week appeared to produce a significant increase in the liver fat of the newborn. Concomitantly, liver pantothenic acid level was lower than normal, both at birth and at seven days of age. Young whose mothers had received the deficient diet during the ninth, the seventh, or the sixth weeks of gestation showed no significant changes in liver fat at birth, but liver pantothenic acid concentration was lower than normal. No gross morphological abnormalities were observed in any of the offspring of deficient guinea pigs, but one young animal showed behavioral disturbances (postural difficulties and some tremor) in the six days it lived. These experiments suggested that the greatest need for pantothenic acid during fetal development of the guinea pig is in the period shortly before birth, when concentration of pantothenic acid and coenzyme A in fetal liver rises sharply in this species (see Chapter 5).

Pantothenic acid deficiency also produced abnormal development in swine. If the deficiency was extreme, infertility, resorptions, and abortions also occurred.

VITAMIN B_{12}

The importance of vitamin B_{12} in the prenatal development of mammals has been studied in rats. The major effect of this deficiency in the pregnant animal is to produce hydrocephalus in the offspring. Since folic acid and vitamin B_{12} are often closely associated, much of the early work on this subject was difficult to clarify because of the inability to separate the two deficiencies. However, the hydrocephalus that is found when both folate and vitamin B_{12} are inadequate appears to be caused by deficiency of vitamin B_{12}, since the development of hydrocephalus produced by a vitamin B_{12}-deficient diet is the same with or without an added folate antagonist.

Rats deficient in vitamin B_{12} gave birth to a high proportion of young with hydrocephalus and other congenital anomalies. There was also a slight increase in the number of brain cells containing a normal amount of DNA but reduced RNA. At weaning, the hydrocephalic rats had an elevated cerebrospinal fluid pressure. Anomalies of the eye were frequent and seemed to be associated with hydrocephalus. There was also decreased myelination of nerve fibers, most pronounced in the peripheral nerves. Bone defects and increased cellularity of the bone marrow were characteristic of the B_{12}-deficient newborn rat. The alterations of the bone marrow were associated with a macrocytic anemia.

Recent studies have shown that even a marginal intake of vitamin B_{12} during gestation in the rat has important effects on the offspring. The progeny of rats given a diet marginally deficient in vitamin B_{12} were studied for one year after birth. Their birth weight was low and their body weight continued to be significantly lower than normal after 21 days, three months, and one year. In addition, activity of liver glucose-6-phosphatase and aminopyrine demethylase and B_{12} concentration were low in the newborns. There was also lower resistance to Salmonella infection. These findings suggest that an apparently mild deficiency of B_{12} may have subtle consequences on the differentiation and functional development of the fetus. Furthermore, as in the case of other nutrients already described, the effects of a marginally deficient nutrient supply at this phase of development may not be noticed at birth and may become evident only later in life when the organism is subjected to a stressful stimulus or situation.

Although little information is available on vitamin B_{12} deficiency in the human fetus, there are known genetic disorders called vitamin B_{12} dependencies. The term *vitamin dependency* describes certain types of gene-dependent nutritional disorders in which the nutritional intake of a vitamin required for normal function is much greater than the usual amount. These abnormal requirements may result from disorders of vitamin absorption or utilization. The vitamin B_{12} dependencies are thought to involve disturbances in the uptake of the vitamin precursor or its conversion to the active coenzyme form, or in the interaction of the coenzyme with the two apoenzymes that require it (methyl transferase and hydrogen transferase). In children with vitamin B_{12} dependency the amount of the vitamin required may be as high as 1000 μg per day, as compared with 1 μg per day needed by the normal adult human. A human fetus with such a disorder has been treated prenatally by feeding large amounts of vitamin B_{12} to the mother.

Several genetic disorders of B_{12}-dependent metabolism are now known. The metabolism of methylmalonic acid is affected in several of these diseases. Vitamin B_{12} nutrition can also be impaired by a deficiency of intrinsic factor, which results in pernicious anemia and may produce retarded mental and physical development in childhood.

CHOLINE

The importance of choline for reproduction of mammals was first shown in pigs in 1947. In sows given a choline-deficient diet during pregnancy, survival of the offspring to weaning was poor. Some abnormalities, such as kinked tails, spraddled hind legs, and incoordination, were observed. On postmortem and microscopic examination the young showed fatty livers, hemorrhages of the kidney, and other kidney abnormalities.

In mice given choline-deficient diets from the time of weaning, growth was normal, but fertility was decreased and difficulty of parturition was observed. The offspring that were born had a high mortality rate during the third and fourth months of life.

The effect of choline deficiency during pregnancy on maternal and fetal liver lipids was studied in rats. In animals fed a normal diet there was no lipid, as determined histochemically in the livers of pregnant and fetal rats. In the choline-deficient animals, however, there was a marked accumulation of fat in both maternal and fetal livers at term.

A prenatal maternal deficiency of choline also produced postnatal effects. When rats were given a choline-deficient diet during pregnancy only, their offspring were found to have hypertension when they were 35 to 58 days of age. However, by the time they reached the age of 86 to 108 days, blood pressure was normal. These results were thought to be due to the hypertensive effects of kidney damage in choline deficiency. It seemed that the formation of new tissue after weaning could compensate for the prenatally damaged tissue.

A diet low in choline and methionine, but supplemented with vitamin B_{12}, was given to pregnant rats as a marginally deficient diet. This was found to support conception, implantation, and fetal growth normally, and no congenital malformations were seen. Although the marginally deficient newborn offspring appeared clinically normal, biochemical measurements indicated that they had small brain cells and abnormal protein synthesis.

References and Supplementary Readings

GENERAL

GIROUD, A. "Nutrition of the embryo." In: *Symposium on Nutrition and Prenatal Development. Fed. Proc.* **27**: 163–184 (1968).

GIROUD, A. *The Nutrition of the Embryo*. Springfield, Ill.: Charles C Thomas, 1970.

HURLEY, L. S. "Nutritional deficiencies and excesses." In: J. G. WILSON AND F. C. FRASER, eds., *Handbook of Teratology*, Vol. 1, pp. 261–308. New York: Plenum Publishing Corp., 1977.

ASCORBIC ACID

MARTIN, M. P., E. BRIDGFORTH, W. J. MCGANITY, AND W. J. DARBY. "The Vanderbilt cooperative study of maternal and infant nutrition. X. Ascorbic acid." *J. Nutr.* **62**: 201–224 (1957).

NORKUS, E. P., AND P. ROSSO. "Changes in ascorbic acid metabolism of the offspring following high maternal intake of this vitamin in the pregnant guinea pig." *Ann. N. Y. Acad. Sci.* **258**: 401–409 (1975).

RIVERS, J. M., L. KROOK, AND A. CORMIER. "Biochemical and histological study of guinea pig fetal and uterine tissues in ascorbic acid deficiency." *J. Nutr.* **100**: 217–227 (1970).

TEEL, H. M., B. S. BURKE, AND R. DRAPER. "Vitamin C in human pregnancy and lactation." *Am. J. Dis. Child.* **56**: 1004–1010 (1938). Copyright 1938.

RIBOFLAVIN

AKSU, O., B. MACKLER, T. H. SHEPARD, AND R. J. LEMIRE. "Studies of the development of congenital anomalies in embryos of riboflavin-deficient, galactoflavin fed rats. II. Role of the terminal electron transport systems." *Teratology* **1**: 93–102 (1968).

MILLER, Z., I. PONCET, AND E. TAKACS. "Biochemical studies on experimental congenital malformations: Flavin nucleotides and folic acid in fetuses and livers from normal and riboflavin-deficient rats." *J. Biol. Chem.* **237**: 968–973 (1962).

MUTTART, C., R. CHAUDHURI, J. PINTO, AND R. S. RIVLIN. "Enhanced riboflavin incorporation into flavins in newborn riboflavin-deficient rats." *Am. J. Physiol.* **233**: E397–E401 (1977).

THIAMIN

Brown, M. L., and C. H. Snodgrass. "Effect of dietary level of thiamine on reproduction in the rat." *J. Nutr.* **85**: 102–106 (1965).

Nelson, M. M., and H. M. Evans. "Relation of thiamine to reproduction in the rat." *J. Nutr.* **55**: 151–163 (1955).

Van Gelder, D. W., and F. U. Darby. "Congenital and infantile beriberi." *J. Pediatr.* **25**: 226–235 (1944).

NIACIN

Chamberlain, J. G., and M. M. Nelson. "Congenital abnormalities in the rat resulting from single injections of 6-aminonicotinamide during pregnancy." *J. Exp. Zool.* **153**: 285–300 (1963).

VITAMIN B_6

Alton-Mackey, M. G., and B. L. Walker. "Graded levels of pyridoxine in the rat diet during gestation and the physical and neuromotor development of offspring." *Am. J. Clin. Nutr.* **26**: 420–428 (1973).

Bayoumi, R. A., and W. R. D. Smith. "Some effects of dietary vitamin B_6 deficiency on γ-aminobutyric acid metabolism in developing rat brain." *J. Neurochem.* **19**: 1883–1897 (1972).

Lumeng, L., R. E. Cleary, R. Wagner, P. Yu, and T. Li. "Adequacy of vitamin B_6 supplementation during pregnancy: a prospective study." *Am. J. Clin. Nutr.* **29**: 1376–1383 (1976).

FOLIC ACID

Baumslag, N., T. Edelstein, and J. Metz. "Reduction of incidence of prematurity by folic acid supplementation in pregnancy." *Brit. Med. J.* **1**: 16–17 (1970).

Gross, R. L., P. M. Newberne, and J. V. O. Reid. "Adverse effects on infant development associated with maternal folic acid deficiency." *Nutr. Reports Inter.* **10**: 241–248 (1974).

Hibbard, B. M. "Folates and the fetus." *S. Afr. Med. J.* **49**: 1223–1226 (1975).

Hibbard, E. D., and R. W. Smithells. "Folic acid metabolism and human embryopathy." *Lancet* **1**: 1254 (1965).

Jaffe, N. R., and E. M. Johnson. "Alterations in the ontogeny and specific activity of phosphomonoesterases associated with abnormal chondrogenesis and osteogenesis in the limbs of fetuses from folic acid-deficient pregnant rats." *Teratology* **8**: 33–50 (1973).

Kitay, D. Z. "Folic acid deficiency in pregnancy." *Am. J. Obstet. Gynec.* **104**: 1067–1107 (1969).

Nelson, M. M., H. W. Wright, C. W. Asling, and H. M. Evans. "Multiple congenital abnormalities resulting from transitory deficiency of pteroylglutamic acid during gestation in the rat." *J. Nutr.* **56**: 349–369 (1955).

Stone, M. L., A. L. Luhby, R. Feldman, M. Gordon, and J. M. Cooperman. "Folic acid metabolism in pregnancy." *Am. J. Obstet. Gynec.* **99**: 638–648 (1967).

VITAMIN B_{12}

AMPOLA, M. G., M. J. MAHONEY, E. NAKAMURA, AND K. TANAKA. "Prenatal therapy of a patient with vitamin-B_{12}-responsive methylmalonic acidemia." *N. Eng. J. Medicine* **293**: 313–317 (1975).

WOODARD, J. C., AND P. M. NEWBERNE. "The pathogenesis of hydrocephalus in newborn rats deficient in vitamin B_{12}." *J. Embryol. Exp. Morph.* **17**: 177–187 (1967).

13

Major mineral elements

CALCIUM AND PHOSPHORUS

The fetus contains little calcium until the latter part of gestation, and the greatest accumulation of the element occurs during the last trimester (see Table 13–1).

DEFICIENCY

The effects of calcium deficiency during pregnancy are similar to those of vitamin D deficiency in both animals and man. Probably the earliest

TABLE 13–1 CALCIUM ACCRETION IN THE DEVELOPING FETUS OF MAN, CATTLE, AND THE RAT

Man			*Cattle*			*Rat*[a]		
Age, months	*Weight, g*	*Calcium, g*	*Age, months*	*Weight, kg*	*Calcium, g*	*Age, days*	*Weight, g*	*Calcium, mg*
1	0.04	—	5	2.56	10.1	14	0.10	0.018
2	3.0	0.032	6	6.505	43.2	15	0.14	0.042
3	36.0	0.25	7	16.46	140	16	0.25	0.088
4	120.0	1.1	8	31.8	375	17	0.62	0.46
5	330.0	3.3	9	49.3	673	18	1.5	1.5
6	600.0	7.5				19	2.7	5.2
7	1000.0	11.6				20	3.8	8.1
8	1500.0	20.4				21	4.9	8.7
9	2200.0–3200.0	—				22	5.6	12.3

[a]Per fetus.

From Comar, 1956.

experiment demonstrating the importance of maternal nutrition for the fetal development of mammals concerns calcium (see Chapter 6). In experiments published between 1911 and 1924, it was found that when cows were fed a wheat ration, their offspring were prematurely born and were either stillborn or, being extremely weak and undersized, died soon after birth. When the ration was supplemented with bone meal (supplying calcium phosphate), fetal development was improved, but the addition of cod liver oil (providing vitamins A and D) was necessary to produce normal reproduction and fetal development (Figures 13–1 and 13–2).

If calcium deficiency is mild or of short duration, no abnormal effects are seen in the fetus. In rats, fetal development and calcification were found to be normal under such conditions of mild calcium deficiency in pregnant females. If the maternal diet contains an insufficient quantity of calcium to provide for the needs of the offspring, calcium is removed from the maternal skeleton under stimulation from the parathyroid glands. An early study showed that when pregnant rats were given a diet containing a low level of calcium, their fetuses contained more calcium than had been consumed by the mother during the pregnancy. The pregnant rats were thus mobilizing calcium from their own skeletons, which was used for the benefit of the developing fetuses when the dietary calcium level was low.

In Chapter 6 we discussed the old idea that the mammalian fetus was a parasite on the mother and would draw from her body the nutrients it needed for itself. Calcium is an example of a nutrient for which the fetus may be thought of as a parasite, since the fetal need for calcium is supplied at the expense of the maternal skeleton. The mechanism by which this is brought about, however, is probably related more to maternal physiology than to fetal requirements. The level of plasma calcium is regulated within very narrow limits, so that it is maintained even when the dietary intake is less than the total of urinary, fecal, and other pathways of excretion of the element. In this case, the lowering of plasma calcium level stimulates the secretion of the parathyroid hormone, which is turn increases the rate of breakdown of bone salt in the skeleton and increases the rate of calcium mobilization from bone. This calcium, circulating in the maternal blood, is of course available to the fetus through the placenta. The availability of calcium to the fetus thus remains at a normal or nearly normal level, even though the dietary intake of the mother may be low. If this process continues, demineralization of bone will occur in the mother.

In rats given a calcium-deficient diet beginning on the day of mating, it was found that their litters were as rich in ash content as were those of controls. However, the ash content of maternal femurs was much lower in the animals receiving the calcium-deficient diet during pregnancy than it was in the normally fed pregnant rats. Thus, the calcification of the fetuses was maintained at the expense of maternal bone.

In contrast to the effects of mild or short-term deficiency of calcium, when the deficiency is severe or prolonged over a long period, normal development and calcification of the fetus do not occur. In rats severely deficient in calcium to the point of losing weight during pregnancy, the young were stillborn. The percentage of ash in these offspring was extremely low at birth, and their bones were almost transparent. Studies on pigs also showed that severe calcium deficiency influenced the calcification of fetal bones, and when cows were fed a low-calcium diet, tissue levels of the element were lower than normal in their fetuses.

Figure 13–1 The results with the balanced ration of 1907. Protein and energy, the sole factors emphasized at that time, were supplied by the use of a ration made from wheat straw, wheat meal, and wheat gluten. Common salt was allowed *ad libitum*. The cow was shaggy coated, slow and sleepy in movement, and had a tendency to drag her hind feet. The calf was born prematurely and died. In other cases the calves were born prematurely, were extremely weak, and died soon after birth.

From Hart et al., 1924.

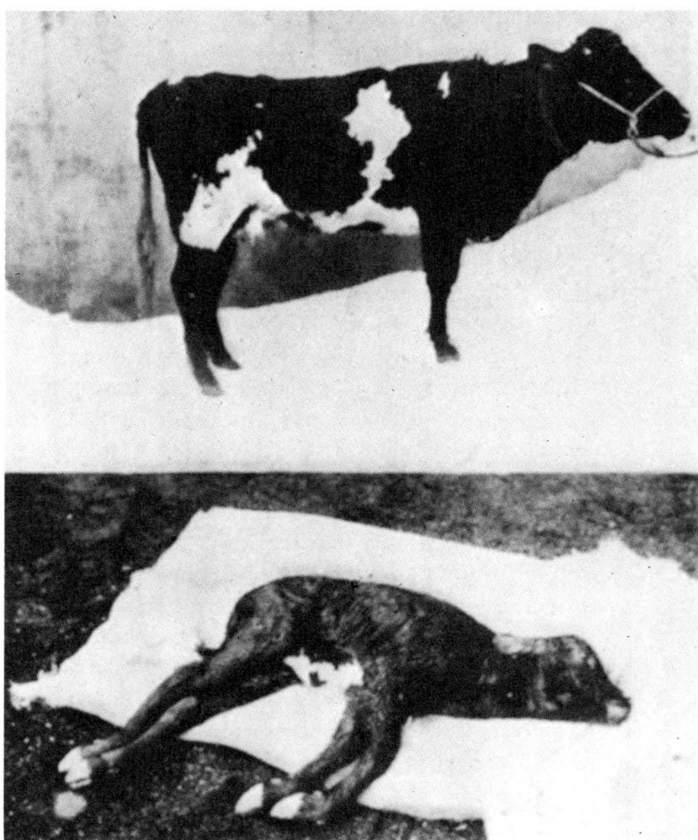

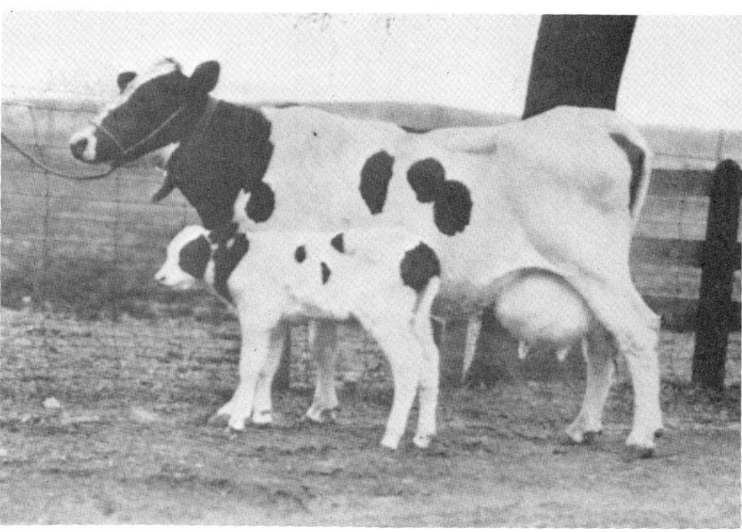

From Hart et al., 1924.

Figure 13–2 The result with the balanced ration of 1924—the same wheat ration proportions as used in 1907, but supplemented with bone meal 2%, common salt 1%, and raw cod liver oil 2%. The cow was sleek in appearance, active, and apparently in normal nutritive condition. A normal strong calf (115 pounds at birth) was the result from this ration.

PLACENTAL TRANSFER

The transfer of calcium across the placenta is not passive. Studies of placental transfer using radioactive calcium have demonstrated the rapidity of transfer across the placental barrier, the avidity of the fetal bones for calcium, and the high rate of transfer as compared with the amount of calcium in the blood. Furthermore, the fetal plasma calcium level is higher than the maternal plasma calcium concentration, so that active transport must be involved (see Figure 13–3).

In pregnant ewes, the rate of absorption of calcium from the intestine increased steadily throughout pregnancy but was insufficient to meet the requirements of late pregnancy and early lactation. During this period, when the extra calcium was supplied by increased bone resorption, maternal calcium balance became negative (Figure 13–4).

Studies of placental transfer have also demonstrated that the dietary level of calcium influences the amount of the element available to the fetus. Investigations of the movement of radioactive calcium in the maternal-fetal organism have indicated that maternal needs influence the movement of calcium and its transfer to the fetuses. Studies of this type, in both rats and

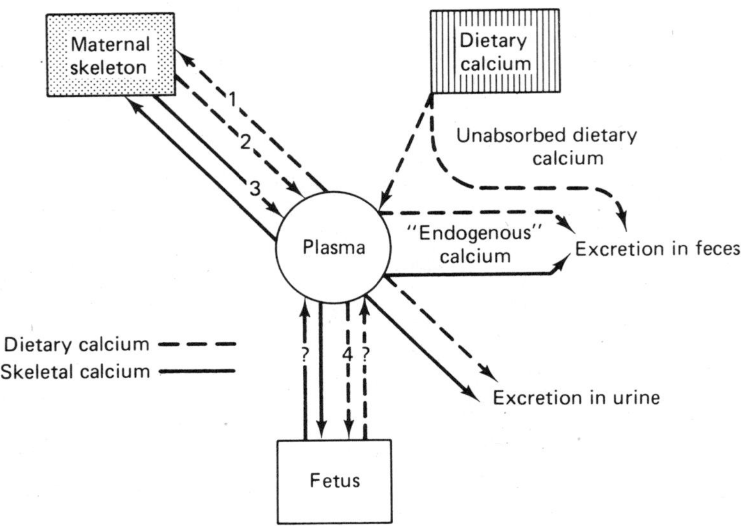

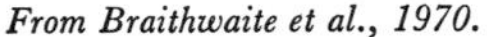

From Bawden and Osborne, 1962, modified from Comar, 1956.

Figure 13–3 Calcium transfer.

Figure 13–4 Calcium balance of ewes with twin lambs at different stages of pregnancy and lactation.

From Braithwaite et al., 1970.

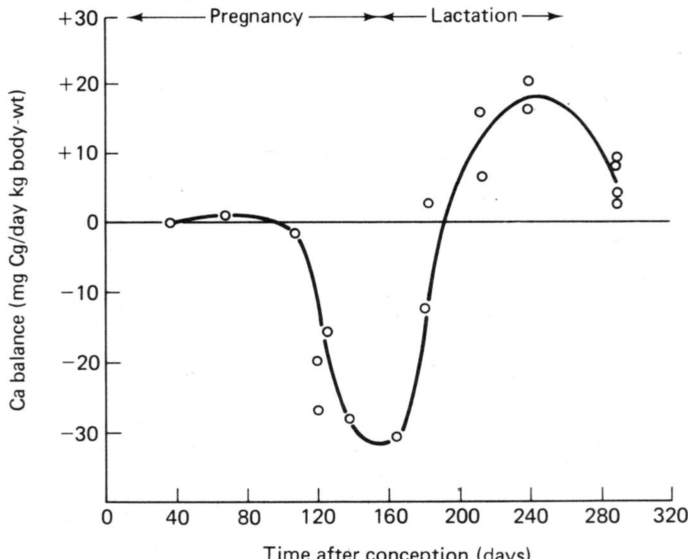

swine, showed that the equilibrium levels of calcium between fetal and maternal blood were lower than normal when dietary calcium was restricted. When maternal pools were already saturated by an adequate previous intake of dietary calcium, more absorbed ^{45}Ca was transferred directly to the fetus and somewhat less was deposited in maternal bones than under conditions of dietary calcium restriction. In maternal soft tissues, however, specific activity (absorbed ^{45}Ca) and calcium concentration were maintained at somewhat higher levels in adequately fed than in calcium-restricted females. Although more radiocalcium was absorbed and less total calcium and ^{45}Ca were transferred to fetuses of low-calcium-fed sows than to those of normal sows, the percentage distribution of the calcium retained by the fetuses was not significantly affected by low dietary intake. Thus, the fetuses of sows given low-calcium diets had less completely calcified bones and were maintained at a lower calcium status than were those of controls.

The ratio of calcium to phosphorus as well as the amount of calcium is important in the development of normal ossification and calcification of the skeleton in the offspring of pregnant animals. In humans, there is ample evidence that good ossification of the fetus depends upon an adequate supply to the mother of dietary calcium and phosphorus as well as vitamin D.

EXCESS

Excessive as well as inadequate amounts of calcium are detrimental to the fetuses of pregnant rats. In one experiment, increasing the dietary calcium to high levels (and keeping the phosphorus concentration constant) produced deleterious effects on the young. In another experiment, a very high level of calcium (3% in the diet as compared with the control level of 0.8%) resulted in hypercalcemia in pregnant rats, who showed an elevation of the plasma calcium level at parturition. These hypercalcemic females produced small litters with offspring of low birth weight. However, despite the hypercalcemia of the mothers, the plasma calcium levels in the offspring were significantly lower than normal at birth, but returned to normal 24 hours later. The females were fed the high-calcium diet during lactation as well as during pregnancy, and their offspring showed poor growth and short, sparse fur with patchy alopecia (Figure 13–5).

MAGNESIUM

As early as 1938, a study of magnesium deficiency in rats indicated that magnesium was necessary for normal pregnancy. More recently, the effect of magnesium deficiency on reproduction and fetal development in rats has been studied extensively by Hurley and her colleagues. A diet severely defi-

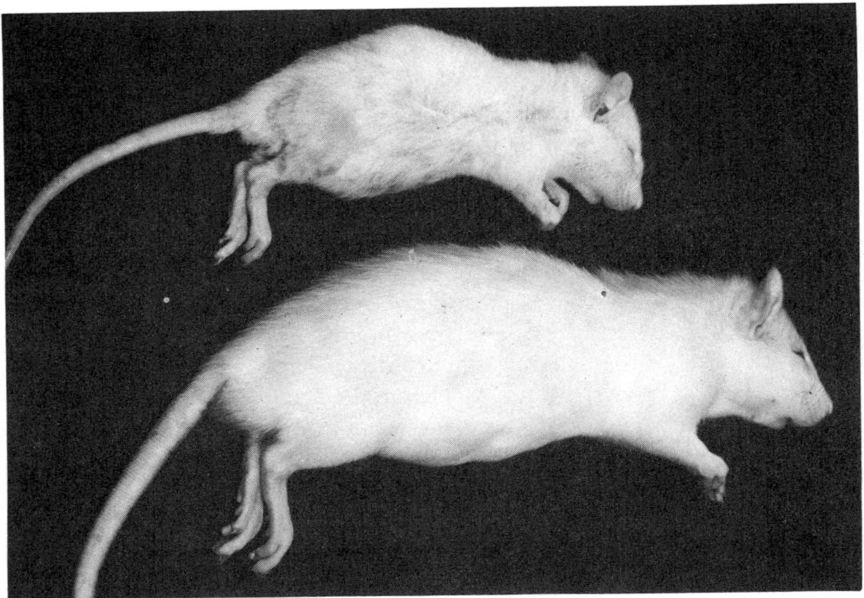

From Fairney and Weir, 1970.

Figure 13–5 Five-week-old rats: the one above was born to a rat fed on a high-calcium diet throughout pregnancy and lactation. The rat below was from a larger litter born to a rat fed a normal diet throughout pregnancy and lactation.

cient in magnesium (0.2 mg magnesium/100 g diet) produced a very rapid fall in maternal plasma magnesium levels in both pregnant and nonpregnant rats (see Figure 13-6). By the second day of this deficiency regimen the plasma magnesium was one-half, and on the fourth day it had fallen to about one-third its initial value. Thus the nonpregnant as well as the pregnant rat is unable to mobilize magnesium from its skeleton and other tissues at a rate sufficient to maintain plasma levels and requires an adequate dietary intake in order to do so.

Under these conditions of magnesium deficiency, no pregnancies were carried to term. When pregnant females were given a diet severely deficient in magnesium from day 6 to day 14 of pregnancy, the incidence of resorptions was extremely high (50 to 90%), and many of the surviving fetuses were malformed. Thus, most of the implantation sites were affected by the maternal dietary deficiency. When the deficient diet was given from days 6 to 12 of gestation, both resorptions and malformations were reduced but were still significantly higher than in controls. Malformations produced by magnesium deficiency included cleft lip, short tongue, hydrocephalus, micrognathia or agnathia, club feet, polydactyly, syndactyly, short or curly tail, herniations, and heart, lung, and urogenital anomalies.

Dietary magnesium deficiency also caused a decreased maternal weight gain, possibly associated with reduced food consumption. Short periods of magnesium deficiency during pregnancy had a lesser effect on plasma magnesium levels at term and on food consumption but still dramatically influenced the ability of female rats to maintain pregnancy. Diets containing either casein or soybean protein appeared to have the same effects on these parameters, although the casein-fed rats were not as severely affected. The rapid effects of dietary magnesium deficiency on the developing rat embryo are probably related to the low maternal plasma level that occurred after only a few days of dietary deficiency.

Figure 13–6 Plasma magnesium levels of pregnant or nonpregnant rats fed either a magnesium-deficient or control diet. Each point represents the mean ±S.E. of samples from five rats.

From Hurley et al., 1976.

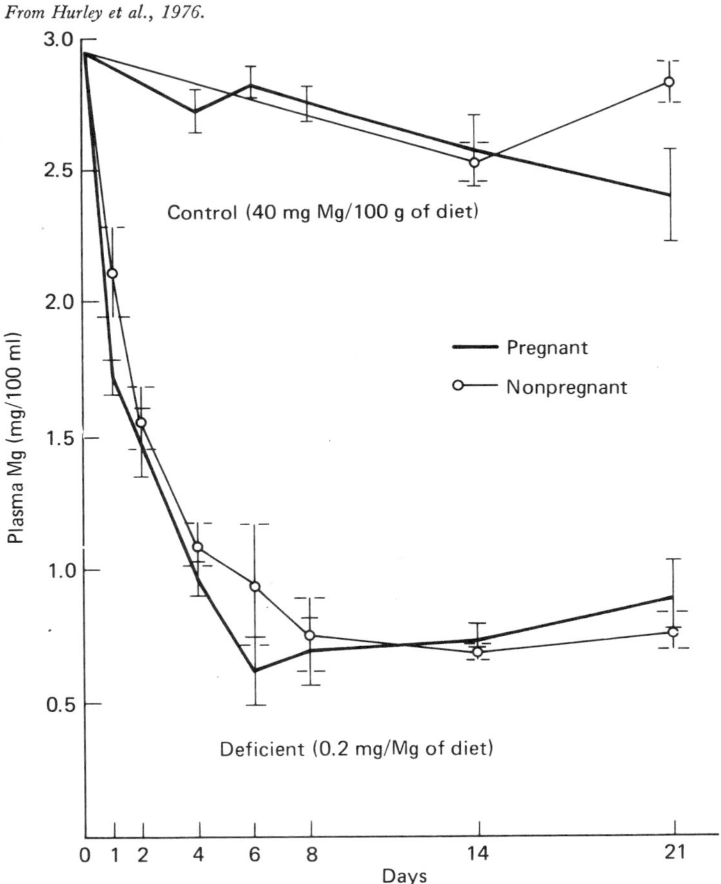

The concentrations of magnesium, calcium, and zinc of maternal and fetal tissues were measured in rats given a diet mildly deficient in magnesium (5 mg/100 g) during pregnancy, and their controls. In females fed the magnesium-deficient diet, kidney calcium was higher and femur magnesium was lower at term than in controls. The magnesium content of the fetuses as well as its concentration in the ash was lower in fetuses from magnesium-deficient females than in controls. Calcium concentration in the ash, however, was unchanged in the magnesium-deficient fetuses. The zinc content in these animals, both total zinc per fetus and its concentration in the ash, were significantly lower in magnesium-deficient fetuses than in controls.

In a different study by Schwartz and her colleagues, pregnant rats were fed magnesium-deficient diets containing 8 mg/100 g. There was a high incidence of stillbirths, and over 90% of the offspring alive at birth died during the first week of life. Body weight and magnesium content of offspring were significantly reduced.

When rats were given a magnesium-deficient diet from day 5 to day 12 of pregnancy, their offspring showed high neonatal mortality and abnormal histological findings in the brain, including necrosis. There was also a significant decrease in potassium concentration in the magnesium-deficient fetuses. Newborn rats showed swelling of the mitochondria and loss of lipid inclusions in the brown adipose tissue. The high neonatal mortality of these animals may be related to these abnormalities, since the brown adipose tissue plays an important role in temperature regulation in the newborn period.

With a relatively mild deficiency of magnesium (approximately 2.5 to 5 mg/100 g) the incidence of resorptions was high, and again malformations occurred. Furthermore, the fetuses alive at term were edematous and severely anemic. The number of red blood cells and the concentration of hemoglobin were markedly reduced in full-term fetuses of females fed a magnesium-deficient diet; hemoglobin was less than half the normal level. This was in contrast to maternal hematology, where these parameters were normal. In neither the mothers nor the fetuses was the concentration of magnesium in the red blood cells reduced by dietary deficiency of the element (Table 13–2).

Maternal dietary magnesium deficiency thus had profound effects on fetal hematopoiesis. In magnesium-deficient fetuses erythropoiesis was significantly greater than normal in liver, adrenal, and spleen. There was a disturbance in the formation of red cells, with many cells abnormally shaped. Stained and unstained smears of peripheral blood revealed extreme alterations in red-cell morphology characterized by abnormality in size, shape, amount of hemoglobin, membrane conformation, and the number and type of nucleated red cells. There was an obvious macrocytosis associated with numerous microcytes and red-cell fragments. Scanning electron microscopy of peripheral red blood cells from magnesium-deficient fetuses showed

TABLE 13–2 FETAL ANEMIA IN MAGNESIUM DEFICIENCY

Diet, mg Mg/100 g	*No. of Rats*	*RBC,[a] No. × 10^6*	*Hgb,[b] g/100 ml*	*RBC Mg, mg/100 ml*
		Maternal		
Control:				
40 mg Mg	13	5.2	10.4	4.3
Deficient:				
2.5 mg Mg	13	4.9	10.7	4.2
		Fetal		
Control:				
40 mg Mg	5	1.6	8.0	12.4
Deficient:				
5 mg Mg	4–12	1.6	9.2	—
2.5 mg Mg	5	1.0[c]	3.6[c]	14.9

[a]Red blood cells.
[b]Hemoglobin.
[c]Significantly different from control, $P < 0.01$.

From Cosens et al., 1977.

abnormalities of shape consisting of budlike excrescences and irregular small pointed fragments, excessive discocytic forms, blebs or protrusions, and holes (Figure 13–7). These flattened discocytic forms were due not to vacuoles but to absence of hemoglobin in the center of the enlarged, flattened red blood cells.

Plasma protein concentration was also significantly lower in fetuses from magnesium-deficient rats than in controls, but in maternal blood, magnesium deficiency did not reduce the concentration of plasma protein. Electrophoresis of plasma proteins showed no differences in protein mobility between normal and magnesium-deficient animals, either fetuses or mothers. Electrophoresis of blood hemolysates showed five identical hemoglobin bands in both mothers and fetuses. Magnesium deficiency also did not influence the electrophoretic pattern of hemoglobin. There was no evidence of alteration in the chemical structure of the hemoglobin molecule.

The anemia of magnesium-deficient fetuses is hemolytic in nature and appears to be the direct result of red-cell malformation. The morphological features of this anemia are consistent with the hypothesis that the most important factor in its development is abnormality of the red-cell membrane due to magnesium deficiency.

Magnesium deficiency also produced abnormalities of chromosomes. Cells of both maternal bone marrow and fetal liver showed significantly more chromosomal anomalies than did those of controls. Chromosomal aber-

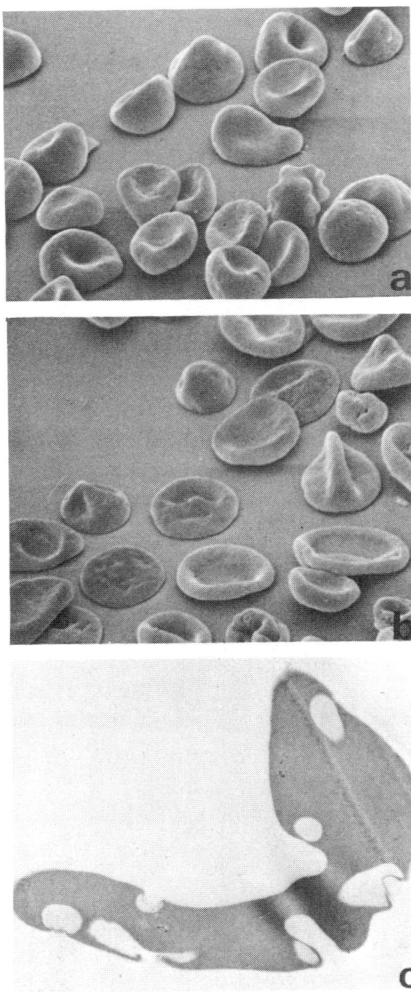

From Cosens et al., 1977.

Figure 13–7 (a) Scanning electron microscopic study of control fetal rat erythrocytes. Magnification × 2450. (b) magnesium-deficient fetal rat erythrocytes showing an abundance of enlarged flattened cells or torocytes. Magnification × 2450. (c) transmission electron microscopic study of a magnesium-deficient erythrocyte from the same fetal sample. Note severe vacuolization and disruption of the outer membrane. (Magnification × 12,500.)

rations occurring in highest incidence were terminal deletions and fragments. "Stickiness" of chromosomes was also observed in cells from magnesium-deficient animals, as had previously been found in magnesium-deficient plants. Magnesium may thus be necessary for the integrity of chromosome structure; however, the relationship of the chromosomal anomalies to congenital malformations is not known.

SODIUM AND POTASSIUM

DEFICIENCY

Relatively few studies have been made of the effect of sodium deficiency during pregnancy on the development of the fetus. In an early experiment, rats were given a sodium-deficient diet from the time of weaning. The fertility of females under this regime was extremely low, and the few young that were born were very small. In later studies, pregnant rats were given a diet low in sodium for one week prior to mating and throughout pregnancy. With this period of sodium deprivation, litter size, incidence of resorptions, and fetal weight at term did not seem to be affected. However, the pregnant females themselves showed abnormal effects, including languor and debility, less weight gain, and smaller retentions of tissue sodium and potassium than in pregnant females receiving higher intakes of sodium. Under these conditions the fetal levels of sodium and potassium in the plasma, the amniotic fluid, total fetal body, or placenta were not significantly influenced by the level of sodium in the maternal diet. However, there were changes in electrolytes of plasma, muscle, bone, and brain of the maternal organism. The changes in water and electrolyte metabolism that were observed resembled those that have been associated with complications of pregnancy in humans.

In sheep, however, the effects of sodium deficiency were quite different. In ewes acutely depleted of sodium during pregnancy the sodium levels of the fetal plasma and amniotic fluid were lower, and the volume of the allantoic fluid was greater, than in those of controls, indicating that sodium depletion of the ewe leads to a deficiency of sodium in the fetus. The apparent discrepancy between the effect of sodium deficiency in rats and in sheep may, however, be a function of the severity of the deficiency rather than a species difference. It would appear that if maternal sodium deficiency is relatively mild, there are few effects on the fetus, although the maternal organism seems to be extremely sensitive to inadequate intakes of this element. In severe sodium deficiency, however, the fetus as well as the mother appears to be affected.

The effect of sodium deficiency during pregnancy on the sodium levels of the fetus was studied in rats. The sodium concentration of fetal plasma

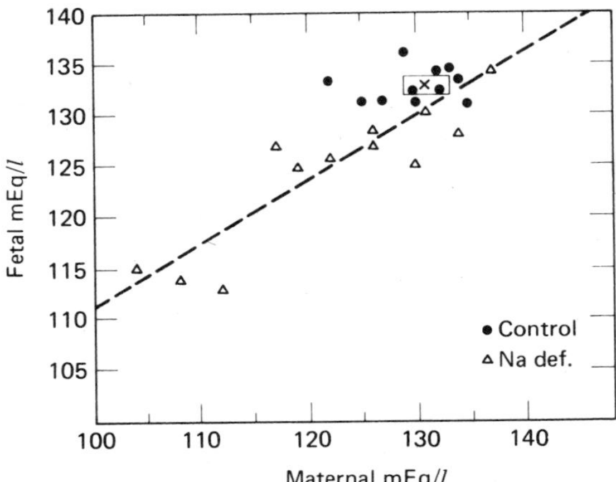

From Dancis and Springer, 1970.

Figure 13–8 Relation of maternal and fetal plasma sodium. Small box indicates mean of control values ± twice the standard error of the mean. Regression line of sodium-deficient fetuses is indicated. Control values do not form a regression line.

was found to be proportional to the plasma level of sodium in the mother when the maternal diet was deficient in the element. However, when the diet contained a normal amount of sodium, the fetal plasma sodium was maintained within a narrow range (see Figure 13–8). The total sodium content of the fetus was also reduced by maternal sodium deficiency.

Fetal homeostasis in rats was also studied in relation to potassium. When rats were given a diet deficient in potassium during pregnancy, the maternal plasma level of the element fell to one-half the normal value, and the concentration in maternal muscle fell by about 30%. However, the potassium concentration in fetal plasma did not change significantly, but in placenta and total fetus the content of potassium decreased by about 10%. A high level of potassium in the maternal plasma, which could be induced either by a sodium-deficient diet or by infusions of potassium, also brought about an increased level of potassium in the fetal plasma.

The effect of potassium deficiency on the development of human embryonic kidneys has been studied in organ culture. When the potassium concentration of the organ culture medium was low, development of the kidney was abnormal. This study suggests that a normal level of fetal plasma potassium must be maintained in order to provide for normal kidney development. It also raises the question of a possible role of potassium insufficiency of fetal plasma as a cause of abnormal development of the kidney in humans.

EXCESS

A few experiments have investigated the effects of excessive amounts of sodium or potassium. The most striking of these is a study on the subcutaneous injection of sodium chloride into pregnant mice. These large amounts of sodium chloride, at levels of 1900 or 2500 mg per kg of body weight, at 10 or 11 days of gestation, produced fetal death and malformations in mice. This experiment is a very good example of the principle that most substances, even those that are essential to life, can be teratogenic if administered in sufficiently large amounts or under appropriate conditions of dosage and administration.

Using milder conditions of excessive sodium, other workers found no adverse effects either on the mother or on the fetus of rats when the maternal diet contained a high sodium intake.

References and Supplementary Readings

CALCIUM AND PHOSPHORUS

BAWDEN, J. W., AND J. W. OSBORNE. "Tracer study on the effect of dietary calcium deficiency during pregnancy in rats." *J. Dent. Res.* **41**: 1349–1358 (1962).

BODANSKY, M., AND V. B. DUFF. "Dependence of fetal growth and storage of calcium and phosphorus on the parathyroid function and diet of pregnant rats." *J. Nutr.* **22**: 25–41 (1941).

BOELTER, M. D. D., AND D. M. GREENBERG. "Effect of severe calcium deficiency on pregnancy and lactation in the rat." *J. Nutr.* **26**: 105–121 (1943).

BRAITHWAITE, G. D., R. F. GLASCOCK, AND S. RIAZUDDIN. "Calcium metabolism in pregnant ewes." *Brit. J. Nutr.* **24**: 661–670 (1970).

COMAR, C. L. "Radiocalcium studies in pregnancy." *Ann. N.Y. Acad. Sci.* **64**: 281–298 (1956).

FAIRNEY, A., AND A. A. WEIR. "The effect of abnormal maternal plasma calcium levels on the offspring of rats." *J. Endocr.* **48**: 337–345 (1970).

HART, E. B., H. STEENBOCK, G. C. HUMPHREY, AND R. S. HULCE. "New observations and a reinterpretation of old observations on the nutritive value of the wheat plant." *J. Biol. Chem.* **62**: 315–322 (1924).

HOWARTH, A. T., D. B. MORGAN, AND R. B. PAYNE. "Urinary excretion of calcium in late pregnancy and its relation to creatinine clearance." *Am. J. Obstet. Gynec.* **129**: 499–502 (1977).

ITOH, H., S. L. HANSARD, J. C. GLENN, F. H. HOSKINS, AND D. M. THRASHER. "Placental transfer of calcium in pregnant sows on normal and limited-calcium rations." *J. An. Sci.* **26**: 335–340 (1967).

KRISHNAMACHARI, K. A. V. R., AND L. IYENGAR. "Effect of maternal malnutrition on the bone density of the neonates." *Am. J. Clin. Nutr.* **28**: 482–486 (1975).

TOVERUD, K. U., AND G. TOVERUD. "Studies on the mineral metabolism during pregnancy and lactation and its bearing on the disposition to rickets and dental caries." *Acta Paediatr.* Suppl. 2, **12**: 1–116 (1931).

MAGNESIUM

Bell, L. T., M. Branstrator, C. Roux, and L. S. Hurley. "Chromosomal abnormalities in maternal and fetal tissues of magnesium or zinc deficient rats." *Teratology* **12**: 221–226 (1975).

Cohlan, S. Q., V. Jansen, J. Dancis, and S. Piomelli. "Microcytic anemia with erythroblastosis in offspring of magnesium-deprived rats." *Blood* **36**: 500–506 (1970).

Cosens, G., I. Diamond, L. L. Theriault, and L. S. Hurley. "Magnesium deficiency anemia in the rat fetus." *Pediatr. Res.* **11**: 758–764 (1977).

Gunther, T., F. Dorn, and H. J. Merker. "Embryo-toxic effects produced by magnesium deficiency in rats." *Z. Klin. Chem. Klin. Biochem.* **11**: 87–92 (1973).

Hurley, L. S. "Magnesium deficiency in pregnancy and its effects on the offspring." In: J. Durlach, ed., *First International Symposium on Magnesium Deficiency in Human Pathology*. I. Volume of Reports, pp. 481–492. Vittel, France: S.G.E.M.V. Publishers, 1971.

Hurley, L. S., G. Cosens, and L. L. Theriault. "Teratogenic effects of magnesium deficiency in rats." *J. Nutr.* **106**: 1254–1260 (1976).

Tufts, E. V., and D. M. Greenberg. "The biochemistry of magnesium deficiency. II. The minimum magnesium requirement for growth, gestation, and lactation, and the effect of the dietary calcium level thereon." *J. Biol. Chem.* **122**: 715–726 (1938).

Wang, F. L., R. Wang, E. A. Khairallah, and R. Schwartz. "Magnesium depletion during gestation and lactation in rats." *J. Nutr.* **101**: 1201–1210 (1971).

SODIUM AND POTASSIUM

Crocker, J. F. "Human embryonic kidneys in organ culture: Abnormalities of development induced by decreased potassium." *Science* **181**: 1178–1179 (1973).

Dancis, J., and D. Springer. "Fetal homeostasis in maternal malnutrition: Potassium and sodium deficiency in rats." *Pediatr. Res.* **4**: 345–351 (1970).

Kirksey, A., and R. L. Pike; and Kirksey, A., R. L. Pike, and J. A. Callahan. "Some effects of high and low sodium intakes during pregnancy in the rat." *J. Nutr.* **77**: 33–51 (1962).

Nishimura, H., and S. Miyamoto. "Teratogenic effects of sodium chloride in mice." *Acta Anat.* **74**: 121–124 (1969).

Phillips, G. D., and S. K. Sundaram. "Sodium depletion of pregnant ewes and its effects on foetuses and foetal fluids." *J. Physiol.* **184**: 889–897 (1966).

Orent-Keiles, E., A. Robinson, and E. V. McCollum. "The effects of sodium deprivation on the animal organism." *Am. J. Physiol.* **119**: 651–661 (1937).

14

Trace elements I: iron, copper, iodine

The importance of trace elements for prenatal or perinatal development has been a subject of speculation for some time, but extensive investigation of this topic has occurred only recently. The earliest recognized example of a relationship between a trace element and early development is probably that of iodine deficiency and the thyroid gland: the development of cretinism (see below). First reports on the essentiality of trace metals for prenatal development appeared in the 1930s with the observations by Orent and McCollum, and Daniels and Everson on debility in offspring of manganese-deficient rats. Lyons and Insko reported on nutritional chondrodystrophy in chick embryos resulting from manganese deficiency, and Bennetts and Chapman presented evidence that enzootic ataxia in lambs was caused by copper deficiency. These pioneer investigations were followed by more extensive inquiries after 1950, when improved methods for measurement of trace substances became available.

IRON

The major proportion of iron in the body is found in hemoglobin in the red blood cells. A deficiency of iron is marked by anemia characterized by low levels of hemoglobin in both animals and man. Although placental transfer of iron from the maternal plasma to the fetus occurs by active transport and takes place readily, nonetheless if iron deficiency in a pregnant female is severe enough to produce anemia, the young will be born with low levels of hemoglobin. The degree of anemia in the offspring as well as other manifestations of iron deficiency depends upon the extent of iron deficiency in the maternal diet.

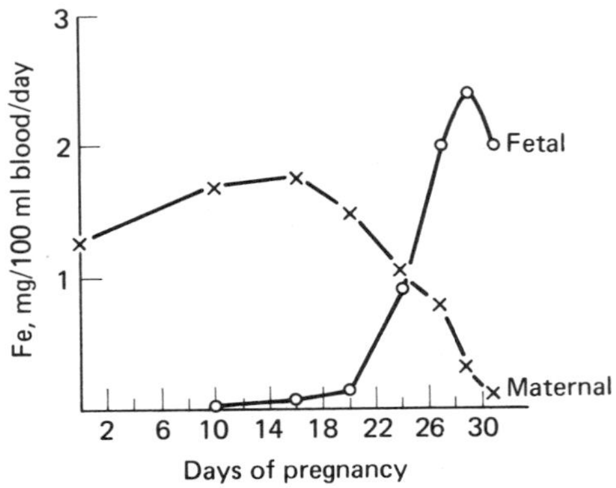

From Bothwell et al., 1958.

Figure 14–1 Plasma iron turnover in pregnant rabbit. The amount of iron assimilated by maternal and by fetal tissues determined at intervals through pregnancy in the rabbit is plotted.

EXPERIMENTAL ANIMALS

Studies on the placental transfer of iron in pregnant rabbits have shown that the amount of iron transported from the maternal plasma to the fetus increases progressively with the age and weight of the fetus. By the end of pregnancy, 90% of the plasma iron turnover was directed to the fetus (Figure 14–1). The major accumulation of fetal iron occurs late in gestation.

In rats, a number of studies have shown that animals raised on a diet deficient in iron, and continued on the iron-deficient regime during pregnancy, gave birth to young that were anemic during the early weeks of life. The degree of iron deficiency in the offspring increased with the number of litters produced by a female. When the mother had a mild deficiency, the blood of the young at birth had a normal hemoglobin content, but there was depletion of the iron stores. More severe deficiency of iron in the mother resulted in anemia in the newborn. Thus, the newborn rat shows the same effects as adult animals; that is, the first evidence of iron deficiency is a decrease in iron reserves, while further depletion of iron results in a decrease in the hemoglobin content of the blood. If the young animals had very severe deficiencies of iron, their neonatal mortality was very high. In later work, a diet more complete in the other nutrients but equally deficient in iron caused a mild anemia in pregnant rats. Their offspring, however, were severely anemic, weak, and almost entirely nonviable.

Offspring of rats deficient in iron during pregnancy and lactation also showed lipidemia with elevated levels of triglycerides, cholesterol, and phospholipids in serum. In the young of animals receiving the iron-deficient diet only during pregnancy, lipidemia was nearly normal in most cases. However, in some reports, severely anemic young that died the first few days after birth also showed lipemia.

HUMANS

The effects of iron deficiency during pregnancy in humans are similar to those observed in experimental animals. Infants of anemic mothers usually share the maternal iron deficiency and are anemic themselves. It appears that the more severe the anemia in the mother, the more severe will be the effects in the infant at birth. In one study, the difference between the mean circulating hemoglobin mass of the nonanemic infants and those of the anemic group represented a deficiency of about 20% of the iron otherwise available to the anemic infants compared with normal newborns. Such a profound effect on the newborn, depriving it of a large proportion of its readily available iron store, may be expected to influence the production of iron-deficiency anemia in later infancy, making these infants more susceptible to this disorder.

COPPER

Copper is extremely important for normal embryonic and fetal development. This has been shown in a number of species, both in the laboratory and in domestic animals under field conditions. There is also increasing evidence that copper is essential for development in humans.

DEFICIENCY

Lambs. Information on the importance of copper for prenatal development arose out of investigations of a disease in lambs called enzootic ataxia or "sway back." This disease occurred in a number of countries, especially Australia and England, and has also been found in parts of the United States, including California. Knowledge of the relationship of copper to enzootic ataxia begins with a report in 1932 from Western Australia. The disorder is characterized by spastic paralysis especially of the hind limbs, severe incoordination, blindness in some cases, and anemia. The wool of the animals is also abnormal; the fibers straighten and the normal crimp disappears. The brains of newborn lambs with this condition are smaller than normal and have collapsed cerebral hemispheres and shallow convolutions. The cerebellum is particularly small, and throughout the brain there is a marked insufficiency of normal myelin. The abnormalities in the brain and

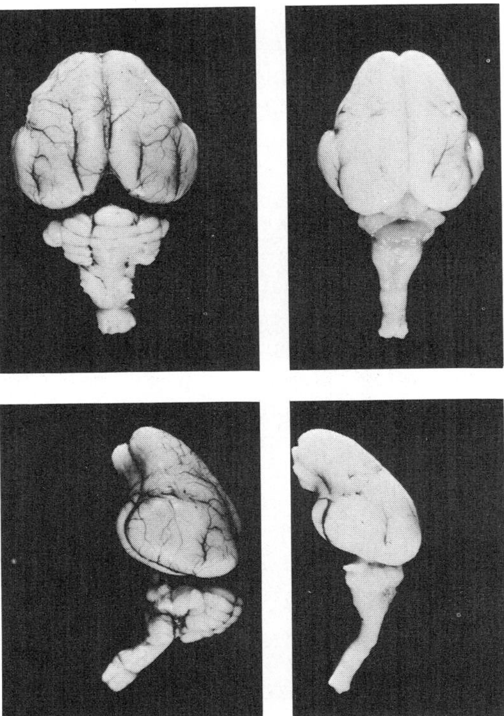

From Everson et al., 1967.

Figure 14–2 Brain of a control guinea pig at birth (left) and a copper-deficient animal (right); top, dorsal view; bottom, lateral view.

nervous system are apparently responsible for the ataxia (incoordination and lack of equilibrium) that these animals exhibit (see Figure 14–2). Lambs with enzootic ataxia die within a short time after birth or are born dead.

A relationship of enzootic ataxia to copper deficiency was suggested when it was found that the copper content was very low in liver of newborn ataxic lambs and in the blood and milk of their mothers. Both the anemia of the ewes and the incidence of enzootic ataxia in these geographical areas could be prevented by copper administration to the pregnant sheep during the gestation period. The primary lesion in the lambs is a low copper content of the brain, leading to a deficiency of cytochrome oxidase in the motor neurons. Cytochrome oxidase, a terminal respiratory enzyme, contains copper as a part of its molecule. The biochemical evidence suggests abnormal myelin synthesis rather than excessive myelin degeneration.

Copper deficiency in the pregnant ewe may also be induced by conditions other than a low intake of dietary copper. For example, a high intake of sulfate and molybdate also results in enzootic ataxia, both in the field and in experiments, by producing a conditioned copper deficiency. In newborn lambs of ewes receiving such rations, there was a low level of copper in the brain and a deficiency of cytochrome oxidase in the motor neurons. Other dietary intakes that apparently result in conditioned copper deficiency in pregnant ewes have also been reported. In Iceland, offspring of ewes fed on seaweed showed the symptoms and the morphological characteristics of enzootic ataxia. The lambs had demyelination of the cerebrum and other abnormal development of the brain. Although the copper intake itself was not low, the pregnant females showed low levels of blood copper, and the copper content of livers from the affected lambs was very low. The disorder could be largely prevented by giving a supplement of copper to the pregnant ewes.

Copper deficiency in dairy cows has resulted in infertility, decreased numbers of young, and retarded growth and development of the calves, including stunting in the young stock.

Rats. Copper deficiency in rats during pregnancy has extremely deleterious effects on embryonic and fetal development. When a copper-deficient diet (containing less than 0.4 ppm of copper) was given for one month before pregnancy and during pregnancy, very few young survived to term.

In later work, in which the diet was less severely deficient and contained approximately 1 ppm of copper, there was reasonably good reproduction. No signs of anemia were seen in adult rats fed this diet. However, the offspring of pregnant animals even in the first litters had a high incidence of edema, anemia, and subcutaneous hemorrhages. Many had skeletal abnormalities and abdominal hernias. Abnormal elastin was seen in histological examination of the aortas from these animals. In addition, abnormal changes in the skin were apparent on histological examination. The skin was thin, and there was a decreased number of hair follicles. Newborn animals suffered a high rate of neonatal mortality. Neural lesions have also been found in the offspring of female rats fed a copper-deficient diet from the time of weaning.

Guinea pigs. In the guinea pig, copper deficiency produced abnormalities of the nervous system similar to those seen in lambs with enzootic ataxia. Female guinea pigs were given a copper-deficient diet during growth and pregnancy. Their offspring showed a high incidence of ataxia and gross abnormalities of the brain at birth (see Figure 14–2). The brains of the copper-deficient newborn guinea pigs appeared pale and translucent or hemorrhagic. In some cases the lack of development of the cerebellum was especially striking. The cerebral cortex also was not well developed. Morphologically immature kidneys were seen in the newborn animals. Their liver copper values were abnormally low. Throughout the brain there was underdevelopment of myelin. If the animals were allowed to live and were given the copper-deficient diet during the neonatal period, aneurisms of the aortic arch and the abdominal aorta developed within the first month of life.

COPPER MUTANTS

An influence of copper during prenatal development of mammals has also been demonstrated in some genetic states. Certain mutant genes in mice have been shown to be related to copper metabolism. Mice homozygous for the mutant gene *crinkled* (*cr*) have a smooth coat, thin skin, delayed pigmentation, and early mortality. Development of the hair bulbs in the skin is retarded and abnormal. Only one type of hair is formed (straight) rather than four types, of which some are bent or crimped, as occurs in normal mice. Because of the similarities of the phenotypic characteristics to those of copper deficiency in sheep and rats (see above), the possibility of a relationship between the mutant gene *crinkled* and copper was investigated by supplementing the mice during pregnancy and lactation with a high level of copper. This supplementation treatment increased the survival of mutant mice in the neonatal period. Although only 22 to 32% of crinkled young of females fed control diets survived to weaning, 59% of those fed a high-copper diet survived to this age (Figure 14–3). A high dietary level of copper also

Figure 14–3 Postnatal survival in offspring of mice fed stock diet, control (purified) diet, and high copper diet during pregnancy and lactation. Solid bars represent nonmutant controls (+/?); cross-hatched bars represent littermates homozygous for mutant gene *crinkled* (*cr*/*cr*). Numbers represent percent survival, from day 0 to day 14 on left, from day 11 to day 30 on right.

From Hurley, 1976.

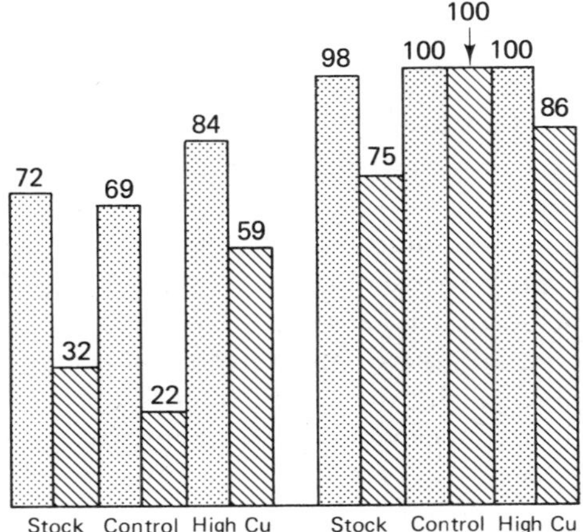

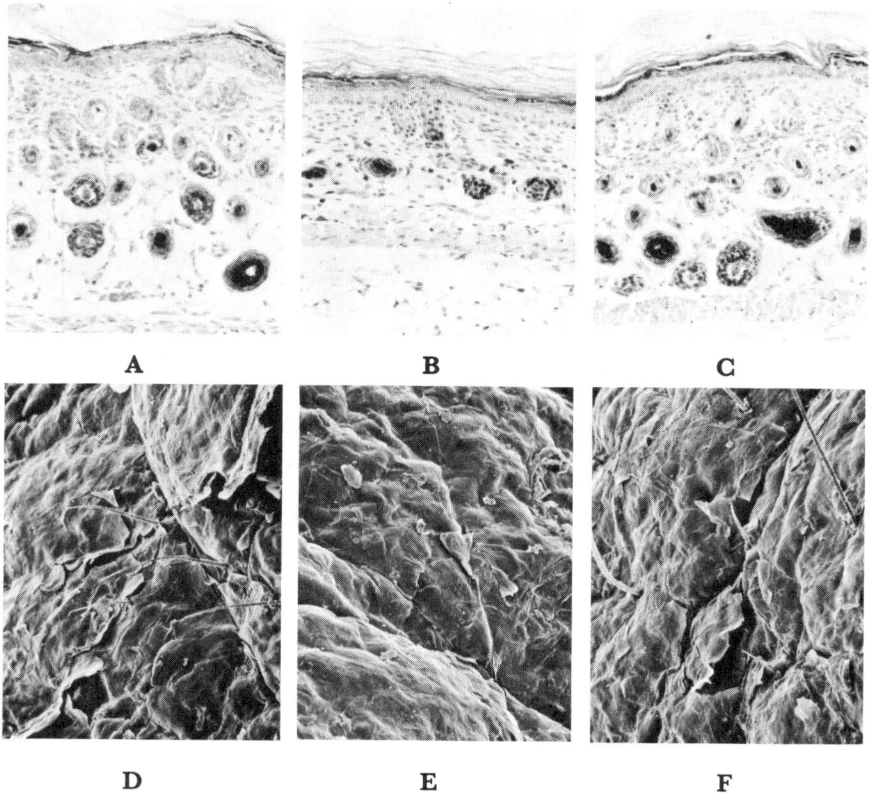

From Hurley and Bell, 1975.

Figure 14–4 Photomicrographs of dorsal skin from six-day-old mice. (A) Nonmutant from the stock diet group, (B) crinkled mutant from stock or control diet groups, and (C) crinkled mutant from the high-copper diet show the increases in pigmentation, hair-bulb development, and skin thickness of mutants after dietary copper treatment. Pieces of the same skin (D, E, F): dried using the critical point (liquid CO_2) technique, metal coated, and viewed with the scanning electron microscope show the increase in hair growth of crinkled mice from the high copper diet group. (× 124)

prevented the lag in pigment development characteristic of the mutant. Furthermore, skin and epidermal thickness and hair-bulb development were nearly normal in the high-copper group, in contrast to the thin skin and sparse hairs in mutants from females fed the normal diet (Figure 14–4). This experiment showed that increased availability of copper favorably altered the expression of the mutant gene, and it demonstrated the interaction of a gene and the trace metal copper in perinatal development.

Crinkled mutants also show abnormalities of lipid composition in the brain. Sulfatides were higher than normal in young mutants, and cerebrosides were higher in old adults. The brains of crinkled mice contained cholesterol esters, not normally found in mouse brain. Microscopically, the brains of mutant mice showed abnormalities in myelin structures of varying degrees of severity. The chemical findings, in connection with the microscopic changes, suggest that the myelin disruption found in these mutant mice is secondary to axonal degeneration rather than due to a primary defect of the myelin itself.

Another mutant in mice that is related to copper metabolism is the gene *quaking* (*qk*). This gene produces in homozygotes an intermittent axial body tremor that is first seen about day 10 after birth and persists throughout life. These mice also show abnormalities of myelin and reduced levels of brain cerebrosides and sulfatides. When mice homozygous for the mutant gene *quaking* were given a diet containing a high level of copper during pregnancy and lactation, the frequency of tremors in their offspring was markedly reduced (Figure 14–5). Thus, copper supplementation was effective in ameliorating the deleterious effects of this gene.

The copper concentration of the brain in the mutant mice was abnormal. In quaking mice fed a normal diet, the copper content of the brain was lower than in their nonmutant littermates, but feeding the high-copper diet brought the brain copper to normal levels (see Table 14–1). Thus it appears that the mutant gene *qk* brings about an abnormality of copper metabolism.

The *mottled* mutants of mice also have defects of copper metabolism. These X-linked mutants consist of a number of different alleles at the mottled locus. In the case of many of the alleles, the male hemizygote does not survive beyond birth. In all cases where it does, the animals show a severe

Figure 14–5 Polygraph recordings of tremors from 27-day-old quaking mice over a ten-second period. (A) Quaking mouse from the control purified diet group (6 ppm of Cu). (B) Quaking mouse from the copper-supplemented diet group (250 ppm of Cu), showing a reduction in tremor frequency.

From Keen and Hurley, 1976.

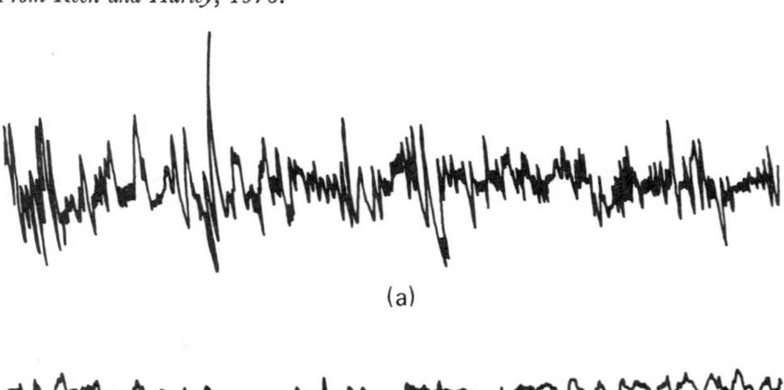

TABLE 14–1 BRAIN WEIGHT AND COPPER CONCENTRATION IN 21-DAY-OLD QUAKING (qk/qk) AND NONQUAKING (+/?) MICE

Group	Dietary Copper, ppm	Geno-type	No. of Ani-mals	Brain Weight,[a] g	Copper Concentration, ppm
Purified control	6	+/?	5	0.358 ± 0.019[b,c]	1.735 ± 0.197
	6	*qk/qk*	5	0.374 ± 0.197[c]	1.097 ± 0.048[d]
Copper	250	+/?	5	0.398 ± 0.008[c]	2.025 ± 0.040
supplemented	250	*qk/qk*	5	0.398 ± 0.006[c]	1.998 ± 0.097

[a]Wet weight.

[b]Mean ± standard error of the mean.

[c]No significant differences (by Student's *t*-test).

[d]Significantly lower (by Student's *t*-test) than nonquaking animals on control diet ($P < .02$) and quaking and nonquaking mice fed the copper supplemented diet ($P < .001$). There were no significant differences among the other three groups.

From Keen and Hurley, 1976.

dilution in hair pigmentation and a persistent neurological disturbance consisting of a mild sustained tremor and general inactivity. Copper levels in liver and brain are low in these mice, while copper in the intestinal wall is higher than normal. Thus a deficiency in copper transport is likely. The mice also have a defect in collagen and elastin cross-linking leading to aortic aneurisms, which is also true of copper-deficient animals. Probably the most interesting aspect of the mottled mutants is the similarity of their symptoms to those of the human genetic disease, Menkes' kinky hair syndrome (see below), which is also X-linked. Mottled mice are therefore being used as animal models to gain some insight into the human disorder.

Humans. Menkes' kinky hair syndrome. A genetic disease observed in infants was first described in 1962 by Menkes. This disorder produces progressive degeneration of the brain and is also characterized by abnormal structure of the hair and an X-linked inheritance. It usually causes death before three years of age. There are also changes in the long bones, resembling those in scurvy, and tortuosity of the cerebral and other arteries. The blood-vessel abnormalities are similar to the changes in elastic fibers of blood vessels seen in collagen and elastin structures of copper-deficient animals (Figure 14-6).

Danks, an Australian pediatrician and human geneticist, and his coworkers showed in 1972 that patients with this disorder (also called Menkes' steely hair syndrome) had a defect in copper transport. The consequent failure of many copper enzyme systems appears to explain the features of

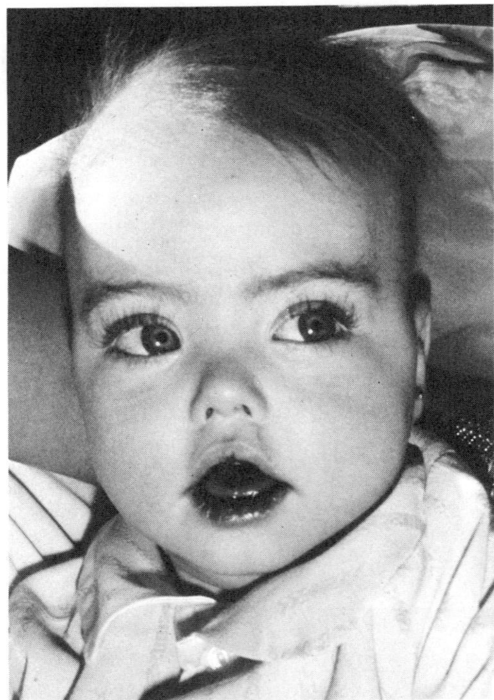

From Hambidge and Walravens, Trace elements in nutrition, Practice of Pediatrics, *Vol. 1, chapter 29, 1975.*

Figure 14–6 Steely hair disease in nine-month-old infant. Characteristic features include pudgy cheeks and straight eyebrows; hair resembles steel wool.

the disease. The evidence both from patients with Menkes' steely hair syndrome and from mottled mutant mice (see above) suggests that the primary defect involves increased affinity of a copper-binding molecule for copper, which causes increased accumulation of copper in a form inadequately available to copper enzymes in the same cell. Danks has suggested that such a molecule exists in most cells, but not in those of the liver. Regardless of the validity of this hypothesis, the information provided by patients with this genetic disorder gives ample proof of the importance of copper for normal fetal and neonatal development.

It is also possible that conditioned copper deficiency can occur in humans. One case has been reported in which a young woman was treated with penicillamine during pregnancy and gave birth to an abnormal child. The child had a connective tissue defect including lax skin, hyperflexibility of the joints, fragility of the veins, varicosities, and impairment of wound healing. The physicians reporting the case concluded that the penicillamine taken by the mother was the cause of the defect in the child. Penicillamine is used clinically to remove copper from certain patients (for example, in Wilson's disease), so it is possible that the treatment produced copper deficiency in the fetus, since the symptoms described are similar to those of this deficiency. However, the investigators reporting the case did not mention this possibility. It should be noted, however, that penicillamine also removes other trace elements, such as zinc, so the effect of the compound in this case may involve other metals besides copper.

IODINE

DEFICIENCY

Iodine functions as part of the thyroid hormone thyroxine. Thus, iodine deficiency results in hypothyroidism, and the effects of iodine deficiency are those of an insufficient quantity of thyroxine. When this occurs in the growing individual or adult, a condition called goiter results. Because iodine deficiency in certain geographical areas is related to the iodine content of the soil, "endemic goiter" occurs there. The term "endemic goiter" is used because under conditions of iodine deficiency in a geographical area, endemic goiter affects a specific portion of a given population. Endemic goiter refers to the enlargement of the thyroid gland that occurs when the iodine intake is inadequate.

In certain areas where endemic goiter occurs with high incidence, there is also a high frequency of cretinism. Cretinism has been recognized as an entity for hundreds of years; it was described as early as the sixteenth century. By the beginning of the nineteenth century its association with goiter was realized. A connection between iodine and goiter was postulated soon after this time. In the middle of the nineteenth century the idea was proposed that endemic goiter and, by implication, endemic cretinism were due to iodine deficiency. It is now clear that endemic goiter is a direct result of iodine deficiency, but the causative connection between iodine deficiency and endemic cretinism is still under discussion. The major question relates to the fact that endemic cretinism does not always occur in areas where there is a high incidence of endemic goiter.

Endemic cretinism is only one of the types of cretinism. Other forms are (1) congenital thyroid aplasia, (2) genetic defects of thyroxine metabolism, and (3) juvenile hypothyroidism.

The cretinous child presents a clinical picture of mental and physical retardation with a potbelly, large tongue, and facial characteristics resembling those of Down syndrome (Figure 14–7). The skin is coarse and thick

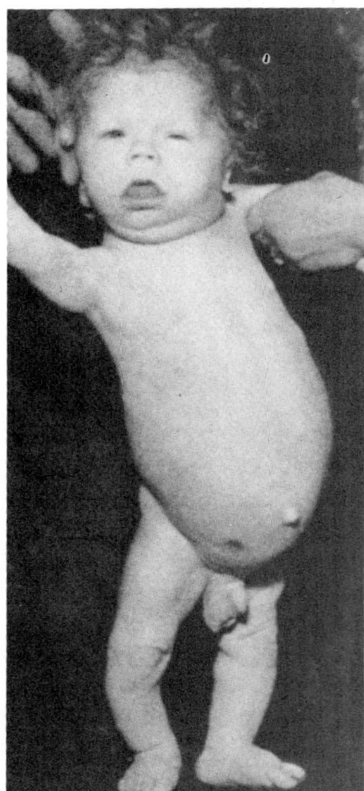

From Crile, G. Jr., 1949 (courtesy of Dr. E. Perry McCullagh). Practical Aspects of Thyroid Disease, *W. B. Saunders, Philadelphia.*

Figure 14–7 Cretin.

(myxedematous). Neurological disorders such as squint and spasticity are often found. There is abnormal development of bones (delayed appearance of ossification centers leading to short stature, abnormal gait, and changes in the skull). Retarded dentition and delayed epiphyseal development are characteristic. Deafness, deafmutism, or impaired speech often occur. Mental retardation, which may be extreme, is also usually present. In highland Ecuador, where iodine deficiency is severe, a study of the clinical pattern of cretinism showed that there was a wide range of variation in the various signs and symptoms of the disease.

In regions where the incidence of endemic cretinism was high in the past, a marked decline took place after the introduction of iodine prophylaxis. In certain valleys of the Swiss Alps, for example, where both endemic goiter and endemic cretinism were of high frequency, endemic cretinism has virtually disappeared after the introduction of iodized household salt. Records show that cretinism has not recurred after endemic goiter has been effectively eliminated by the use of iodized salt.

Additional confirmatory evidence that endemic cretinism is related to iodine deficiency comes from a study in the New Guinea highlands. This research was carried out in a valley where the incidence of both endemic cretinism and endemic goiter was high. In this region, a change occurred in the type of salt that was consumed after contact with outsiders in 1953. Previously, a native salt had been used, which came from salt springs rich in iodine, but the imported rock salt was low in this element. Thus, the high incidence of cretinism in this population appeared to result from a change in the type of salt used by the poeple. To establish whether endemic cretinism in this group was in fact the result of iodine deficiency, alternate families in the valley were injected intramuscularly with either iodized oil or (as a control) saline solution. Out of the total of 534 children born over the next few years to mothers who had not received iodized oil, 26 were endemic cretins. In comparison, only seven cases of endemic cretinism occurred among 498 children born to mothers who had been treated with iodized oil (see Table 14–2). In six of these seven cases the mother was pregnant when the trial began. These results indicate that severe iodine deficiency in the mother produced cretinism during fetal development. It would also appear that iodine, at least when administered as intramuscular iodized oil, must be given prior to conception.

It seems clear beyond doubt that iodine deficiency is an important factor in the development of endemic cretinism, but it is likely that other factors, either environmental or genetic, may also be involved. Genetic factors certainly appear to be implicated, since high rates of endemic cretinism are associated with specific geographic regions, usually mountain valleys where, because of isolation, consanguinous marriages occur.

TABLE 14–2 CHILDREN BORN IN JIMI RIVER SUBDISTRICT CLASSIFIED ACCORDING TO TREATMENT RECEIVED BY MOTHER

Treatment Received by Mother	*Total No. of New Births*	*No. of Children Examined*	*No. of Deaths Recorded*	*No. of Endemic Cretins*
Iodized oil	498	412	66	7[a]
Untreated	534	406	97	26[b]

[a]Six already pregnant when injected with oil.
[b]Five already pregnant when injected with saline solution.

From Pharaoh et al., 1971.

Nutritional factors other than iodine deficiency may also be involved, such as goitrogenic substances in food. Perhaps other nutritional deficiencies may also play a role. One expert on this subject has pointed out that, as far as is known, endemic cretinism occurs only in poor and backward societies whose inhabitants are poorly nourished, either qualitatively or quantitatively or both. There thus may be an interaction of various factors, genetic and environmental, in the production of cretinism. The possibility also exists that differential responses to low levels of iodine may occur because of differences in genetic factors. Thus, certain genes in certain populations may cause more extreme responses to iodine deficiency than would be the case with other population groups and other genetic backgrounds (see also the section on manganese in Chapter 15).

There is some suggestion that in areas where severe endemic goiter and endemic cretinism exist, less severe changes than those apparent in the cretins may also be present in a larger proportion of the population. Since all the residents in such communities are potentially exposed to a suboptimal supply of thyroxine during their development, there may be subtle but serious effects on the community as a whole. It might be speculated that adequate iodine prophylaxis in these regions could lead to a desirable change in the physical and mental characteristics of the entire community.

In regions where endemic goiter and cretinism exist, the birth of defective young exhibiting abnormalities similar to those of cretins has been well documented in field animals. Such abnormal young have also been produced in experimental animals by iodine deficiency.

EXCESS

An excessive amount of iodine during pregnancy, as well as a deficiency, is deleterious to the developing offspring. Women who took large amounts of iodides during pregnancy, mostly as treatment for asthma or bronchitis, have given birth to abnormal infants. Congenital goiter and hypothyroidism were obvious in these newborns. The neonatal mortality of this group was high, and many of the survivors were mentally retarded.

Similarly, use of radioactive sodium iodide (^{131}I) therapy during pregnancy has led to the birth of infants with cretinism. Presumably, the radioactive iodide caused damage to the fetal thyroid, and the severe hypothroidism resulted in the abnormal development of the embryo and fetus. The same effects were seen in dogs treated experimentally with radioactive iodide during pregnancy. Experimental cretinism was produced in the dogs by administration of ^{131}I to the pregnant female or to the puppies during the first few months of life. Cretinism in dogs was characterized by impairment of growth and skeletal development, obesity, leathery coarse dry skin and hair, and in some cases protruberant tongues. In the litters treated with ^{131}I *in utero*, instinctive functions such as nursing and moving toward the mother were absent. The neonatal mortality was very high.

References and Supplementary Readings

GENERAL

HURLEY, L. S. "Interaction of genes and metals in development." *Fed. Proc.* **35**: 2271–2275 (1976).

O'DELL, B. L., B. C. HARDWICKE, AND G. REYNOLDS. "Mineral deficiencies of milk and congenital malformation in the rat." *J. Nutr.* **73**: 151–157 (1961).

UNDERWOOD, E. J. *Trace Elements in Human and Animal Nutrition*, 4th ed. New York: Academic Press, 1977.

IRON

ALT, H. L. "Iron deficiency in pregnant rats." *Am. J. Dis. Child.* **56**: 975–984 (1938).

BOTHWELL, T. H., W. F. PRIBILLA, W. MEBUST, AND C. A. FINCH. "Iron metabolism in the pregnant rabbit. Iron transport across the placenta." *Am. J. Physiol.* **193**: 615–622 (1958).

GUTHRIE, H. A., M. FROOZANI, A. R. SHERMAN, AND G. P. BARRON. "Hyperlipidemia in offspring of iron-deficient rats." *J. Nutr.* **104**: 1273–1278 (1974).

SISSON, T. R. C., AND C. J. LUND. "The influence of maternal iron deficiency on the newborn." *Am. J. Clin. Nutr.* **6**: 376–385 (1958).

COPPER

BENNETTS, H. W., AND F. E. CHAPMAN. "Copper deficiency in sheep in Western Australia: A preliminary account of the aetiology of enzootic ataxia of lambs and an anaemia of ewes." *Aust. Vet. J.* **13**: 138–149 (1937).

CARLTON, W. W., AND W. A. KELLY. "Neural lesions in the offspring of female rats fed a copper-deficient diet." *J. Nutr.* **97**: 42–52 (1969).

DANKS, D. M. "Steely hair, mottled mice and copper metabolism." *New Eng. J. Med.* **293**: 1147–1148 (1975).

EVERSON, G. J., R. E. SHRADER, AND T. WANG. "Chemical and morphological changes in the brains of copper-deficient guinea pigs." *J. Nutr.* **96**: 115–125 (1968).

EVERSON, G. J., H. C. C. TSAI, AND T. WANG. "Copper deficiency in the guinea pig." *J. Nutr.* **93**: 533–540 (1967).

HALL, G. A., AND J. M. HOWELL. "The effect of copper deficiency on reproduction in the female rat." *Brit. J. Nutr.* **23**: 41–45 (1969).

HOLTZMANN, N. A. "Menkes' kinky hair syndrome: a genetic disease involving copper." *Fed. Proc.* **35**: 2276–2280 (1976).

HURLEY, L. S., AND L. T. BELL. "Amelioration by copper supplementation of mutant gene effects in the crinkled mouse." *Proc. Soc. Exp. Biol. Med.* **149**: 830–834 (1975).

HURLEY, L. S., AND C. L. KEEN. "Teratogenic effects of copper." In: J. D. Nriagu, ed., *Copper in the Environment*. John Wiley and Sons, Inc., New York, 1979.

KEEN, C. L., AND L. S. HURLEY. "Copper supplementation in quaking mutant mice: Reduced tremors and increased brain copper." *Science* **193**: 244–246 (1976).

MILLS, C. F., AND B. F. FELL. "Demyelination in lambs born of ewes maintained on high intakes of sulphate and molybdate." *Nature* **185**: 20–22 (1960).

MJOLNEROD, O. K., S. A. DOMMERUD, K. RASMUSSEN, AND S. T. GJERULDSEN. "Connective-tissue defect probably due to D-penicillamine treatment in pregnancy." *Lancet* **1**: 673–675 (1971).

PALSSON, P. A., AND H. GRIMSSON. "Demyelination in lambs from ewes which feed on seaweeds." *Proc. Soc. Exp. Biol. Med.* **83**: 518–520 (1953).

SOLOMON, L., G. ABRAMS, M. DINNER, AND L. BERMAN. "Neonatal abnormalities associated with D-penicillamine treatment during pregnancy." *New Eng. J. Med.* **196**: 54–55 (1977).

THERIAULT, L. L., D. D. DUNGAN, S. SIMONS, C. L. KEEN, AND L. S. HURLEY. "Lipid and myelin abnormalities of brain in the crinkled mouse." *Proc. Soc. Exp. Biol. Med.* **155**: 549–553 (1977).

IODINE

CARSWELL, F., M. M. KERR, AND J. H. HUTCHISON. "Congenital goitre and hypothyroidism produced by maternal ingestion of iodides." *Lancet* **1**: 1241–1243 (1970).

CLEMENTS, F. W., ed. *Endemic Goitre*. Geneva: World Health Organization, 1960.

FIERRO-BENITEZ, R., I. RAMIREZ, J. GARCES, C. JARAMILLO, F. MONCAYO, AND J. B. STANBURY. "The clinical pattern of cretinism as seen in highland Ecuador." *Am. J. Clin. Nutr.* **27**: 531–543 (1974).

GILLIE, B. "Endemic goiter." *Scientific American*, June 1971, pp. 93–101.

GREEN, H. G., F. J. GAREIS, T. H. SHEPARD, AND V. C. KELLEY. "Cretinism associated with maternal sodium iodide I 131 therapy during pregnancy." *Am. J. Dis. Child.* **122**: 247–249 (1971).

PHARAOH, P. O. D., I. H. BUTTFIELD, AND B. S. HETZEL. "Neurological damage to the fetus resulting from severe iodine deficiency during pregnancy." *Lancet* **1**: 308–310 (1971).

SMITH, C. A., H. A. OBERHELMAN, JR., E. H. STORER, E. R. WOODWARD, AND L. R. DRAGSTEDT. "Production of experimental cretinism in dogs by the administration of radioactive iodine." *Arch. Surg.* **63**: 807–820 (1951).

STANBURY, J. B., AND A. QUERIDO. "On the nature of endemic cretinism." *J. Clin. Endocrin. Metab.* **17**: 803–804 (1957).

15

Trace elements II: manganese and zinc

MANGANESE

Manganese is a required nutrient for every species in which it has been studied, including rats, mice, guinea pigs, rabbits, pigs, chickens, turkeys, ducks, cattle, sheep, and goats. There can be no doubt that manganese is also essential for man.

SKELETAL ABNORMALITIES

In growing animals, manganese deficiency produces abnormalities of skeletal growth and development, and these occur in all species. With manganese deficiency during prenatal life, abnormal skeletal growth and development results in chondrodystrophy—disproportionate abnormal skeletal growth. Nutritional chondrodystrophy resulting from manganese deficiency was first reported in 1937 in chick embryos. The condition in chicks is characterized by short, thick legs and wings, "parrot beak" (from a disproportionate shortening of the lower jaw), globular contours of the head (due to anterior bulging of the skull), and high mortality.

Similarly, in the offspring of manganese-deficient rats there is also chondrodystrophic skeletal development. In this species, severe shortening of the radius, ulna, tibia, and fibula takes place (in proportion to body length), as well as disproportionate growth of the skull. The skulls of manganese-deficient rats are significantly shorter, wider, and higher than those of controls in relation to skull length, resulting in doming of the skull. These changes in skeletal proportions are especially pronounced at birth, demonstrating the necessity of adequate availability of manganese for normal skeletal growth in the prenatal period (see Chapter 2). The shortening of the skull in the newborn was not due to a proportional depression of growth in the cranial bones: length of the interparietal and parietal bones in newborn deficient young was similar to that of controls, and the length of the

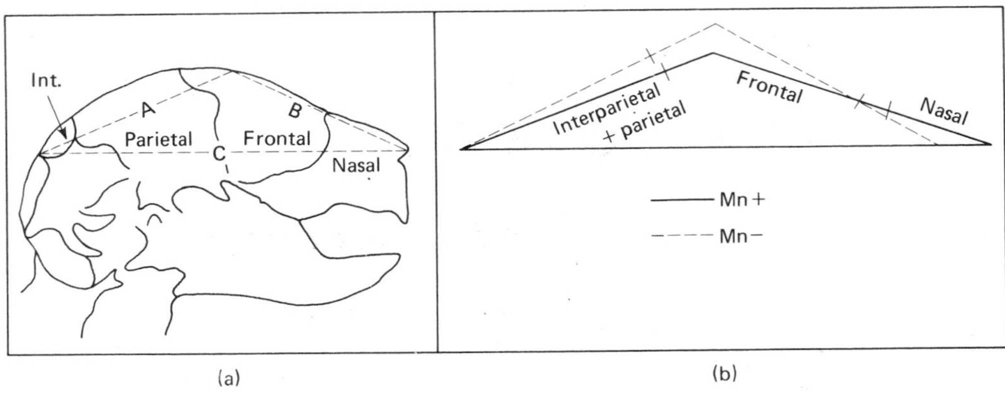

From Hurley et al., 1961.

Figure 15–1 (A) Diagram of rat skull showing dimensions measured in midline in newborn rats. "A" is the distance from the base of the interparietal bone to the point of highest curvature of the skull. "B" is the distance from the point of highest curvature of the skull to the tip of the nasal bone. "C" is the distance from the base of the interparietal bone to the tip of the nasal bone. (B) A diagrammatic representation of the results of skull measurements made in midline in newborn young. Each triangle is drawn to scale using the mean values for the respective group. The solid lines represent the skull measurements of normal (manganese-supplemented) animals; the broken lines represent the skull measurements of manganese-deficient rats. The short lines perpendicular to those representing dimensions "A" and "B" indicate the lengths of the cranial bones: interparietal + parietal, frontal, and nasal.

frontal bone was less reduced than that of the nasal bone or the skull as a whole (see Figure 15–1).

The shortening of the skull appears to be due largely to an inhibition of growth in its basal portion, and this, together with dissimilar growth rates in the cranial bones, results in doming of the frontal portion. These changes in skull growth in manganese-deficient animals, concomitant with the disproportionate shortening of the long bones, indicate that endochondral osteogenesis is abnormal in this deficiency.

Manganese deficiency during prenatal development also causes abnormal and delayed ossification of the otic capsule (the bony covering of the inner ear) and failure of calcification of the otoliths (the calcified structures necessary for the vestibular reflexes controlling balance). If manganese deficiency is continued through the growth period of postnatal life, abnormal development of the knee joint occurs, and curvature of the spine is also seen.

The types and analysis of abnormalities observed in the skeleton suggested that the basic defect produced by manganese deficiency was in the formation of the matrix of cartilage or of bone. In addition, the metabolism of calcium was found to be normal in manganese-deficient rats, while the synthesis of mucopolysaccharides in skeletal cartilage was decreased by the deficiency. *In vitro* studies of fetal cartilage in rats showed that the uptake of radiosulfur (^{35}S) in tibia from manganese-deficient fetuses was both slower and of smaller magnitude than in those of controls, indicating a depressed synthesis of sulfomucopolysaccharides in the fetuses as well as in older animals.

NEONATAL ATAXIA

The first report that manganese deficiency was essential during prenatal life was published in 1931 by Orent and McCollum, who showed that the offspring of manganese-deficient rats had high neonatal mortality. These investigators ascribed the poor viability of the newborn animals to a lack of maternal care. Later work showed, however, that female rats deficient in manganese were capable of raising normal foster young, although their own young died, and the investigators concluded that the high death rate was due to a congenital debility. Many of the deficient offspring exhibited neonatal ataxia with incoordination and lack of equilibrium.

Congenital ataxia is probably the most striking effect of manganese deficiency. Neonatal ataxia resulting from a deficiency of manganese during prenatal development was first reported in the chick by Norris and Caskey in 1939. These investigators also showed that the ataxia was irreversible; that is, such chicks were not cured by administration of manganese after hatching, either by injection or by feeding.

Critical period. Congenital ataxia is characterized by incoordination, lack of equilibrium, and retraction of the head (Figure 15–2). Hurley and her coworkers have carried out extensive studies of this subject. Supplementation with manganese of manganese-deficient pregnant rats increased the postnatal survival of the offspring and decreased the incidence of ataxia, depend-

Figure 15–2 Typical head retraction in ataxic manganese-deficient rat (on right) as compared with normal posture of control (on left).

From Hurley, 1968.

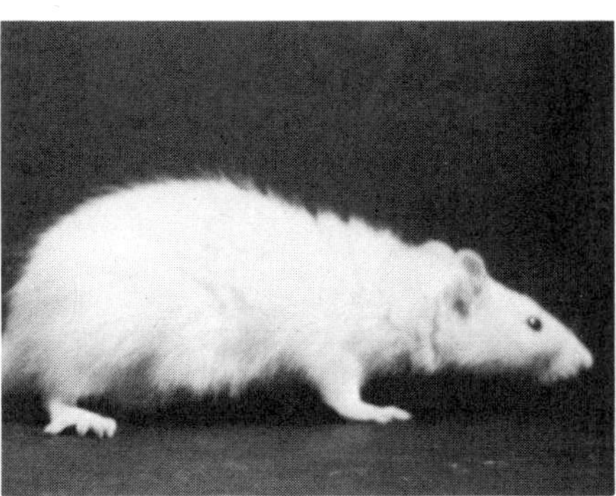

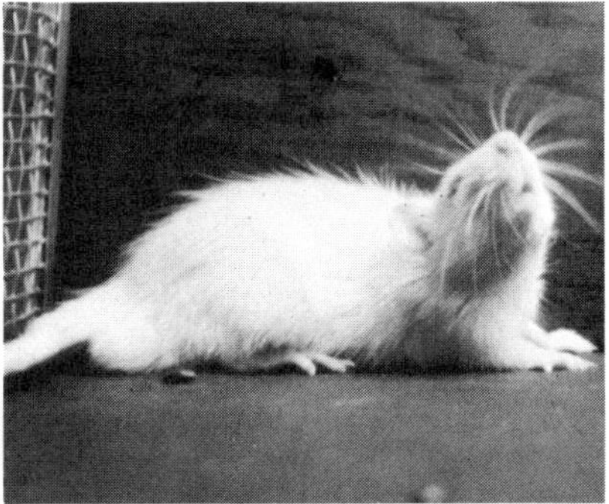

ing upon the time during gestation that manganese was given (see Table 15–1). Manganese supplementation begun on or before the 14th day of gestation was completely effective in preventing ataxia in the young. However, when manganese was withheld until the 18th day of gestation, even if it was continued thereafter throughout life, neonatal survival was low and all of the surviving young were ataxic. Manganese supplementation begun on the 15th or 16th days of gestation resulted in the birth of young of which about half were ataxic. Thus it was shown that an irreversible congenital defect resulting in ataxia occurred between the 14th and 18th days of gestation in manganese-deficient rats. Offspring of manganese-deficient rats also exhibited a marked delay in development of the reflexes responsible for body-righting reactions, but the number of young born and their birth weight were not affected by the deficiency.

Even a short period of supplementation with manganese could prevent the ataxia of manganese-deficient newborns (Table 15–2). Deficient females supplemented with manganese for only 24 hours on day 14 gave birth to young whose survival to weaning approached that of normal controls, and none of these young were ataxic. In contrast, only 11% of the offspring of unsupplemented rats survived to this age, and 81% were ataxic. One day of supplementation, if it occurred on day 14 of gestation, was sufficient to prevent ataxia in the young, but this was not the case when manganese was given on days 16 or 18. Supplementation on day 16 for only 24 hours also resulted in normal survival of the young, but 62% of the survivors were severely ataxic. Supplementation on day 18 for 24 hours improved survival

TABLE 15–1 EFFECT OF MANGANESE SUPPLEMENTATION AT VARIOUS TIMES DURING GESTATION

		No. of Young Born		*Survival to 28 Days*	
Initiation of Supplementation	*No. of Litters*	*Total*	*Per Litter*	*Percent of Live Young*	*Percent Ataxic*
Day of gestation[a]					
7–12	14	105	7.5	53	0
14	6	42	7.0	87	0
15	8	60	7.5	36	48[b]
16	8	54	6.8	44	46[b]
18	8	65	8.1	26	100

[a]Day of finding sperm considered first day of gestation.
[b]Mild.

From Hurley et al., J. Nutr. 66: *309–320, 1958.*

TABLE 15–2 EFFECT OF SHORT-TERM MANGANESE SUPPLEMENTATION ON OFFSPRING OF MANGANESE-DEFICIENT RATS

Group	No. of Litters	Young at 28 Days	
		Survival, %	*Ataxic, %*
Control	61	54	0
Mn Deficient	30	11	81
	Ration Supplemented for 24 Hours During Gestation		
Day: 14	23	51	0
16	29	51	62
18	36	39	84

From Hurley and Everson, 1963.

to 39% with a high incidence (84%) of ataxia. Congenital ataxia and neonatal mortality of manganese-deficient young were differentiated by this treatment, indicating that these two manifestations of prenatal manganese deficiency may develop through different pathways. The basic biochemical defect responsible for these two effects of manganese deficiency may not be the same.

No lesions of the brain or spinal cord that could account for the congenital ataxia of manganese-deficient animals were seen in histological examination, and assays of various tissues for a number of enzymes have not shown any relevant biochemical abnormalities. Cerebral spinal fluid pressure was not significantly different from normal in manganese-deficient young.

The most stringent test for the neonatal ataxia of manganese deficiency is swimming. The normal mouse or rat can swim for long periods without any problem, but the ataxic mouse cannot maintain its body-righting reflexes and will drown if not removed from the water (Figure 15–3). The abnormal swimming response demonstrating congenital ataxia results from anomalous development of the otoliths of the inner ear. These structures, which are essential for the vestibular reflexes important for balance and body-righting mechanisms, are composed of small crystalline structures, the otoconia, embedded in an amorphous mucopolysaccharide-rich matrix. The lack of development of the otoliths in prenatal manganese deficiency was first shown in mice, and later in the chick, the rat, and the guinea pig. The degree of development of the otoliths can be correlated very closely with the ability of the animal to swim (see Table 15–3).

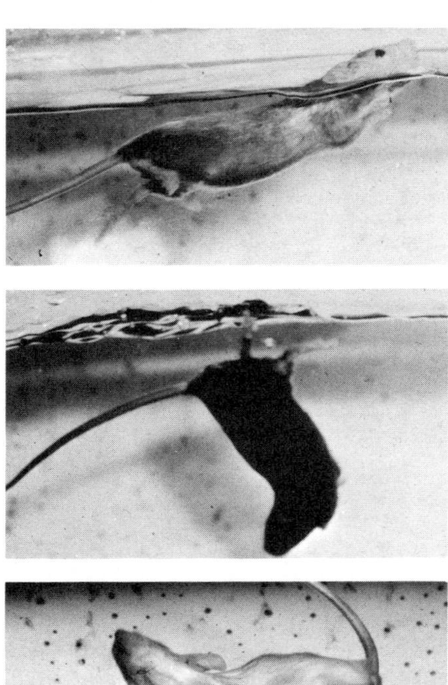

From Erway et al., 1970.

Figure 15–3 Normal and ataxic mice tested for swimming ability. A normal mouse (top) does not spontaneously lower its head beneath the surface of the water. Many of the manganese-deficient mice (middle, black mouse and bottom, albino mouse) were unable to maintain balance and could not avoid swimming beneath the surface of the water.

Genetic interactions. A condition similar to that produced by prenatal manganese deficiency, that is, ataxia caused by missing or absent otoliths, occurs as a result of a mutant gene in mice called *pallid* (*pa*). This gene also affects pigmentation, giving the animals their pale color. When pregnant mice, homozygous for the gene *pa*, are given a diet containing a high level of manganese (1000 ppm) during pregnancy, their offspring are perfectly normal with respect to swimming behavior and do not show ataxia. A similar group of females fed a normal diet (containing about 50 ppm manganese) had offspring of which 68% were unable to swim (see Table 15–4). This

TABLE 15–3 CORRELATION BETWEEN STATE OF OTOLITH FORMATION AND ABILITY TO SWIM IN CONTROL AND MANGANESE-DEFICIENT MICE[a]

	State of Otolith Formation		Ability to Swim	
	u/s	*u/s*[b]		
1.	+/+	+/+	684 normal:	none affected
2.	0/+	+/+	5 normal:	1 partially affected
3.	0/0	+/+	26 normal:	9 partially affected, 7 severely affected
4.	0/0	0/+	2 normal:	4 severely affected
5.	0/0	0/0	None normal:	107 severely affected

[a]Mice for which both swimming and otolith scores were available.

[b]The code: u = utricular otolith of either ear, s = saccular otolith of either ear, + = any otolithic crystals present, 0 = no otolithic crystals present. For example, no. 2 indicates that only one utricular otolith was absent, the others being normal or nearly so; no. 3 indicates that both the utricular and saccular otoliths of one ear were absent, whereas those of the other ear were normal, or nearly so.

From Erway et al., 1970.

TABLE 15–4 EFFECT OF MANGANESE SUPPLEMENTATION ON INCIDENCE OF EAR DEFECT IN PALLID MICE

Group	*No. of Litters*	*No. of Offspring*	*Percent Unable to Swim*
Stock diet control	29	162	68
Mn-supplemented (1000 ppm)	7	45	0

From Erway et al., Science 152: *1766–1768, 1966.*

observation showed an interaction between the gene *pallid* and the nutrient manganese (Figure 15–4). Manipulation of a single agent (the nutrient manganese) could, through its deprivation, alter the expression of the wild type gene to produce a phenocopy of the mutant. On the other hand, administration of large amounts of the agent (the nutrient manganese) altered the expression of the mutant allele to produce the normal phenotype.

The occurrence of a mutant gene analogous to *pallid* has recently been reported in mink. Approximately one-fourth of the animals with the recessive mutation *pastel* have an ataxic condition caused by reduction or absence of otoliths. The ataxia and the abnormal development of the otoliths can be prevented by manganese supplementation of pregnant females.

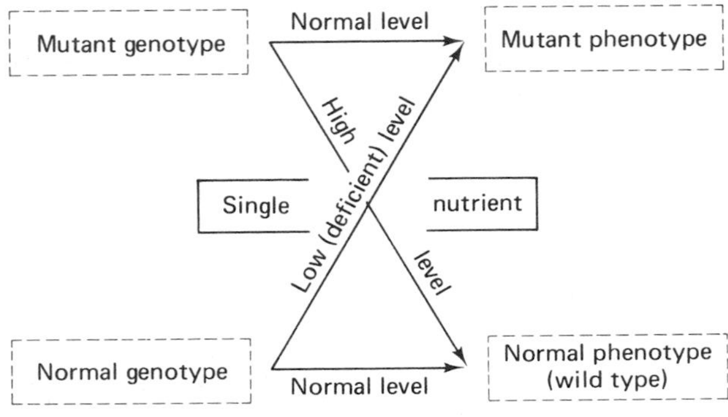

From Hurley, 1976.

Figure 15–4 Interaction of a nutrient and a gene during development. Giving the normal (usual) level of the nutrient to the mutant carrier results in offspring with the mutant genotype and phenotype, while giving a high level of the nutrient results in offspring with a normal phenotype. On the other hand, depriving animals of the normal genotype of the nutrient results in a phenocopy of the mutant.

Another type of interaction of genetic factors with manganese nutrition has been studied. The influence of the genetic background of various strains of mice on their response to manganese deficiency during prenatal development was examined by measuring otolith development. The response to low dietary levels of the element varied considerably among various genetic strains. These findings suggest that at low or borderline levels of dietary intake of essential nutrients, the response of individuals may vary quite significantly depending upon their genetic background. However, with the usual normal dietary amount of the nutrient, normal responses occur (Table 15–5). Thus, in the case of genetic backgrounds susceptible, for example, to low levels of iodine, it may be possible that under circumstances in which the normal amount of iodine is present, no adverse effects such as cretinism will occur. However, if the diet is low in iodine, there may be an exaggerated response to the low dietary level, and cretins will be born. Thus, an interaction between the genetic background and the level of the nutrient may occur in which extreme responses to low dietary intakes are seen (see also the section on cretinism in Chapter 14).

BIOCHEMICAL DEFECTS

To explain the mechanism of the failure of otolith development in manganese-deficient or *pallid* mutant fetuses, there appeared to be two possibilities. Failure of calcification can occur through abnormal metabolism of calcium or through abnormal development of the matrix upon which calci-

TABLE 15–5 EFFECT OF MANGANESE LEVEL DURING PREGNANCY ON BIRTH WEIGHT AND OTOLITH DEVELOPMENT OF PROGENY

Strain	*Diet (Mn conc., ppm)*	*No. of Litters*	*Mean Newborn Weight,[a] g*	*MOS[b], %*
C57B1/10J	3	6	1.26	31.1 ± 7.71[c]
	45	5	1.20	100.0
DBA/2J	3	9	1.34	4.4 ± 2.41
	45	7	1.13	100.0
SEC/REJ	3	14	1.27	5.5 ± 0.90
	45	9	1.32	98.3 ± 0.30
C57B1/10J-pa/pa	1	5	1.18	0.0
	3	9	1.23	0.0
	45	14	1.23	5.8 ± 2.20
	1500	6	1.26	93.6 ± 0.04
	2000	8	1.25	92.8 ± 3.64
Hybrid	1	17	1.36	22.1 ± 7.86
	3	20	1.33	33.8 ± 6.49
	45	17	—[d]	99.6 ± 0.04
	Stock[e]	10	—	100.0

[a]All animals were weighed in litters, not individually.

[b]MOS, % = mean otolith score calculated as

$$\frac{\text{otolith score observed per litter}}{\text{otolith score expected per normal litter}} \times 100$$

[c]S.E.M.

[d]Newborn weights were not taken, nor were males left in the cages for further breeding.

[e]Manganese concentration of stock diet approximately 45 ppm.

From Hurley and Bell, 1974.

fication (in this case, of the otolithic crystals) takes place. Calcium metabolism per se was not abnormal in manganese-deficient rats, but the abnormal skeletal development and the defective mucopolysaccharide synthesis suggested that aberrant development of the inner ear, like that of the skeleton, was also caused by depressed synthesis of mucopolysaccharides.

This hypothesis was tested by injecting radioactive sulfate into pregnant mice, both manganese-deficient and *pallid*, and comparing the uptake of sulfur into the otolithic matrix of the fetuses with that of controls. In the inner ear of normal fetuses, radioactive sulfur was seen in the epithelial cells of the macula upon which one of the otoliths rests, and in the otolithic matrix. In contrast, in both manganese-deficient and *pallid* fetuses, no otoliths and no sulfur uptake were apparent. The distribution of ^{35}S in cartilage cells and matrix was also different in manganese-deficient and *pallid* fetuses from that of controls. In normal animals, the proportion of sulfur in the matrix was higher than it was in the cells, while in manganese-deficient and in *pallid* mice, the relationship was reversed. However, the difference from normal was much smaller in *pallid* than it was in manganese-deficient fetuses. The relatively smaller change from normal in *pallid* mice may explain the lack of obvious skeletal abnormalities in the mutant.

An additional biochemical change in manganese-deficient animals was depression of mitochondrial function. In isolated mitochondria from manganese-deficient rats, P/O ratios were normal, but oxygen uptake was reduced. The changes in mitochondrial structure produced by manganese deficiency may be related to the role of manganese in superoxide dismutase, a mitochondrial enzyme that inactivates excess oxygen, since similar mitochondrial abnormalities have been produced with excessive amounts of oxygen. Furthermore, in young chicks deficient in manganese, activity of the mitochondrial manganese-containing superoxide dismutase was low.

ULTRASTRUCTURAL DEFECTS

The abnormal development of the inner ear leading to congenital irreversible ataxia, as well as the skeletal abnormalities characteristic of manganese deficiency, appear therefore to be caused by abnormal synthesis of sulfomucopolysaccharides. Ultrastructural findings are consistent with such an explanation. In liver, pancreas, kidney, and heart, electron microscopy showed alterations in the integrity of cell membranes in manganese-deficient mice. Mitochondria were found with elongated, stacked cristae. In addition, disorganization and dilation of the rough endoplasmic reticulum (RER) was seen, the vascular portion of the liver-cell reticulum was increased, and the Golgi apparatus was enlarged. Since the RER and the Golgi are considered to be sites of mucopolysaccharide synthesis, the abnormalities observed in these organelles are particularly pertinent to the hypothesis that both skeletal and otolith development in manganese deficiency are affected through mucopolysaccharide synthesis.

Mitochondria were especially abnormal, often clumped, with cristae parallel to the outer membrane instead of perpendicular to it. In some, the outer mitochondrial membrane was missing. The abnormalities of mitochondrial structure are consistent with the observed depression of mitochondrial function.

BRAIN FUNCTION

Manganese appears to play an important role in the central nervous system, and either its deficiency or its excess can affect the brain. Manganese-deficient rats, whether ataxic or not, were more susceptible to convulsions than were normal animals. They also had abnormal electroencephalograms. These epileptiform aberrations, in addition to the higher convulsability of these rats, demonstrated that manganese is required for normal function of the brain.

Abnormal neurological function related to manganese has also been found in humans. Of the people studied, about one-third of those with convulsive disorders had low manganese concentration in their plasma. In some cases, the mothers of epileptic children who were found to have low blood manganese, also showed the condition.

Pallid mutant mice, with a genetic propensity for manganese deficiency, seem insensitive to the cerebral effects of L-dopa, a precursor of catecholamines, and also show decreased accumulation and transport of L-dopa and L-tryptophan in the brain, suggesting connections between the metabolism of manganese and that of catecholamines. Cotzias has considered that this mutant may provide a model for genetic variations among patients with Parkinsonism or those suffering from chronic manganese poisoning. Manganese toxicity produces profound neurological disturbances similar to those of Parkinson's disease.

The positive correlation between cerebral dopamine and cerebral manganese in adult mice also holds for neonatal animals, suggesting that maturation of the dopaminergic apparatus might be manganese dependent. Possible connections between manganese, L-dopa, tryptophan, and melanin are of special interest in relation to the role of manganese in the metabolism of biogenic amines and brain function, but their relationship to prenatal development is obscure.

ZINC

The importance of zinc for embryonic development was first demonstrated in chicks in 1960. Gross malformations in embryos from zinc-deficient hens included skeletal defects, brain abnormalities, microphthalmia, and visceral herniations. More recently, an extensive series of investigations into the effects of zinc deficiency in the prenatal development of mammals has been carried out in rats.

CONGENITAL MALFORMATIONS IN RATS

A deficiency of zinc in the maternal diet produces a wide variety of gross congenital malformations in this species. When normal female rats, fed a complete diet before mating, were given a zinc-deficient diet during pregnancy (days 0 to 21), about half the implantation sites were resorbed. The full-term young weighed about half of controls, and 90% of fetuses showed gross congenital malformations. Food intake controls had normal young. Shorter periods of deficiency were also teratogenic. When the zinc deficiency occurred from day 6 to day 14 of gestation, about half of the young were abnormal. Even when the deficiency lasted for only the first ten days of pregnancy, 22% of the full-term fetuses were malformed (see Table 15–6 and Figure 15–5). Many investigators have confirmed the finding of congenital malformations in zinc-deficient rats. In rats deficient in this metal throughout gestation, almost all implantation sites were affected (either the fetus was resorbed or a malformed fetus was produced), while in control females only 2 to 5% of implanted embryos died or were abnormal.

The congenital malformations produced were varied; they affected

TABLE 15–6 EFFECT OF SHORT-TERM AND TRANSITORY ZINC DEFICIENCY ON REPRODUCTION IN RATS

Period of Deficiency, Days of Gestation	*No. of Rats*[a]	*Net Wt. Change During Gestation, g*	*Rats with Living Young, %*	*Implantation Sites Dead or Resorbed, %*	*Implantation Sites Affected,*[b] *%*	*Full-Term Fetuses*			
						No.	*Mean Number/Litter*[c]	*Mean Wt.,*[d] *g*	*Malformed, %*
None (control)	15	+76±5[e]	100	4.3	4.9	176	11.7±0.5	5.2	0.6
0–6	14	+66±4	100	5.9	7.0	160	11.4±0.6	5.1	1.2
0–8	13	+58±5	100	5.5	7.3	155	11.9±0.6	5.0	1.9
0–10	17	+63±4	82	25	42	133	7.8±1.2	4.8	22
0–12	15	+47±5	93	49	77	97	6.5±1.0	4.1	56
0–14	20	+42±3	70	55	89	103	5.2±1.0	3.6	76
0–16	20	+29±4	70	57	91	103	5.1±1.0	3.6	80
0–18	17	+18±4	76	52	92	96	5.6±1.0	3.4	82
0–21	15	−21±7	93	41	94	101	6.7±1.0	2.7	90
4–10	10	+71±5	100	9.5	18	105	10.5±0.6	5.1	10
6–10	10	+84±5	100	1.6	9.0	120	12.0±0.8	5.0	8
4–12	11	+56±3	100	12	38	106	9.6±1.0	4.5	29
6–12	15	+50±5	87	24	37	129	8.6±1.2	4.8	18
8–12	15	+66±5	73	37	43	116	7.7±1.3	5.0	9
4–14	12	+46±8	92	24	79	103	8.6±1.0	4.2	73
6–14	13	+61±4	100	5.6	49	151	11.6±0.9	4.4	46
8–14	14	+65±5	86	27	43	128	9.1±1.2	4.9	22

[a]Number of rats with implantation sites.
[b]Implantation sites with either a resorption or a malformed fetus.
[c]Means include all females with implantation sites.
[d]In every instance the S.E. was less than ±0.1 g.
[e]Mean ± S.E.

From Hurley et al., 1971.

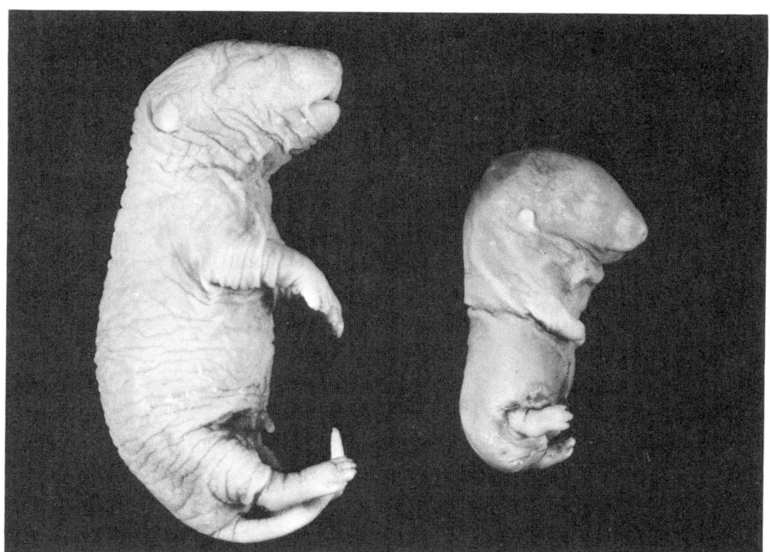

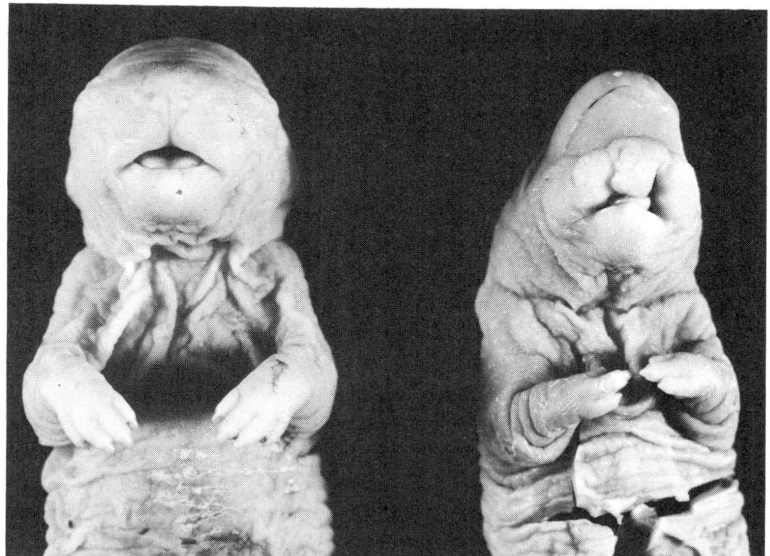

From Hurley, 1968.

Figure 15–5 (Upper) Typical appearance of full-term fetus from zinc-deficient rat (on right) as compared with control (on left). Note small size, abnormal shape of head and body, short limbs (micromelia), fused or missing digits (syndactyly), short lower jaw (micrognathia), and absence of tail in zinc-deficient fetus. (Lower) Cleft lip and domed skull (due to hydrocephalus) in full-term rat fetus from zinc-deficient female (on right) as compared with control (on left). Note also syndactyly in deficient fetus.

TABLE 15–7 TYPES AND INCIDENCE OF CONGENITAL MALFORMATIONS IN ZINC-DEFICIENT RAT FETUSES[a]

Malformations	*Percent of Fetuses*
Cleft lip	7
Cleft palate	42
Brain[b]	47
Micro- or anophthalmia	42
Micro- or agnathia	14
Spina bifida	3
Clubbed legs	38
Fore	10
Hind	35
Syndactyly	64
Tail	72
Dorsal herniation	1
Diaphragmatic herniation	8
Umbilical herniation	7
Heart[c]	2
Lung[d]	54
Urogenital	21

[a]Based on 101 full-term fetuses from 14 litters.
[b]Hydrocephalus, anencephalus, hydranencephalus, and some exencephalus.
[c]Primary transposition of great vessels and abnormal position of heart.
[d]Small or missing lobes.

From Hurley et al., 1971.

every organ system and occurred in high incidence (Table 15–7). A large number of skeletal malformations as well as soft tissue anomalies were seen. Malformations included cleft palate, cleft lip, short or missing mandible, curvature of the spine, club feet, syndactyly (fused or missing digits), curly or stubby tail, various brain malformations (such as hydrocephaly, anencephaly, or exencephaly), microphthalmia or anophthalmia (small or missing eyes), herniations, spina bifida, and heart, lung, and urogenital abnormalities. Frequencies ranged from 3 to 72% of living young at term. The malformations of the nervous system were especially noteworthy (Table 15–8). In full-term fetuses of rats given the zinc-deficient diet from the beginning of pregnancy to term, 47% had brain anomalies, 3% had spina bifida, and 42% had microphthalmia or anophthalmia. In addition, the spinal cord and olfactory tract also showed defects. Prenatal zinc deficiency affected many derivatives of the primitive neural tube.

When the deficiency period of zinc was limited to three days in pregnant

TABLE 15–8 EFFECT OF SHORT-TERM AND TRANSITORY ZINC DEFICIENCY ON INCIDENCE OF GROSS MALFORMATIONS OF THE NERVOUS SYSTEM

	Period of Deficiency (Days of Gestation)																
	None (Control)	*0–6*	*0–8*	*0–10*	*0–12*	*0–14*	*0–16*	*0–18*	*0–21*	*4–10*	*6–10*	*4–12*	*6–12*	*8–12*	*4–14*	*6–14*	*8–14*
No. of litters	15	14	13	14	14	14	14	13	14	10	10	11	13	11	11	13	12
No. of fetuses	176	160	155	133	97	103	103	96	101	105	120	106	129	116	103	151	128
Malformations, % fetuses:																	
Brain (total)[a]	0	1.2	1.3	3.8	9.3	38	34	24	47	2.9	3.3	2.8	4.7	4.3	18	11	0
Hydrocephalus	0	0.6	0.6	3.8	6.2	38	29	22	42	2.9	3.3	2.8	3.1	4.3	18	11	0
Anencephalus	0	0	0.6	0.8	4.1	22	16	16	36	0	0	0	1.6	0	11	0	0
Exencephalus	0	0.6	1.3	0.8	2.1	6.8	3.9	4.2	11	0	0	0	2.3	0	0	0	0
Spina bifida[a]	0	0	0.6	0.8	1.0	1.9	1.0	3.1	3.0	1.0	0	0	0	0	1.0	0	0
Micro- or anophthalmia	0	0.6	1.3	15	29	20	39	27	42	8.6	7.5	20	5.4	0	14	0	0

[a]Hydrocephalus, anencephalus, hydranencephalus, and some exencephalus.
[b]Does not include spina bifida occulta.

From Hurley and Shrader, 1972.

rats, from the tenth to the 12th days of gestation, a small but significant number of young were abnormal and had important malformations of the brain.

The zinc-deficient rat fetuses with a high incidence of congenital malformations showed a histological mucosal lesion of the esophagus. This lesion is sufficiently characteristic to serve as an indicator of the deficiency state and is the fetal counterpart of the esophageal lesion seen in zinc-deficient adult animals. It is characterized by hyperplasia of the esophageal mucosa, with an increase in the number of cells in the basal layer. The hyperplasia, occurring as it does in a severely stunted fetus, suggests that there is epithelial stimulation with increased cell division in this particular site. This is in contrast to the generalized hypoplasia occurring in the rest of the animal. Somewhat similar lesions of mucosa were found in the tongue, pharynx, and fore stomach of zinc-deficient fetuses.

Because of the high incidence of lung malformations, morphologic and biochemical maturation of the lung was studied in zinc-deficient fetuses. Growth of the lung was specifically inhibited; that is, lungs were smaller relative to body weight than in controls. In addition, phosphatidyl choline (lecithin) concentration of lungs was lower than normal at term. Lecithin is an important constituent of surfactant, which is necessary for normal respiratory function, and the depression of lecithin synthesis was correlated with morphological evidence that showed the lungs of zinc-deficient fetuses to be unexpanded and immature. In humans the ratio of lecithin to sphingomyelin (L/S) in the amniotic fluid is used as an indication of fetal maturity. In zinc-deficient rats, the L/S ratio, as in premature human fetuses, was lower than normal.

RAPID EFFECT OF DIETARY DEFICIENCY

The effect of dietary deficiency of zinc in the pregnant rat is extremely rapid. Zinc deficiency during the first few days of pregnancy results in abnormal cleavage and blastulation in preimplantation eggs, as early as day 3 of gestation. On day 4 of gestation, 98% of eggs recovered from control females had formed normal blastocysts, but only 17% of eggs from zinc-deficient females were in this stage (see Figure 15–6). It is thus possible for a nutritional deficiency to affect the embryo even before implantation into the uterus occurs.

The rapid effect of zinc deficiency arises from the need for a constant source of zinc in order to maintain plasma levels of the element. When rats were given a zinc-deficient diet at the beginning of pregnancy, plasma zinc concentration dropped sharply (Figure 15–7). After only 24 hours of the deficiency regime, plasma zinc had fallen by approximately 40%. This rapid change was brought about by lack of mobilization of zinc from maternal

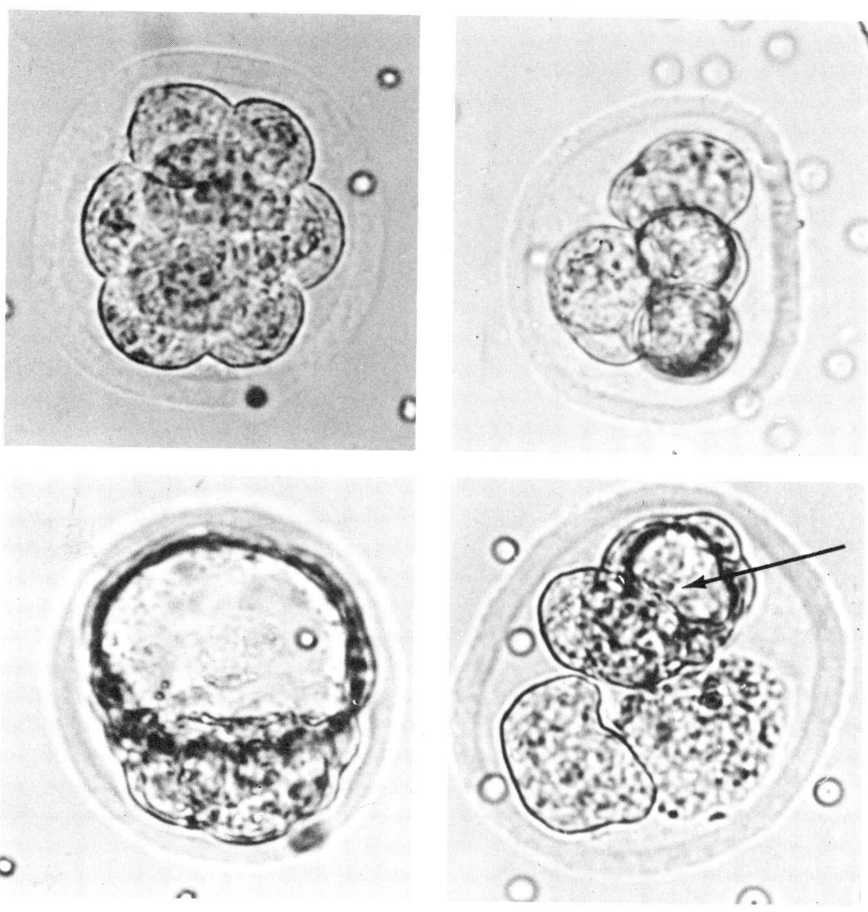

From Hurley and Shrader, 1975.

Figure 15–6 Examples of embryos obtained from the oviducts of control (a and b) and zinc-deprived (c and d) female rats on day 3 (a and c) and day 4 (b and d) of gestation. (a) Control, day 3, eight-cell stage; (b) Control, day 4, normal blastula. (c) Zinc deprived, day 3, abnormal seven-cell embryo containing one excessively large blastomere. (d) Zinc-deprived, day 4, abnormal blastulation with dissociated blastomeres and a degenerating mass of cytoplasm. Blastocoel indicated by arrow.

stores. After 21 days of a zinc-deficient diet, the zinc content of bone (which contains the major portion of the body's zinc) was the same in pregnant as it was in nonpregnant rats, although the zinc content of the fetuses was abnormally low and they were malformed. Thus, the pregnant rat cannot mobilize zinc from maternal tissues in amounts sufficient to supply the needs of normal fetal development.

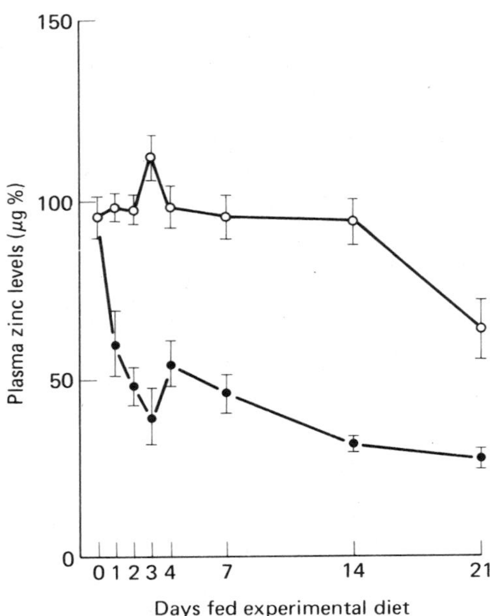

From Dreosti et al., 1968.

Figure 15–7 Plasma zinc levels in pregnant adult rats; open circles, zinc-supplemented controls; closed circles, zinc-deficient rats. Points represent the mean ± S.E. of five animals in each group.

The hypothesis was therefore developed that zinc could be released from the maternal skeleton only under conditions in which there is breakdown of the bone itself. This hypothesis was tested by comparing the effects of a diet lacking calcium as well as zinc with those of a diet deficient in zinc alone. In accordance with the hypothesis, the teratogenic effects of zinc deficiency were alleviated by lack of dietary calcium (Table 15–9). Female rats fed the diet deficient in both calcium and zinc had larger litters, fewer resorptions, and fewer malformed fetuses than did those fed the diet deficient in zinc alone. Furthermore, the ash, zinc, and calcium concentrations of bone were also reduced in rats receiving neither calcium or zinc during pregnancy. However, alleviation of the teratogenic effect of zinc deficiency by calcium deficiency did not occur in parathyroidectomized rats, providing further evidence in support of the hypothesis. In a dietary deficiency of calcium, resorption of bone is accelerated through the action of parathyroid hormone, in order to maintain plasma levels of calcium within the narrow limits compatible with life. The increased breakdown of bone releases zinc at the same time as calcium, thus increasing the availability of maternal skeletal zinc to the developing fetuses.

TABLE 15–9 EFFECT OF ZINC AND CALCIUM DEFICIENCY ON REPRODUCTION IN RATS

	Zn Deficient	*Zn and Ca Deficient*
Females:		
No.[a]	25	23
No. with live young	17	23
Initial body wt., g	234	229
Percent with live young	68	100
Percent implantation sites dead or resorbed	56	17
Percent implantation sites affected[b]	93	65
Fetuses:		
No. at term	121	221
Avg. no. per litter	4.8	9.6
Mean wt., g	2.7	3.2
Percent living young malformed	83	57
Malformations, percent fetuses:		
Cleft lip	7	0.4
Cleft palate	12	13
Brain[c]	14	12
Micro- or agnathia	7	2
Micro- or anophthalmia	25	11
Clubbed feet	44	13
A- or syndactyly	46	12
Curly or stubby tail	71	52
Dorsal herniation	4	0.4
Heart[d]	5	0.6
Lung[e]	18	12
Urogenital[f]	40	35

[a]Only females with at least one implantation site were included.
[b]Implantation sites with dead, resorbed, or malformed fetuses.
[c]Hydrocephalus, anencephalus, or exencephalus.
[d]Abnormal position.
[e]Missing lobes.
[f]Hydronephrosis, missing kidney, or abnormal position.

From Hurley and Tao, 1972.

A similar effect occurs when a higher rate of breakdown of maternal soft tissue is brought about by giving pregnant females a diet deficient in protein as well as in zinc. In this case, with zinc-deficient diets containing either 8% or 5% of protein (compared with the normal level of 30%), the percentage of implantation sites affected was markedly lower than in rats receiving a diet deficient only in zinc. As with calcium deficiency (in relation to breakdown of maternal tissues in order to maintain the animals, see the section on protein in Chapter 18), and at the same time, tissue catabolism released the zinc present in all cells, which was then available to the fetuses through the maternal plasma.

MECHANISM OF ACTION

Zinc is a known constituent of a number of important metalloenzymes and is a necessary cofactor for other enzymes. One of the most obvious approaches to investigation of the mechanisms bringing about these disturbances of morphogenesis was therefore to examine enzyme activity. A number of enzymes were assayed both histochemically and chemically in rat fetuses and in young animals. In most cases, little if any differences were apparent between normal and zinc-deficient animals. There were some differences in cellular localization of enzyme reactivity, but, in general, when specific cell types were present in an organ, the enzyme activity associated with that cell type was normal.

An example may be given from studies of malic dehydrogenase activity in testes of weanling rats. There were no differences between control and zinc-deficient rats in the biochemical assay of enzyme activity. Histochemically, it was clear that the testes of control rats, carrying out normal spermatogenesis, were composed of a different population of cells from those of zinc-deficient rats in which spermatogenesis had been arrested. Thus, the cellular localization of enzyme reactive sites was different in the two tissues. Intensity of enzyme activity was related to the cell types present, which were in turn a function of the stage of spermatogenesis. In embryos, of course, the cell types present at any one time would be related to the stage of development of the tissue. If the cell containing the enzyme was present, the enzyme was present. If, however, development was abnormal so that the cell type was not present, then that particular enzyme was not present either. Enzyme changes were, therefore, probably not causative factors in producing the congenital malformations of zinc deficiency.

Prenatal zinc deficiency affects many derivatives of the neural tube as well as those of other systems. The nature of these malformations, as well as their diverse origins, suggests that the action of zinc is on fundamental rather than on secondary processes. One of the generally accepted observations regarding zinc deficiency in pregnant animals, as well as in nonpregnant and juvenile animals, is that it affects primarily rapidly proliferating tissues—the embryo, the gonads, and the skin, where cell division is occurring at a rapid rate. Present evidence suggests that congenital malformations in zinc-deficient embryos as well as lesions of the gonads and skin are brought about by impaired synthesis of nucleic acids. It is thought at present that the effect of zinc deficiency on nucleic acid synthesis produces an asynchrony of mitotic rhythms. This is manifested by the large numbers of cells observed in mitotic arrest, which can then produce asynchronous growth patterns. Prolongation of the mitotic interval and reduction in the number of neural tube cells early in development could combine to produce a wide range of abnormalities. Asynchrony in histogenesis and organogenesis could therefore result from alterations in differential rates of growth.

Experiments with a number of systems, *in vitro* as well as *in vivo*, and with various species, have shown a requirement for zinc in DNA synthesis. In zinc-deficient rat embryos at 12 days of gestation, incorporation of tritiated thymidine into DNA was much lower than normal, suggesting that DNA synthesis was depressed. Autoradiographs of the cerebral cortex were consistent with this observation. The head region was more vulnerable than the body, but both could be brought to normal by prior injection of zinc into the pregnant female (see Table 15–10).

The activity of thymidine kinase was also depressed in zinc-deficient embryos. The thymidine kinase pathway for the production of thymidine nucleotides is not prominent in normal adult cells, but it becomes important for DNA synthesis in tissues undergoing rapid cell division. Since the effect of zinc deficiency on cell division has been found to be most extreme in rapidly proliferating tissues, the relationship of zinc to thymidine kinase in the developing embryo might be of critical importance. Another enzyme involved in DNA synthesis is also depressed in zinc-deficient embryos. DNA polymerase activity was lower in embryos from dams given a zinc-deficient diet than in controls. The normal increase with embryonic age of both these

TABLE 15–10 INCORPORATION OF ^{3}H-THYMIDINE INTO DNA OF EMBRYO HEAD

Group	*Counts of $^{3}H^{a}$*
	dpm[b]/μg DNA
Untreated:	
Control, ad libitum	$1527 \pm 281^{\alpha}$
Control, pair-fed	$1170 \pm 190^{\alpha}$
Zinc-deficient	$793 \pm 76^{\beta}$
Zinc-injected:	
Control, ad libitum	$1737 \pm 121^{\alpha}$
Control, pair-fed	$1953 \pm 182^{\alpha}$
Zinc-deficient	$1815 \pm 172^{\alpha}$

[a]Numbers are means of six embryos ± standard error of the mean.
[b]dpm = disintegrations per minute (counts of radioactivity).
$^{\alpha,\beta}$Differing Greek letter superscripts indicate significantly different groups.

Adapted from Eckhert and Hurley, 1977.

TABLE 15–11 EFFECT OF ZINC DEFICIENCY AND DAY OF GESTATION ON ACTIVITY OF THYMIDINE KINASE AND DNA POLYMERASE IN RAT EMBRYOS

	Groups							
	Control Ad Libitum		*Control Restricted Intake*		*Zinc-Deficient*		*Zinc-Deficient to Restricted Intake Control*	
Day of Gestation	*Thymidine Kinase*[a]	*DNA Polymerase*[b]	*Thymidine Kinase*	*DNA Polymerase*	*Thymidine Kinase*	*DNA Polymerase*	*Thymidine Kinase, %*	*DNA Polymerase, %*
9	79 ± 9[d]	2.32 ± 0.12[d]	81 ± 14[d]	2.19 ± 0.24[d]	64 ± 6[c,d]	1.44 ± 0.30[c,d]	79	67
10	323 ± 66[d]	2.68 ± 0.25[d]	351 ± 52[d]	2.51 ± 0.22	196 ± 32[c,d]	1.62 ± 0.25[c,d]	56	66
11	665 ± 95	2.96 ± 0.28	659 ± 101[d]	2.62 ± 0.42	372 ± 76[c]	1.88 ± 0.25[c]	56	72
12	729 ± 101	3.06 ± 0.35	950 ± 48	2.59 ± 0.38	356 ± 79[c]	1.97 ± 0.26[c]	37	76

[a]Thymidine kinase activity expressed as pM^{3}H-thymidine incorporated/mg protein/hr.
[b]DNA polymerase activity expressed as nM^{3}H-TTP incorporated/mg protein/hr.
[c]$p < 0.05$ compared to ad libitum and restricted intake controls.
[d]$p < 0.05$ compared to activity in one-day-older embryos in the same group.

Adapted from Duncan and Hurley, 1978.

enzymes did not occur in the zinc-deficient rats (Table 15–11). Thus, decreased activity of thymidine kinase and DNA polymerase may lead to depression of nucleic acid synthesis in zinc deficiency. However, recent work with the microorganism *Euglena gracilis* indicates that zinc may be required at every stage of the cell cycle, and thus thymidine kinase and DNA polymerase are probably not the only factors involved.

Additional findings consistent with the hypothesis that zinc deficiency causes aberrations of DNA synthesis come from cytogenetic studies. Chromosome spreads from fetal liver of zinc-deficient fetuses showed chromosomal aberrations, especially gaps and terminal deletions. Such chromosomal abnormalities were also seen in maternal bone marrow and occurred in significant incidence in both maternal and fetal tissue.

MILD OR MARGINAL ZINC DEFICIENCY

Relatively mild states of zinc deficiency may be more relevant to human problems than the extreme zinc deficiency described so far. Marginal zinc deficiency has also been studied in pregnant rats. One approach was to correlate the level of zinc in the diet with the incidence of malformations in rats and to determine the concentration of dietary zinc that would prevent such malformations. With diets containing less than 9 ppm zinc during pregnancy, there was a high incidence of fetal death and malformation. Both total litter weight and fetal weight at term correlated with the level of dietary zinc up to 14 ppm, but there was no correlation between the incidence of malformations and the fetal zinc content or the maternal plasma zinc level at term. However, maternal plasma zinc during the second third of pregnancy (the second week in the rat) was correlated with frequency of malformations.

One of the nutritional concerns related to pregnant women is the evaluation of their zinc status. How can we best determine the level of zinc nutriture, especially in regard to its relation to fetal development? It may be, as suggested by the experiment described, that analysis of maternal plasma zinc level during the second trimester of pregnancy would provide a more useful index than such measurements at term.

A transitory deficiency of zinc during prenatal life was also used as a means of examining the effects of mild rather than severe zinc deficiency. When normal pregnant rats were given a zinc-deficient diet from day 6 to day 14 of gestation, maternal plasma zinc levels fell rapidly, but they returned quickly to original values after zinc was refed. Young born to these females showed a high rate of stillbirths, a high incidence of congenital malformations, low birth weight, and very poor survival to weaning, although postnatal growth of survivors was normal. Most of the postnatal mortality occurred in the first week. None of these effects was seen in control groups,

TABLE 15–12 EFFECT OF TRANSISTORY GESTATIONAL ZINC DEFICIENCY ON POSTNATAL SURVIVAL

Group.	*No. of Young*	*Percent of Young Alive at Birth*		
		Day 7	*Day 14*	*Day 21*
Control, ad libitum	107	97	91	87
Control, restricted intake	105	91	90	89
Experimental, Zn-deficient (days 6–14 gest.)	57	30	28	28

Adapted from Hurley and Mutch, 1973.

either ad libitum fed or with restricted food intakes (Table 15–12). Concentration of zinc in postpartum maternal plasma and milk, as well as in plasma of the pups was normal, suggesting that postnatal zinc nutriture of the young was adequate (Figure 15–8). Poor survival of young born to

Figure 15–8 Blood plasma zinc levels in female rats and their offspring. Means and standard errors for maternal zinc levels were: gestation day 8: experimental 53 ± 5 ($N = 8$), control 138 ± 12 (6); day 14: experimental 41 ± 6 (8), control 124 ± 8 (8); day 16: experimental 171 ± 17 (8), control 136 ± 8 (8); day 21: experimental 97 ± 6 (16) control 91 ± 6 (14); lactation day 0: experimental 162 ± 19 (3), control 146 ± 14 (4); day 1: experimental 186 ± 9 (6), control 170 ± 12 (7); day 7: experimental 164 ± 14 (5), control 151 ± 15 (8).

From Hurley and Mutch, 1973.

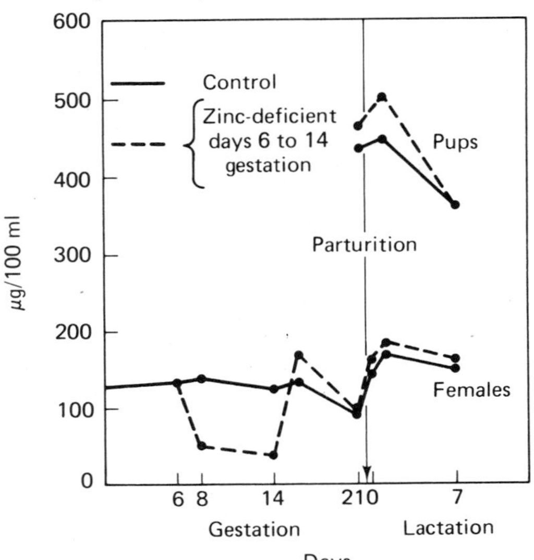

females fed a zinc-deficient diet for a short period may be due to congenital abnormalities or to failure to suckle because of weakness at birth. A short period of zinc deficiency during prenatal life thus caused an irreversible change that subsequently affected postnatal development.

Another way of studying the effects of mild deficiency was to feed rats a diet only marginally deficient in zinc (9 ppm) during pregnancy. At parturition they were given a normal diet. The survival of offspring was significantly lower than in animals fed the normal diet throughout. Eighty-one percent of living young born to stock-fed females survived to weaning, but only 46% of living young born to females fed the marginally deficient diet survived to this age. Cross-fostering studies were carried out with appropriate controls; that it, offspring of females that received the marginally deficient diet during pregnancy were suckled by females normally fed during pregnancy, and pups of females normally fed during pregnancy were suckled by females fed the marginally deficient diet during pregnancy (Table 15–13). It was evident that the decreased survival was due to both maternal and fetal factors.

The survival of pups from females marginally deficient during pregnancy was the same whether they were suckled by their own mothers or by foster mothers normally fed during pregnancy. Conversely, the pups of females normally fed during pregnancy showed depression of postnatal survival when they were fed by females given the marginally deficient diet during pregnancy. Thus, the maternal diet during pregnancy affected both the development of the offspring and the ability of the female to suckle her young. The offspring suffered from some irreversible effects of prenatal zinc deficiency, and the female's ability to suckle and/or care for her young also was diminished by the deficiency during pregnancy.

TABLE 15–13 MARGINAL ZINC DEFICIENCY: EFFECT ON SURVIVAL

Maternal Diet		*Percent Survival*	
Gestation	*Lactation*	*One Week*	*6 Weeks*
Stock	Stock[a]	(124) 94	(106) 80[b]
Stock	Stock	(203) 89	(160) 70
9 ppm Zn	9 ppm Zn	(156) 63	(127) 51
9 ppm Zn	Stock	(102) 62	(74) 45
9 ppm Zn	9 ppm Zn	(37) 54	(31) 46

[a]Not cross-fostered; all other groups fostered.
[b]Males only at six weeks. Nos. of rats in parenthesis.

From Hurley, 1977.

ZINC DEFICIENCY IN PREGNANT MONKEYS

Zinc is an essential element for the reproduction of monkeys. Zinc-deficient females of the species *Macaca radiata*, the bonnet monkey, showed abnormal ovarian development. No pregnancies resulted from 32 matings, although about 20% of matings in this species yielded pregnancies in control monkeys. Thus in monkeys as well as in rats zinc deficiency during early stages of gestation has deleterious effects on development.

ZINC DEFICIENCY IN HUMANS

The occurrence of zinc deficiency in humans in the Middle East, resulting in hypogonadal dwarfism, is now well established. More recently, zinc deficiency has also been found in children in the United States (see Chapters 18 and 19). Since this condition can occur in humans, it has been suggested that zinc deficiency may also be a factor in congenital abnormalities in man. There is some evidence that zinc deficiency is in fact teratogenic for humans. Epidemiological data may support a relationship between zinc deficiency and malformations of the central nervous system in humans, since the two countries in which zinc deficiency has been found in people, Egypt and Iran, both have high rates of such malformations.

Another type of evidence comes from women with the disease acrodermatitis enteropathica, a genetic disorder of zinc metabolism (see also Chapter 18). Until it was learned, in the early 1970s, that the signs and symptoms of the condition could be cured with oral zinc therapy, patients were treated with a drug that permitted survival and growth but was not able to maintain plasma zinc at normal levels. Thus, women with the genetic trait who became pregnant had an abnormally low concentration of zinc in their blood plasma. The outcome of these pregnancies was extremely poor. The number of miscarriages and infants with malformations was very much higher than in a normal population. Out of seven pregnancies there were two infants with major congenital malformations and one spontaneous abortion.

If zinc deficiency is teratogenic for man, then it is possible that marginal levels of deficiency, perhaps in combination with other factors such as genetic traits or medicinal or other drugs, could provoke abnormalities of development in humans (see also Chapter 16).

In Sweden, a correlation was found between low zinc in pregnant women and various complications of pregnancy. Women who gave birth to malformed infants, or to post-term infants, or who had abnormal deliveries, had significantly lower serum zinc levels than women whose deliveries and infants were normal, or whose infants were of low birth weight.

Calculations of the zinc content of American diets have suggested that the zinc nutrition of many Americans may be marginal. More information is needed concerning the possibility of deleterious effects on the outcome of pregnancy because of marginal zinc deficiency and its prevalence in various human populations.

INDUCED ZINC DEFICIENCY

Zinc deficiency may also be induced by means other than an inadequate dietary intake. For example, ingestion of a chelating agent, EDTA, during pregnancy impaired reproduction in rats and resulted in congenitally malformed young. When EDTA was fed from days 6 to 21 of gestation, all of the full-term young had gross congenital malformations. The full-term fetuses were markedly stunted in size and had a high incidence of various types of malformations. For example, 44% of the young had severe brain malformations, 57% had cleft palate, and nearly all had clubbed legs and malformed tails. These anomalies could be completely prevented by giving a high intake of zinc with the chelating agent. The similarity in the types of malformations and their frequency to those of females given diets severely deficient in zinc suggests that the severe effects of EDTA were due to an induced deficiency of zinc. Such effects are important in the use of chelating agents such as EDTA or NDTA in the therapeutic removal of metal ions in cases of heavy-metal poisoning.

Other conditions are known to induce zinc deficiency, for example, alcoholism in humans, but their relationship to pregnancy and congenital abnormalities can only be conjectured (see Chapter 16).

ZINC EXCESS

High levels of zinc in an otherwise normal diet appear to have little effect on embryonic development in rats. Without copper added to the diet, however, excess zinc tended to decrease reproduction and increase the frequency of stillbirths, but did not decrease survival in the first week after birth.

ZINC AND CADMIUM

Zinc metabolism may also be involved in the effects of another metal, cadmium. Injection of cadmium into pregnant animals has teratogenic effects on the offspring as well as toxic effects on the mother. Simultaneous administration of zinc with cadmium protects against the deleterious action of cadmium on the embryo. The mode of action of cadmium toxicity and its interaction with zinc are not understood, but it may be that the toxicity of cadmium is mediated through antagonistic effects on the biochemical role of zinc, such as in zinc metalloenzymes.

References and Supplementary Readings

GENERAL

Hurley, L. S. "Approaches to the study of nutrition in mammalian development." In: *Symposium on Nutrition and Prenatal Development. Fed. Proc.* **27**: 193–199 (1968).

Hurley, L. S. "Trace elements and teratogenesis." In: *Symposium on biochemical and nutritional aspects of trace elements.* AAAS, New York. *Med. Clinics of N. America* **60**: 771–778 (1975).

Hurley, L. S. "Interaction of genes and metals in development." In: *Symposium on Interaction of Nutritional and Genetic Factors. Fed. Proc.* **35**: 2271–2275 (1976).

Underwood, E. J. *Trace Elements in Human and Animal Nutrition,* 4th ed. New York: Academic Press, 1977.

MANGANESE

Daniels, A. L., and G. J. Everson. "The relation of manganese to congenital debility." *J. Nutr.* **9**: 191–203 (1935).

de Rosa, G., R. M. Leach, and L. S. Hurley. "Influence of dietary Mn^{++} on the activity of mito-chondrial superoxide dismutase." *Fed. Proc.* **37**: 594 (1978).

Erway, L., L. S. Hurley, and A. Fraser. "Neurological defect: Manganese in phenocopy and prevention of a genetic abnormality of inner ear." *Science* **152**: 1766–1768 (1966).

Erway, L., L. S. Hurley, and A. Fraser. "Congenital ataxia and otolith defects due to manganese deficiency in mice." *J. Nutr.* **100**: 643–654 (1970).

Hurley, L. S. "Manganese and other trace elements." In: D. M. Hegsted, ed., *Present Knowledge in Nutrition,* pp. 345–355. 4th ed. Washington, D.C.: The Nutrition Foundation, 1976.

Hurley, L. S., and L. T. Bell. "Genetic influence on response to dietary manganese deficiency." *J. Nutr.* **104**: 133–137 (1974).

Hurley, L. S., and G. J. Everson. "Influence of timing of short-term supplementation during gestation on congenital abnormalities of manganese-deficient rats." *J. Nutr.* **79**: 23–27 (1963).

Hurley, L. S., E. Wooten, and G. J. Everson. "Disproportionate growth in offspring of manganese-deficient rats. II. Skull, brain, and cerebrospinal fluid pressure." *J. Nutr.* **74**: 282–288 (1961).

Orent, E. R., and E. V. McCollum. "Effects of deprivation of manganese in the rat." *J. Biol. Chem.* **92**: 651–678 (1931).

Shrader, R. E., L. Erway, and L. S. Hurley. "Mucopolysaccharide synthesis in the developing inner ear of manganese-deficient and pallid mutant mice." *Teratology* **8**: 257–266 (1973).

ZINC

Dreosti, I. E., S. Tao, and L. S. Hurley. "Plasma zinc and leukocyte changes in weanling and pregnant rats during zinc deficiency." *Proc. Soc. Exp. Biol. Med.* **127**: 169–174 (1968).

DUNCAN, J. R., AND L. S. HURLEY. "Thymidine kinase and DNA polymerase activity in normal and zinc deficient developing rat embryos." *Proc. Soc. Exp. Biol. Med.* **159**: 39–43 (1978).

ECKHERT, C. D., AND L. S. HURLEY. "Reduced DNA synthesis in zinc deficiency: Regional differences in embryonic rats." *J. Nutr.* **107**: 855–861 (1977).

HURLEY, L. S. "Zinc deficiency in prenatal and neonatal development." In: G. J. BREWER AND A. S. PRASAD, eds., *Zinc Metabolism. Current Aspects in Health and Disease.* Alan R. Liss, Inc., New York, 1977, pp. 47–58.

HURLEY, L. S., AND P. B. MUTCH. "Prenatal and postnatal development after transitory gestational zinc deficiency in rats." *J. Nutr.* **103**: 649–656 (1973).

HURLEY, L. S., AND R. E. SHRADER. "Congenital malformations of the nervous system in zinc-deficient rats." In: C. C. PFEIFFER, ed., *Neurobiology of the Trace Metals Zinc and Copper. Intl. Rev. Neurobiol.*, Suppl. 1, pp. 7–51. New York: Academic Press, 1972.

HURLEY, L. S., AND R. E. SHRADER. "Abnormal development in preimplantation rat eggs after three days of maternal dietary zinc deficiency." *Nature* **254**: 427–429 (1975).

HURLEY, L. S., AND S. TAO. "Alleviation of teratogenic effects of zinc deficiency by simultaneous lack of calcium." *Am. J. Physiol.* **222**: 322–325 (1972).

HURLEY, L. S., J. GOWAN, AND H. SWENERTON. "Teratogenic effects of short-term and transitory zinc deficiency in rats." *Teratology* **4**: 199–204 (1971).

VOJNIK, C., AND L. S. HURLEY. "Abnormal prenatal lung development resulting from maternal zinc deficiency in rats." *J. Nutr.* **82**: 862–872 (1977).

WARKANY, J., AND H. G. PETERING. "Congenital malformations of the brain produced by short zinc deficiencies in rats." *Am. J. Ment. Defic.* **77**: 645–653 (1973).

16

Alcohol

Alcohol is not generally thought of as a nutrient or a food, but because it provides calories (approximately 7 kcal/g), it does affect nutritional intake. Consequently, an examination of the effect of alcohol consumption in pregnant women on the development of their offspring is pertinent here. It is now well established that alcoholic women have a high risk of giving birth to abnormal children.

The modern rediscovery of the deleterious effects of alcoholism during pregnancy on the development of the offspring was reported independently by the French workers Lemoine and associates in 1968 and by Jones and Smith and their co-workers of Seattle, Washington, in 1973. The close similarity between the reports, described independently by two research groups in different parts of the world, and later by others as well, suggests strongly the validity of the observations. The Seattle workers named the condition the Fetal Alcohol Syndrome (FAS). The major features of the syndrome are growth retardation, small head size, anomalies of the face, eyes, heart, joints, and external genitalia, and mental deficiency. Other anomalies include micrognathia, epicanthic folds, and hypoplastic midfacial structures, including broad nasal ridge, upturned nares, and long upper lip. There are abnormalities of the ears, and the palpebral fissures (opening of eyelids) are small (Figure 16–1).

The small palpebral fissures may actually be secondary to microphthalmia. Other ocular defects common in the FAS are ptosis (drooping of the eyelids) and strabismus (cross-eyedness). A wide mouth, prominent ears, and a narrow bifrontal diameter are also common features of the syndrome. Other malformations include cleft palate, visceral anomalies, and small hemangiomas.

The growth failure in these children occurs both prenatally and postnatally. At the time of birth the deficit is often greater in body length than in body weight. Postnatally, FAS babies usually gain weight poorly, and the body weight is more affected than the body height. There is no catch-up in

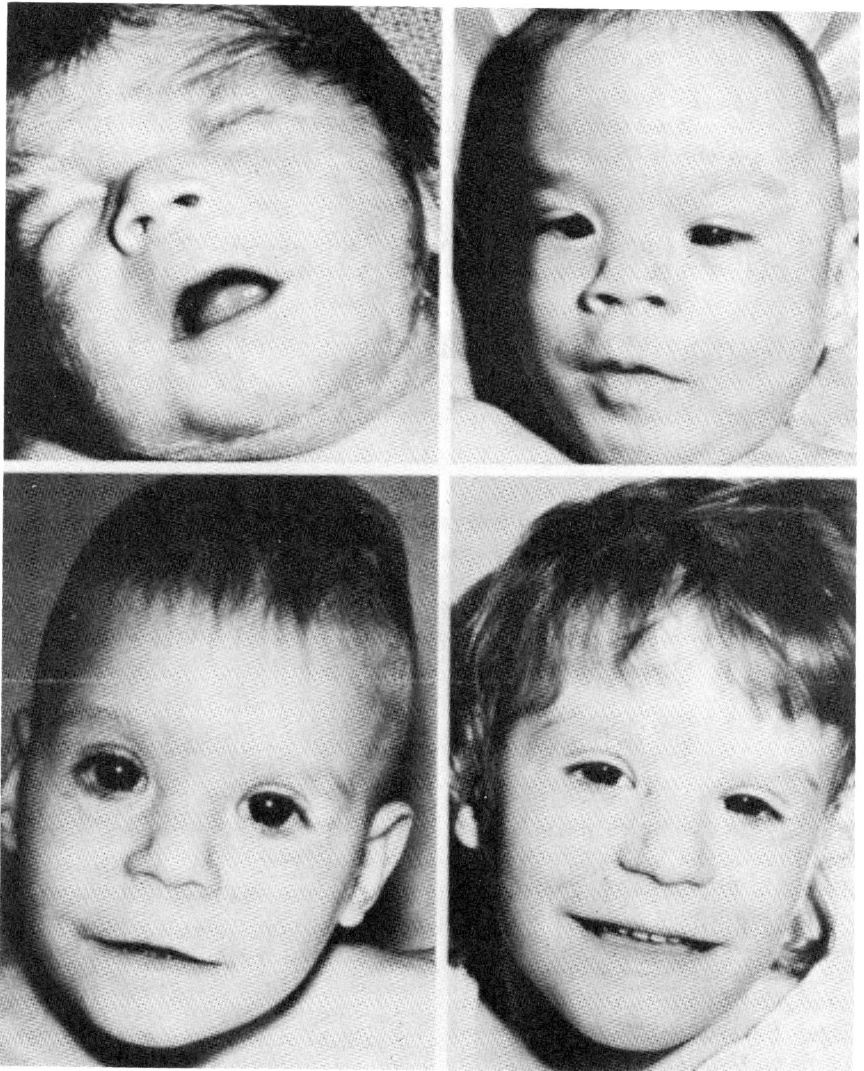

From Hanson et al., 1976.

Figure 16–1 Top, Boy with fetal alcohol syndrome at birth (left, from Jones and Smith) and at age 6 months (right). Bottom, Girl with fetal alcohol syndrome at age 16 months (left) and 4 years (right). Note short palpebral fissures, low nasal bridge with short or upturned nose, epicanthic folds, midface hypoplasia, and long convex upper lip with narrow vermilion border. A narrow bifrontal diameter, ocular ptosis, strabismus, wide mouth, prominent ears, and decreased periocular zone of hair inhibition are common features.

growth during infancy and early childhood. The persisting deficiency of growth appears not to be the consequence of the postnatal environment, since affected babies raised in foster care from early infancy in general show no better growth or performance than those raised by the alcoholic mother. Even infants hospitalized for failure to thrive have not shown catch-up growth.

The perinatal mortality of infants with FAS is high, and those who survive show neurological difficulties. During the neonatal period there is often tremulousness, hyperactivity, and irritability. Although some of these symptoms might result from alcohol withdrawal after birth, the tremulousness frequently persists for a long time, even years, and the fine motor dysfunction and developmental delay may be permanent. Mental deficiency of varying severity also occurs in these children and, in a necropsy study, considerable malformation of the central nervous system was found. Thus it seems that much of the abnormal performance in the early period, as well as the persistent mental deficiency, is secondary to alterations in brain development and function resulting from the prenatal effect on morphogenesis of the central nervous system.

The incidence of the fetal alcohol syndrome in children of chronically alcoholic women appears from present evidence to be in the range of 30 to 50%. Prenatal and postnatal growth failure, developmental delay, and microcephaly occur in about 90 to 97% of the infants with FAS. Incidence of other defects is also shown in Table 16–1.

Description of the syndrome is based on the outcome of pregnancy of chronically aud severely alcoholic women. Little is known about the risk and possible consequences of lower intakes of alcohol. Neither are the critical factors involved understood. For example, in relation to alcohol consumption, is it the continuous alcohol level in the maternal blood that is important, or maximum concentrations during binge drinking? The effect of lower levels of alcohol intake on fetal development, perhaps producing only part of the syndrome, is relatively unexplored. One study suggests that even moderate drinking during early pregnancy may result in alterations of growth and morphogenesis in the fetus.

Congenital abnormalities have also been produced in experimental animals given alcohol during pregnancy, and an animal model of FAS has been developed in mice.

POSSIBLE MECHANISMS

What are the possible mechanisms that could bring about the abnormal development resulting in the FAS? There may be a direct effect of alcohol itself on the developing embryo, since alcohol taken by the mother is trans-

TABLE 16–1 COMMON ABNORMALITIES IN FETAL ALCOHOL SYNDROME[a]

Abnormality	*No. Affected/No. Observed* (%)
Growth and performance:	
Prenatal growth deficiency[b]	38/39 (97)
Postnatal growth deficiency[b]	37/38 (97)
Microcephaly[b]	38/41 (93)
Developmental delay or mental deficiency[b]	31/35 (89)
Fine motor dysfunction	28/35 (80)
Craniofacial:	
Short palpebral fissures	35/38 (92)
Midfacial hypoplasia	26/40 (65)
Epicanthic folds	20/41 (49)
Limb:	
Abnormal palmar creases	20/41 (49)
Joint anomalies (mostly minor)	17/41 (41)
Other:	
Cardiac defect (mostly septal defects)	20/41 (49)
External genital anomalies (minor)	13/41 (32)
Hemangiomas (mostly small, raised, strawberry angiomas)	12/41 (29)
Ear anomalies (minor)	9/41 (22)

[a]Data taken from 41 patients, including 11 whose cases were previously reported.

[b]2 S.D. or more below the normal for age; equivalent to below the 2.5 percentile.

From Hanson et al., 1976.

ported across the placenta. In sheep, a positive correlation was found between maternal and fetal blood alcohol concentration during a one- or two-hour infusion of alcohol into the pregnant ewe (Figure 16–2).

There could also be an indirect effect of chronic alcoholism that might alter the maternal metabolism in such a way as to produce teratogenic effects on the child. However, there are several confounding factors involved in cases of chronic alcoholism among pregnant women. Heavy drinking is often associated with other risk factors for congenital abnormalities, such as heavy smoking, use of other drugs, emotional stress, injury from falls or violence, and poor prenatal medical care.

It seems reasonable to suspect that nutritional deficiencies may contribute to the development of the fetal alcohol syndrome. Although many nutritional deficiencies are teratogenic, three nutrients, folate, magnesium, and zinc, seem most likely to be involved. All three of these nutrients have been recognized as problems in the nutritional status of alcoholics. Furthermore, deficiencies of these substances are highly teratogenic in experimental

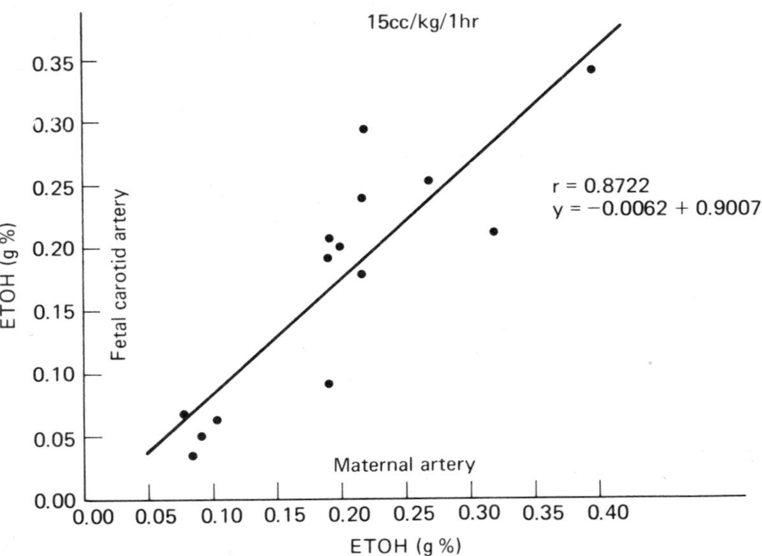

From Mann et al., 1975.

Figure 16–2 Correlation of maternal with fetal blood alcohol concentrations during 1 hour infusion.

animals, and there is at least some evidence of similar effects in humans (see Chapters 12, 13, and 15).

The proposal that deficiencies of one or more specific nutrients may be involved in the production of the FAS is at present based on only indirect evidence. This hypothesis should be investigated by studies both in experimental animal models and in pregnant alcohol-drinking women and their children.

References and Supplementary Readings

CLARREN, S. K., E. C. ALVORD, JR., S. M. SUMI, A. P. STREISSGUTH, AND D. W. SMITH. "Brain malformation related to prenatal exposure to alcohol." *J. Pediatr.* **92**: 64–67 (1978).

CHERNOFF, G. F. "The fetal alcohol syndrome in mice: An animal model." *Teratology* **15**: 223–229 (1977).

HANSON, J. W., K. L. JONES, AND D. W. SMITH. "Fetal alcohol syndrome, experience with 41 patients." *J. Am. Med. Assoc.* **235**: 1458–1460 (1976).

HANSON, J. W., A. P. STREISSGUTH, AND D. W. SMITH. "The effects of moderate alcohol consumption during pregnancy on fetal growth and morphogenesis." *J. Pediatr.* **92**: 457–460 (1978).

JONES, K. L., D. W. SMITH, C. N. ULLELAND, AND A. P. STREISSGUTH. "Pattern of malformation in offspring of chronic alcoholic mothers." *Lancet* **1**: 1267–1271 (1973).

MANN, L. I., A. BHAKTHAVATHSALAN, AND M. LIU. "Placental transport of alcohol and its effect on maternal and fetal acid-base balance." *Am. J. Obstet. Gynecol.* **122**: 837–844 (1975).

STREISSGUTH, A. P., C. S. HERMAN, AND D. W. SMITH. "Intelligence, behavior, and dismorphogenesis in the fetal alcohol syndrome: A report on 20 patients." *J. Pediatr.* **92**: 363–367 (1978).

TZE, W. J., AND M. LEE. "Adverse effects of maternal alcohol consumption on pregnancy and foetal growth in rats." *Nature* **257**: 479–480 (1975).

WARNER, R., AND H. ROSETT. "The effects of drinking on offspring: An historical survey of the American and British literature." *J. Studies on Alcohol* **36**: 1395–1420 (1975).

17

Principles of developmental nutrition

In previous chapters we have considered specific effects of nutritional deficiencies and excesses in the maternal diet upon development of the embryo and fetus. This chapter summarizes the principles relating to developmental nutrition, especially in the prenatal period.

MANIFESTATIONS OF ABNORMAL DEVELOPMENT

It may be well to recall at this point that manifestations of abnormal prenatal development are (1) death, (2) malformation, (3) growth retardation, and (4) functional abnormality. Such evidences of abnormal development may be apparent at birth (before birth in the case of prenatal death), or they may not be noticeable at all until well into postnatal life, even as late as middle age.

Prenatal influences may have permanent postnatal effects, even though the offspring are apparently normal at birth. Mild zinc deficiency, for example, did not cause congenital malformations in the young but increased the postnatal mortality rate. Hypervitaminosis A also produced permanent deficits in postnatal behavior of the animals despite seeming normality when born. The possible relationship to human health problems of postnatal effects of prenatal insult raises an intriguing and important question. Can mild nutritional deficiencies or excesses during prenatal life have subtle effects that may be manifested only in later life as functional abnormalities or susceptibility to degenerative or other diseases?

MATERNAL-FETAL PARTITION OF NUTRIENTS

There are differences among nutrients in their relative partition between mother and fetus. This principle may be phrased in terms of the question,

"Is the fetus a perfect parasite?" In the past it was thought that the mammalian fetus was not affected by environmental factors and that it could derive all of its required nutrition from the mother by removing essential nutrients from her tissues. For some nutrients, this idea may be considered relatively correct. Certain nutrients seem to go to the fetus at the expense of the mother. This is true for calcium to some extent and probably for protein also. But even in these cases the concept is only partially valid.

In the case of other nutrients the idea of the fetus as a parasite is clearly in error. With zinc, for example, the concentration of the element in maternal tissues remained at a normal level in the face of dietary deficiency and was not released preferentially to supply the fetus. The maternal plasma concentration of zinc fell, and this lower level in turn affected the fetus. Magnesium deficiency also produced approximately the same result.

It is important to remember that any essential nutrient may also be deleterious if given in excessive amounts or by inappropriate means (for example, parenterally as opposed to orally). Essential nutrients may also have undesired effects if they are provided in such a way that they interfere with absorption or metabolism of other nutrients.

DIRECT OR INDIRECT EFFECTS

The effect of nutrition during prenatal development may be either direct or indirect. The indirect effects of nutritional deficiencies or excesses in the maternal diet arise from changes in the metabolism of the maternal organism. These in turn alter the composition or the rate of transfer of materials to the embryo and fetus. For example, if the effect on the mother of less-than-optimal nutrition is to produce a lack of hormones necessary for the maintenance of pregnancy, termination of the pregnancy will usually result. In this case, the effect on the fetus is an indirect one through a primary action on maternal hormonal balance. Thus, in severe protein deficiency and vitamin B_6 deficiency in rats, we know that there are abnormal maternal endocrine relationships, because pregnancy is maintained if estrogen and progesterone are administered.

On the other hand, a direct effect of nutrition on prenatal development occurs when the embryo is provided through the placenta with a nutrient substrate inadequate for its nutritional needs. An example might be zinc deficiency, which produces a rapid and severe drop in the zinc concentration of maternal plasma and causes insufficient zinc to be available to the embryo and fetus. Although the differentiation of a direct from an indirect effect is not always possible in a particular instance, the theoretical difference between the two conditions is clear.

MILDNESS OF TERATOGENIC AGENTS

Another principle of developmental nutrition is that teratogenic effects are more likely to occur with relatively *mild* than with severe deficiencies of specific nutrients. If a nutritional deficiency is very severe, death of the embryo or fetus occurs. When the fetal mortality rate is very high, malformations and other abnormalities may not be observable. On the other hand, if the deficiency is relatively mild, but still severe enough to perturb development, acute effects on morphogenesis or on functional development are apt to occur. Such marked consequences of relatively mild deficiencies are seen with riboflavin, zinc, and vitamin A. Figure 17-1 shows a female rat of obviously normal external appearance who nevertheless gave birth to abnormal young as a result of a mild deficiency of vitamin A. The postnatal manifestations of hypervitaminosis A during gestation are another illustration of this principle.

TIME AND AGENT SPECIFICITY

The timing of the nutritional insult during gestation influences the outcome (see Figures 17–2 and 17–3). For example, with vitamin A deficiency or excess, various malformations occurred depending upon the timing of either the lack of the vitamin or its administration. The same principle was apparent in the studies of the Rotterdam famine during World War II. If

Figure 17–1 Female rat submitted to vitamin A deficient diet; at the 21st day of gestation gave birth to an abnormal litter. Note the externally normal aspect of the mother.

From Roux et al., 1962.

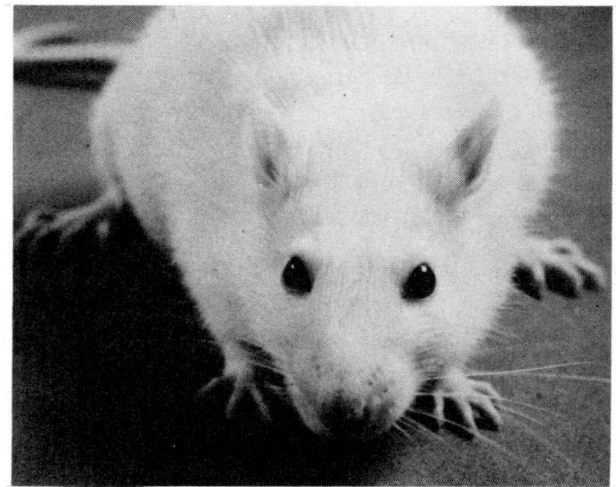

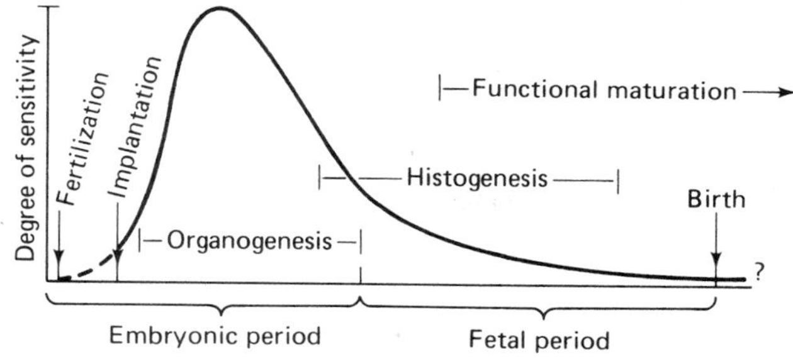

From Wilson, in Pathophysiology of Gestation, *N. S. Assali, ed., Vol. II, pp. 269–320, Academic Press, New York, 1972.*

Figure 17–2 Curve approximating the susceptibility of the human embryo to teratogenesis from fertilization throughout intrauterine development. The highest sensitivity, at least to structural deviation, occurs during the period of organogenesis, from about days 18 to 20 until about days 55 to 60, although the absolute peak of sensitivity may be reached before day 30 postconception. As organogenesis is completed susceptibility to anatomical defects diminishes greatly, but probably minor structural deviation is possible until histogenesis is completed late in the fetal period. Deviations during the fetal period are more likely to involve growth or functional aspects because these are the predominant developmental features at this time.

Figure 17–3 Group of curves representing the susceptibility of particular organs and organ systems in rat embryos to a hypothetical teratogenic agent given on different days of gestation. If the agent were applied on day 10, a syndrome comprised of organs the curves of which are intersected by the vertical line would result, with percentages of incidence corresponding to the points at which the curves were crossed. Shifting the time of treatment from day 10 to another day would alter the composition of the syndrome both qualitatively and quantitatively.

From Wilson, in Teratology: Principles and Techniques, *J. G. Wilson and J. Warkany, eds., Univ. Chicago Press, Chicago, 1965, pp. 251–261.*

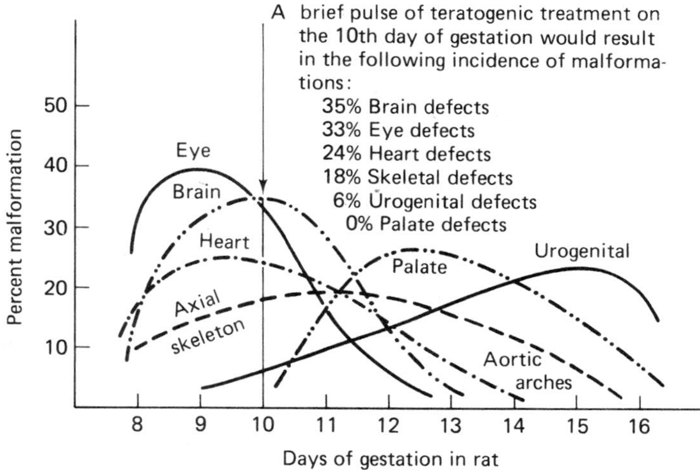

the starvation occurred early in gestation, the offspring showed an increased incidence of congenital malformations of the central nervous system. However, pregnant women subjected to undernutrition during the latter part of gestation had infants of low birth weight. Another example of time specificity was provided by experiments with zinc deficiency. Differences in the frequency of various types of malformations depended on the timing of the maternal dietary deficiency.

In addition to time specificity, there is also some degree of agent specificity. That is, not all nutrient deficiencies or excesses produce the same end results in development. Agent specificity derives from the specific interference of the nutritional insult with the metabolic machinery of either the mother or the embryo.

INTERACTIONS OF NUTRIENTS AND OTHER FACTORS

MATERNAL FACTORS

Maternal factors can influence the effect of nutritional deficiencies or excesses on prenatal development. For example, age of the mother, parity, or metabolic disorders can play a role in development of the embryo and fetus.

GENETIC FACTORS

The response to nutritional abnormality during prenatal life may vary with the genetic background of the developing individual. Thus, response to a less-than-optimal nutritional environment, either nutrient deficiency or excess, may be minimal or it may be very extreme. An example of such an interaction between the dietary level of a nutrient and the genetic background was seen in the effects of manganese deficiency during prenatal life in various strains of mice. Some strains responded with an extreme aberration of normal development, while in others the response was very much less evident.

Genetic influence on the effects of a nutritional deficiency may also explain the variable incidence of endemic cretinism, since this disorder has occurred historically in only a few of the regions where iodine deficiency goiter is endemic. An interaction of iodine intake with genetic factors would seem to be important in this condition.

There may also be interactions of nutritional and genetic factors that may prevent the development of genetic defects. This has been demonstrated in animal models with manganese and copper but remains to be applied to human problems, unless the endemic cretinism example may serve in this connection also.

OTHER INTERACTIONS

Other interactions may also play a role in the production of congenital abnormalities. Nutrients and drugs may interact to produce aberrations of development. For example, certain drugs influence absorption or metabolism of nutrients and may cause a conditioned deficiency at a particular time in gestation.

Nutritional factors may also interact with atmospheric or other environmental toxicants. For example, lead, cadmium, and other trace elements from air pollution may interact with essential trace elements to cause abnormal amounts of these nutrients (either deficiency or excess) to be available to the embryo or fetus. Thus, nutritional deficiencies (or excesses) for the embryo could result despite a normal dietary intake by the mother.

Nutrients may also interact with other essential nutrients or with other components of the diet to influence absorption or metabolism. Such interactions could also result in conditioned deficiencies. An example of such an interaction is the decreased absorption of zinc, iron, and other minerals that occurs in the presence of high-phytate or high-fiber diets, such as the type of diet eaten in the Middle East where zinc deficiency occurs.

Finally, there are undoubtedly multifactorial interactions among nutrients, genes, drugs, environmental components, and various factors in the diet. Such an interplay could produce temporary deficiencies or excesses of essential nutrients for the embryo and fetus and thus lead to abnormal development.

References and Supplementary Readings

ROUX, C., P. FOURNIER, Y. DUPUIS, AND R. DUPUIS. "Carence tératogène en vitamine A." *Biol. Neonat.* **4**: 371–378 (1962).

WILSON, J. G. *Environment and Birth Defects.* New York: Academic Press, 1973.

WILSON, J. G., AND F. C. FRASER, eds. *Handbook of Teratology.* New York: Plenum Publishing Corp., 1977.

18

The maternal organism

In previous chapters we have been concerned with the influence of nutritional factors during prenatal life upon the development of the embryo and fetus. In this chapter we will consider the role of maternal nutrition in terms of the pregnant woman herself. As we have seen from preceding sections, the mammalian embryo and fetus cannot be thought of as a perfect parasite. Furthermore, the developing organism is not attached to an unchanging maternal body. On the contrary, as Thomson and Hytten have pointed out, "The relationship is a complex form of symbiosis in which many aspects of physiology undergo such extensive modification that the pregnant female behaves almost as a distinct species."

PHYSIOLOGICAL ADAPTATION OF THE MATERNAL BODY TO PREGNANCY

PLASMA VOLUME

During pregnancy, there is a marked change in the plasma volume in the mother, with a total increase of about 50%. Figure 18–1 shows the changes in plasma volume that occurred in a group of healthy women in their first pregnancy. Since plasma volume is related to body size, the individual values were adjusted for mean height and weight. The increase in plasma volume shows a peak at about 34 weeks of pregnancy. For multigravidae (second or more pregnancy), the increase in plasma volume is even greater than shown in this figure. Birth weight of the baby correlates with increase in plasma volume of the mother. If the baby has a low birth weight, the increase in plasma volume is usually small. Women with a his-

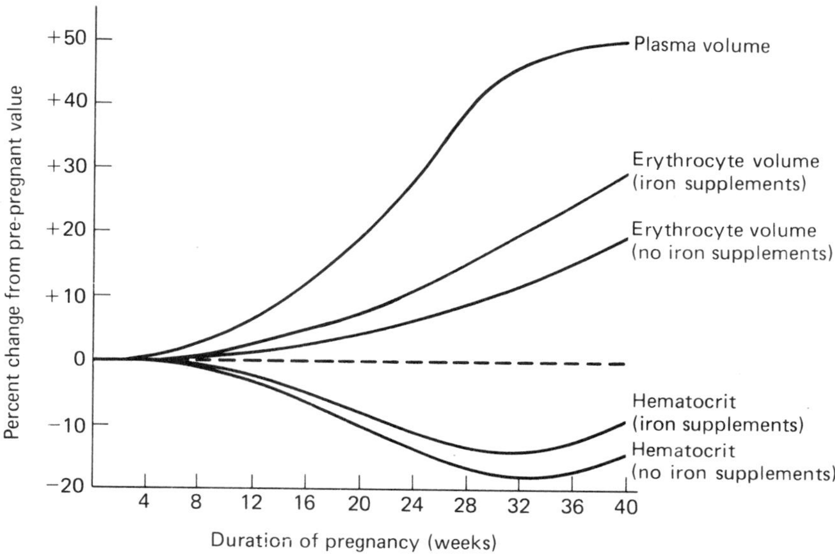

From Pitkin, 1976.

Figure 18–1 Plasma and erythrocyte volume increase and change in hematocrit during pregnancy.

tory of stillbirth, abortion, or low-birth-weight babies also have a smaller increase in plasma volume than do normal mothers.

RED-CELL VOLUME AND HEMOGLOBIN

Changes also occur in the volume of the red cells and in the hematocrit (packed-cell volume). Hemoglobin concentration falls during pregnancy as well, with the minimum concentration reached at about 30 to 32 weeks. This fall in hemoglobin concentration is apparently caused by the relatively greater increase of plasma volume than of red-cell volume. The concentration of hemoglobin in the red cell itself is probably the same in the pregnant as in the nonpregnant state. However, iron supplementation during pregnancy does increase the hemoglobin concentration, sometimes even to nonpregnant levels. Supplementary iron also modifies the usual fall in packed-cell volume and red-cell count seen in pregnant women. It thus seems that the decreased hemoglobin concentration often seen in pregnancy is a sign of iron deficiency.

The composition of the blood changes during pregnancy in other respects as well as those already described. The concentrations of various blood proteins, lipids, and enzymes all are altered during pregnancy.

CARDIAC AND RESPIRATORY FUNCTION

During pregnancy there is increased cardiac output, with enlargement of the heart and increased blood flow. The increased blood flow is regional, so that there is increased circulation to the uterus, kidneys, and skin. Respiratory function also changes, with a rise in ventilation rate and oxygen consumption. The increased oxygen consumption derives from the larger body size. With the greater cardiac output and respiratory work of a larger size, there is augmented use of oxygen (see Figure 18–2). There is also an increase in both the basal metabolic rate and the overall metabolism.

RENAL AND GASTROINTESTINAL FUNCTION

Renal function also undergoes adaptation during pregnancy. Renal blood flow, glomerular filtration rate, and clearance of waste products all are increased during pregnancy. On the other hand, the kidney also seems to excrete many nutrients more readily. Amino acids, glucose, iodine, ascorbic acid, and possibly vitamin B_{12} and folate are all excreted at a more rapid rate in pregnant than in nonpregnant women. Water, however, is not excreted as well during pregnancy as in the nonpregnant state.

In the gastrointestinal tract there is reduced gastric motility, but at the

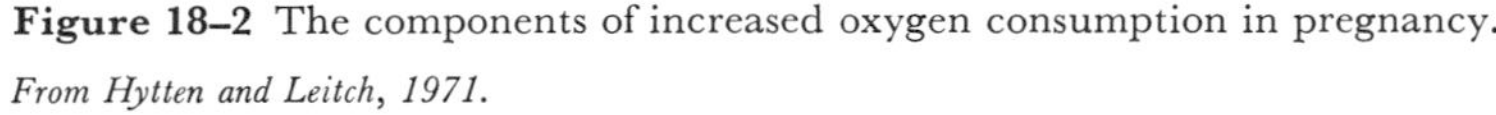

Figure 18–2 The components of increased oxygen consumption in pregnancy. *From Hytten and Leitch, 1971.*

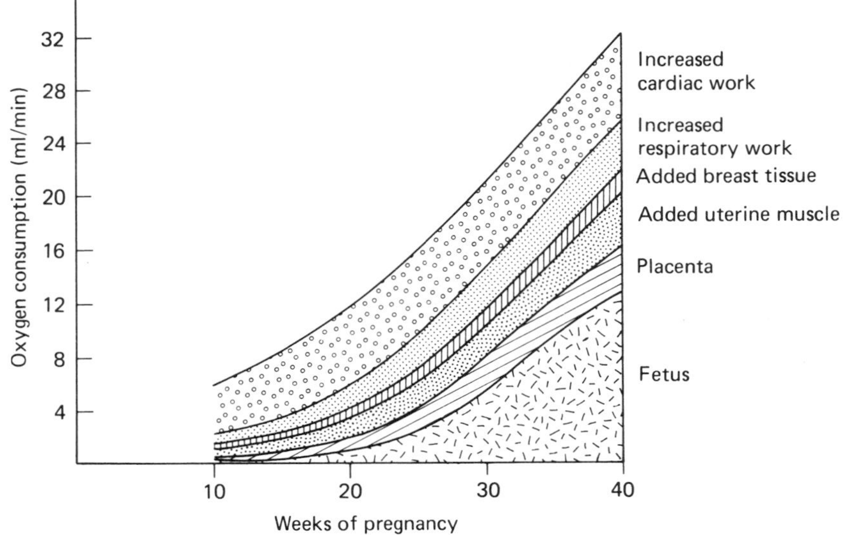

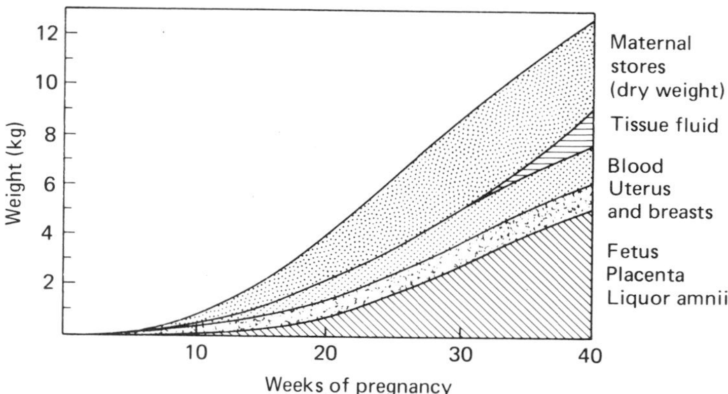

From NRC, Maternal Nutrition and the Course of Pregnancy, *1970.*

Figure 18–3 The components of weight gain in normal pregnancy.

same time, improved intestinal absorption of nutrients is characteristic of pregnancy.

BODY WEIGHT GAIN

During pregnancy there is, of course, an increase in the body weight of the mother. This gain in body weight is derived from both the products of conception and the mother's body tissues. Figure 18–3 summarizes the components of weight gain in normal pregnancy, and Table 18–1 shows the gains made by these various components during the course of pregnancy. At term (40 weeks) the average gain in maternal body weight is 12.5 kg, of which the fetus, placenta, and amniotic fluid, as well as the maternal tissue fluid, account for 7.3 kg. The rest of the body weight gain, which is not accounted for by these increments, represents maternal stores.

Not only is the maternal body producing the fetus and placenta, but many maternal organs are also increasing in size. There is a substantial increase in mass of the uterus and breasts, and, in addition, as noted above, the blood volume is enlarged, the heart increases in size, and other changes occur. Part of the maternal weight gain that is unaccounted for reflects the increased size of the mother's internal organs. However, about 4 kg of maternal weight gain is due to increased storage of fat.

It is interesting that most of the weight gain attributable to the developing new individual occurs during the second half of pregnancy, when the fetus is growing at a very rapid rate. The maternal stores, however, increase in quantity most rapidly before the middle of pregnancy and seem to stop enlarging before term. Measurements of skin-fold thickness in pregnant women have shown progressive increases on the abdomen, back, and upper

TABLE 18–1 ANALYSIS OF WEIGHT GAIN

Tissues and Fluids Accounted for and Total Weight Gained	*Increase in Weight (g) Up to:*			
	10 Weeks	*20 Weeks*	*30 Weeks*	*40 Weeks*
Fetus	5	300	1500	3400
Placenta	20	170	430	650
Amniotic fluid	30	350	750	800
Uterus	140	320	600	970
Mammary gland	45	180	360	405
Blood	100	600	1300	1250
Extracellular extravascular fluid:				
(1) No edema or leg edema	0	30	80	1680
(2) Generalized edema	0	500	1526	4897
Total:				
(1) No edema or leg edema	340	1950	5020	9155
(2) Generalized edema	340	2420	6466	12372
Total weight gained:				
(1) No edema or leg edema	650	4000	8500	12500
(2) Generalized edema	650	4500	10000	14500
Weight not accounted for:				
(1) No edema or leg edema	310	2050	3480	3345
(2) Generalized edema	310	2080	3534	2128

From Hytten and Leitch, 1971.

thighs from weeks 10 to 30 of pregnancy and then remained stationary. These maternal stores seem to be a preparation for possibly insufficient energy intake during the latter part of pregnancy, when the caloric requirement for the rapidly growing fetus is at its highest level. They also provide a safety factor for the subsequently high requirement for calories during lactation. Thus, an increased accumulation of body fat in the pregnant woman could help to protect the late gestational fetus and the newborn infant from undernutrition at these crucial periods.

This hypothesis is consistent with observations from poorly nourished mothers, who showed a much lower increase in body weight gain than occurred in normal pregnancies. The average weight gained by malnourished women in southern India was little more than half that of the average pregnant women shown in Figure 18–4, and the shape of the curve was different. Although birth weight, as well as the weight of placenta and amniotic fluid, were lower than normal, the major difference between the

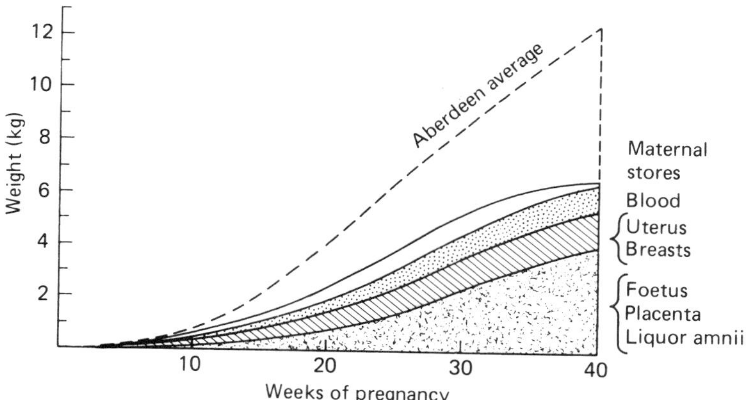

From Hytten and Leitch, 1971.

Figure 18–4 Possible components of weight gained by poor Indian women. Compare with Figure 18–3.

components of weight in the poorly nourished and in the normal women was in the size of the maternal stores. The Indian women were apparently able to store a small amount of fat in early pregnancy, but most of this had been used up by the end of pregnancy.

In a two-year study of pregnant women in Africa, it was found that body weight changes could be related to the season of the year. During the dry season, body weight gain was normal, but in the rainy season, weight gain decreased. The rainy season in this area was the period of heavy agricultural work, for which the women were responsible. Because of a high caloric expenditure together with a limited food supply, the maternal stores were depleted, and the women experienced a decrease in their rate of gain (Figure 18–5).

DIETARY NEEDS IN PREGNANCY

CALORIES

The amount of weight gain during pregnancy that is normal or optimal has received considerable attention. For many years the customary practice was to limit the weight gain of the pregnant woman—in other words, to give her a restricted caloric intake. However, the present recommendation is that caloric intake should not be limited. The Committee on Maternal Nutrition of the National Research Council has recommended that the average weight gain during pregnancy be approximately 24 pounds (11 kg).

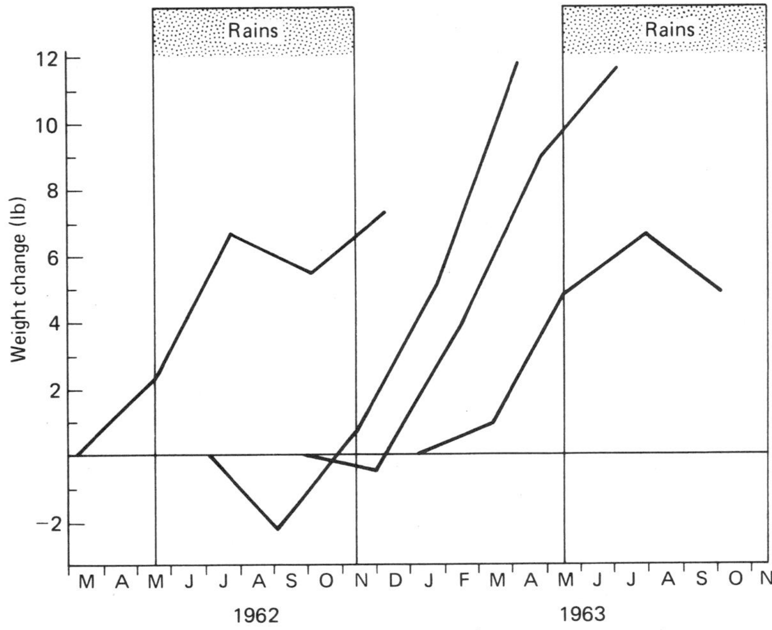

From Hytten and Leitch, 1971.

Figure 18–5 Weight changes during pregnancy in Gambian women by season when parturition occurred.

The weight gain should be in the pattern of a steady increase of one-half to one pound per week.

The relationship of maternal weight gain to birth weight of the infant is now well established, and the likelihood of a low-birth-weight infant is increased substantially if maternal weight gain is inadequate. The past few generations of American physicians have attempted to limit weight gain during pregnancy with the idea that caloric restriction protects against the development of toxemia of pregnancy, as well as preventing the birth of a large baby. This idea, based on an extremely limited study made by a German physician in 1889, has been shown to be erroneous. The original purpose of such procedures was to produce small babies that could be delivered more easily for women with contracted pelvis, a condition quite prevalent at that time.

The recommended dietary allowances (RDA) of the Food and Nutrition Board of the National Research Council for pregnant and nonpregnant women are summarized in Table 18–2. Like all dietary allowances, these are intended only as guides or goals. The RDA's for pregnancy are based on a healthy woman, 58 kg of body weight (128 lb), aged 19 to 22 years. The

RDA's for pregnant women are for semisedentary populations. Obviously, the allowances for women who are more or less active will require appropriate adjustments.

PROTEIN

The need for additional protein during pregnancy is clear, since amino acids from dietary protein are required for the increased synthesis of both maternal and fetal tissues. The current RDA is 30 g of protein per day above the allowance for the nonpregnant woman. For total protein during

TABLE 18–2 RECOMMENDED DIETARY ALLOWANCES

	Nonpregnant Females					
	11–14 yr[a]	*15–18 yr*[b]	*19–22 yr*[c]	*23–50 yr*[c]	*Pregnancy*	*Lactation*
Energy (kcal)	2400	2100	2100	2000	+ 300	+ 500
Protein (g)	44	48	46	46	+ 30	+ 20
Vitamin A (IU)	4000	4000	4000	4000	5000	6000
Vitamin D (IU)	400	400	400	—[d]	400	400
Vitamin E (IU)	12	12	12	12	15	15
Ascorbic acid (mg)	45	45	45	45	60	80
Folacin (μg)	400	400	400	400	800	600
Niacin (mg)	16	14	14	13	+ 2	+ 4
Riboflavin (mg)	1.3	1.4	1.4	1.2	+ 0.3	+ 0.5
Thiamin (mg)	1.2	1.1	1.1	1.0	+ 0.3	+ 0.3
Vitamin B_6 (mg)	1.6	2.0	2.0	2.0	2.5	2.5
Vitamin B_{12} (μg)	3	3	3	3	4	4
Calcium (mg)	1200	1200	800	800	1200	1200
Phosphorous (mg)	1200	1200	800	800	1200	1200
Iodine (μg)	115	115	100	100	125	150
Iron (mg)	18	18	18	18	18+[e]	18
Magnesium (mg)	300	300	300	300	450	450
Zinc (mg)	15	15	15	15	20	25

[a]Weight 44 kg (97 lb), height 155 cm (62 in).

[b]Weight 54 kg (119 lb), height 162 cm (65 in).

[c]Weight 58 kg (128 lb), height 162 cm (65 in).

[d]The requirement for the normal healthy adult seems to be satisfied by nondietary sources.

[e]This increased requirement cannot usually be met by ordinary diets; therefore, the use of supplemental iron is recommended.

NRC, Recommended Dietary Allowances, *1974.*

pregnancy, therefore, the RDA is 1.3 g/kg/day for the mature woman, 1.5 g/kg/day for the adolescent aged 15 to 18, and 1.7 g/kg/day for the pregnant girl under 15.

CALCIUM

The fetus at term contains an average of 27 g of calcium. The placenta contains amounts up to 1 g, and the increased maternal tissues and fluids also contain approximately 1 g of calcium. Thus, the total minimum requirement for this element in pregnancy is about 30 g. Most of the calcium accretion occurs in late pregnancy with calcification of the fetal skeleton, making the daily increment about 300 mg during the third trimester. If the intake of calcium is above minimum requirements, some storage in the maternal skeleton appears to take place, presumably in anticipation of the very high need for calcium during lactation.

Establishment of the minimal or optimal intake of calcium during pregnancy is extremely difficult, and the subject is still very controversial. The RDA for calcium in pregnancy is 1200 mg, which represents an increase of 400 mg above the allowance for the nonpregnant adult.

VITAMIN D

Although vitamin D is important for calcium absorption and metabolism, the vitamin D requirement is not higher during pregnancy than in the nonpregnant state.

IRON

The developing and growing fetus and the increased volume of maternal blood bring about a requirement for additional iron during pregnancy (see Table 18–3). Thus, despite the iron that is no longer lost to the maternal body because of the cessation of menstruation, the pregnant woman needs

TABLE 18–3 IRON BALANCE DURING PREGNANCY

Extra iron (mg) in:	
Product of conception	370
Maternal blood	290
Total	660
Less iron (mg) "saved" by cessation of menstruation	120
Total	540

From NRC, Maternal Nutrition and the Course of Pregnancy, *1970.*

to absorb 540 mg of iron during her pregnancy. Furthermore, the erythrocyte volume and hematocrit of the pregnant woman may be increased above their normally low levels (see the section on red-cell volume and hemoglobin above) by additional provision of iron.

If adequate iron is available, an average of 500 mg will be used for maternal blood during pregnancy. The total requirement for this element during pregnancy is therefore as much as 600 to 800 mg. It is probable that the usual absorption rate of 10% for dietary iron is increased during pregnancy, but it is nevertheless unlikely that the present American diet can provide an adequate intake to meet the needs of pregnancy. Accordingly, it is recommended that pregnant women receive 30 to 60 mg of iron supplementation daily in addition to their dietary iron.

FOLATE

There is now considerable evidence that folate requirements are higher than usual during pregnancy. The increased demand for folate for the synthesis of new tissue represents the most important factor in the higher requirement. The augmented maternal erythropoiesis of pregnancy in itself requires additional amounts of folate. During normal pregnancy the maternal serum folate level declines progressively. At the same time, the incidence of megaloblastic marrow in pregnant women follows a pattern similar to that of the fetal growth curve, suggesting a high incidence of folate deficiency (see also Chapter 12). Dietary survey data suggest that the usual American diet is marginal in folate content, which is consistent with the hematological findings. The RDA for folate is 400 mg/day during pregnancy. Many experts consider folate to be a critical nutrient for pregnant women and recommend supplements of 200 to 400 μg/day.

SODIUM

Sodium, the major electrolyte in extracellular fluid, is retained during pregnancy. This is a normal physiologic adjustment to pregnancy and is related to the increased fluid volume, including the larger amount of blood. In addition, the development of the fetus and the placenta also require sodium. There is thus a required retention of about 25 g of additional sodium. This can be broken down to 100 mg/day in early pregnancy and 200 mg/day near term.

The older and more traditional view of sodium balance in pregnancy was that sodium retention might lead to edema and toxemia. Intake of sodium was therefore restricted, and diuretics were often used. The present view is that since there is a greater need for sodium as well as enhanced sodium excretion during pregnancy, sodium intake should also be increased,

TABLE 18–4 SCREENING CRITERIA FOR WOMEN AT HIGH NUTRITIONAL RISK

I. LIKELY TO NEED THERAPEUTIC DIETS

Maternal Weight
- Obesity
- Low prepregnancy weight
- Insufficient weight gain during pregnancy

Poor Obstetrical History
- History of low-birth-weight infants
- Other poor outcomes:
  - Past difficulty with conception, especially if associated with weight deviation
  - Repeated spontaneous abortion
  - Stillbirth
  - Neonatal death
  - Abruptio placenta
  - Spontaneous premature labor
- Toxemia, preeclampsia, or eclampsia
- Previous cesarian section or therapeutic abortion

Addictions
- Heroin
- Alcohol
- Pica

Preexisting Medical Complications or Those Developing During Gestation
- Diabetes mellitus: overt or gestational diabetes
- Anemia (especially iron deficiency and folate deficiency)
- Preexisting heart disease
- Infectious disease, especially:
  - chronic asymptomatic conditions such as pulmonary and renal tuberculosis
  - asymptomatic bacteruria
- Liver disease:
  - viral hepatitis
  - history of other liver disease
  - drug addiction
- Gastrointestinal disease:
  - cholelithiasis, cholecystitis
  - pancreatitis and pancreatic insufficiency
  - hiatus hernia
  - peptic ulcer
  - gastric atrophy
  - regional ileitis
  - ulcerative colitis
  - protein-losing enteropathy
  - disaccharide intolerance
  - major gastric or bowel resection
  - intestinal parasitism with malabsorption
- Preexisting hypertension or renal disease (including collagen vascular disorders)
- Other:
  - poorly controlled hyperthyroidism
  - hyperlipemias
  - certain inborn errors of metabolism (phenylketonuria, cystinuria, Wilson's disease)

II. LIKELY TO NEED LENGTHY NUTRITION COUNSELING

Age, Parity, and Short Interconceptional Period
- Adolescents, particularly if pregnant and under 17
- Short interconceptional periods or high multiparity

Low Income or Limited Food Budget
- Low income
- Other situations in which food budget is limited, such as

From Dwyer, 1974.

TABLE 18–4 (cont.)

large families or nonsupport, compulsive gambling, drinking or drug addiction by spouse

Ethnic or Language Problems

Unusual Eating Habits
- Vegetarians
- Health food enthusiasts
- Certain religious groups with special food proscriptions

Inadequate Knowledge of Nutrition or Food Resource Management
- Limited knowledge or ability to make required dietary changes with ordinary counseling (e.g., low I.Q., illiteracy, etc.)
- Special family food management problems (e.g., handicapped, one-parent household)
- Inaccessibility or lack of knowledge of food distribution programs among eligibles
- Lack of budgeting or cooking skills
- Lack of infant feeding skill

Poor Somatic Growth Among Offspring

III. LIKELY TO NEED SOME NUTRITIONAL ADVICE OF A SPECIAL NATURE

Smokers Who are Giving Up the Habit
Twin Pregnancy
Out-of-Wedlock Pregnancy
Emotional Stress or Disturbance
Dwellers in Area Where Food Distribution Programs Are Lacking or Badly Operated

which will occur normally through greater food intake. Thus the present recommendation is that sodium intake should neither be restricted nor supplemented during pregnancy.

CRITERIA OF A SUCCESSFUL PREGNANCY

The Committee on Maternal Nutrition of the National Research Council has summarized the criteria of a successful pregnancy as follows:

1. A normal, uneventful pregnancy with a weight-gain average of about 24 lb or 11 kg.
2. Normal hematologic values.
3. Uncomplicated delivery.
4. Normal, healthy, full-term infant.
5. Prompt onset of lactation.
6. Normal growth of the neonatal child.

This Committee has in addition recommended for pregnant women the following:

1. Calories should not be restricted. The woman who is overweight should not be reduced while she is pregnant, but the reduction of body weight should take place after pregnancy is completed.
2. Salt should not be restricted.

3. Diuretics should not be prescribed.
4. An unbalanced weight gain should be avoided.
5. The diet should be supplemented with folate, iron, and iodine (with salt).

Screening criteria for women at high nutritional risk have been tabulated by Dwyer (Table 18–4, page 250).

References and Supplementary Readings

DWYER, J. T., AND H. N. JACOBSON, eds. "Maternal nutrition—its implications for health officers, part two." *Public Health Currents* **14**: 1–5 (1974), Ross Laboratories, Columbus, Ohio.

HYTTEN, F. E., AND I. LEITCH. *The Physiology of Human Pregnancy*, 2nd ed. London: Blackwell Scientific Publications, 1971.

Maternal Nutrition and the Course of Pregnancy. Washington, D.C.: Committee on Maternal Nutrition/Food and Nutrition Board, National Research Council, National Academy of Sciences, 1970, pages 63 and 68.

MOSLEY, W. H., ed. *Nutrition and Human Reproduction*. New York: Plenum Press, 1978.

PIKE, R. L., AND D. S. GURSKY. "Further evidence of deleterious effects produced by sodium restriction during pregnancy." *Am. J. Clin. Nutr.* **23**: 883–889 (1970).

PITKIN, R. M. "Nutritional support in obstetrics and gynecology." *Clin. Obstet. Gynec.* **19**: 489–513 (1976).

Recommended Dietary Allowances, 8th ed. Washington, D.C.: Food and Nutrition Board, National Research Council, National Academy of Sciences, 1974.

THOMSON, A. M., AND F. E. HYTTEN. "Effects of nutrition on human reproduction." *J. Reprod. Fert.*, Suppl. **19**: 581–583 (1973).

III

Nutrition in Infancy and Childhood

19

Nutrition of the infancy period

For some time after birth in mammalian species the only food of the newborn is milk. Even beyond the immediate neonatal period, milk remains a major source of nutrients, and in some human groups throughout childhood. It is therefore important to examine the composition of milk and to consider the influence of nutrition on lactation itself.

LACTATION

COMPOSITION OF MILK

General composition. Milk is composed of water, a fatty fraction, and nonfat solids. The fatty fraction consists of triglycerides and other fat-soluble compounds, including phospholipids, sterols, fat-soluble vitamins, and carotenoids. The nonfat solids are divided into lactose (the carbohydrate of milk) and nitrogenous materials. The latter consist of the proteins casein, albumin, and globulin, proteoses and peptones, and certain enzymes. In addition, milk also contains minerals, water-soluble vitamins, and certain nonprotein compounds (Figure 19–1). Casein is the major protein of milk; albumin, also called lactalbumin, is the protein in second highest concentration. Milk can be distinguished by at least three particular materials that are unique to it: casein, lactose, and butterfat.

Species differences. The composition of milk varies in different species and is correlated with the growth rate of the offspring. Table 19–1 shows the relationship between growth rate and milk composition. The time required for the newborn animal to double its birth weight is shown for a number of species and is compared with the protein and ash concentration of the milk. The amount of protein and ash varies inversely with the time necessary for doubling of birth weight. These variations may be related to differences in

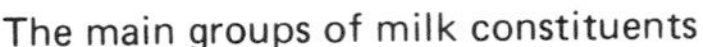

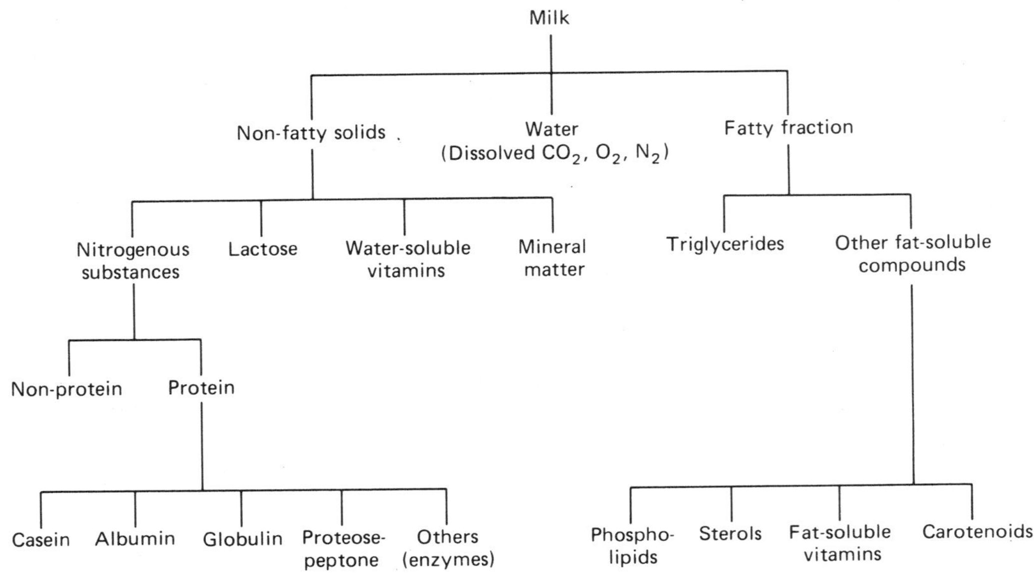

From Ling et al., in Kon and Cowie, 1961.

Figure 19–1 The main groups of milk constituents.

body surface area per body weight rather than to body weight itself. Blaxter has pointed out that although the adult weights range from that of the mare, 800 kg, to that of the cat, 2 kg (Table 19–1), body surface area per kilogram varies by a factor of about 6, and the protein content of the milk varies in the same direction by a factor of 5.

Composition of milk also varies with respect to the general environment of the animal (Table 19–2). For example, the kangaroo rat, a desert animal with very limited water supplies available to it, has a milk low in water concentration, 50% water. The dairy cow, in contrast, produces milk that is 88% water. The fat concentration, conversely, is extremely high in the kangaroo rat's milk, 23.5%, as compared to 3% in cow's milk.

Human milk. Since the natural food of human infants is human milk, it is useful to compare the composition of human milk with that of the commonly used cow's milk. As can be seen in Table 19–3, there are differences in the composition of milk as lactation proceeds. Colostrum (not shown in the table) is secreted by the mammary gland within the first three to five days of lactation and has a composition different from that of mature milk. The caloric value of colostrum as well as its fat and lactose concentrations are lower than those of mature milk, while ash and protein concentrations are almost twice those of mature milk. An important component of colostrum is its rich concentration of antibodies, which provide valuable protection to the infant against infection. During the course of lactation, even after the establishment of mature milk, the composition of milk continues to change. Concentrations of protein, ash, calcium, phosphorus, sodium, potassium, and zinc decrease with the advance of lactation.

TABLE 19–1 BUNGE'S (1898) ORIGINAL TABLE SHOWING THE RELATIONSHIP BETWEEN GROWTH AND MILK COMPOSITION

Species	*Time in Days for Newborn Animal to Double its Birth Weight*	*100 Parts of Milk Contain (parts)*	
		Protein	*Ash*
Man	180	1.6	0.2
Horse	60	2.0	0.4
Ox	47	3.5	0.7
Goat	19	4.3	0.8
Pig	18	5.9	—
Sheep	10	6.5	0.9
Dog	8	7.1	1.3
Cat	7	9.5	—
Additional Fast-Growing Species Not Included in Bunge's Table			
Rabbit	6	14.0	2.2
Rat	6	12.0	2.0

From Blaxter, in Kon and Cowie, 1961.

TABLE 19–2 COMPOSITION OF MILK

	Water, %	*Fat,* %
Kangaroo rat	50	24
Dairy cow	87	4
Camel	88	?
Harp seal	44	43
California sea lion	47	37
Blue whale	47	38

From Kooyman, 1963.

TABLE 19–3 COMPOSITION OF HUMAN MILK AT VARIOUS STAGES OF LACTATION[a]

	Proximate Analysis (g/liter)					*Non-protein*	*Minerals (mg/liter)*						
Stage of Lactation	*Total Solids*	*Protein (N × 6.25)*	*Fat*	*Carbo-hydrate*	*Ash*	*Nitrogen (g/liter)*	*Cal-cium*	*Phos-phorus*	*Mag-nesium*	*Sodium*	*Potas-sium*	*Chlo-ride*	*Zinc*
14th day:													
Mean	126.5	15.4	26.3	83.2	2.32	0.49	278	188	30	204	421	410	3.7
S.D.	12.2	1.8	9.1	9.0	0.28	0.13	45	33	3	58	90	119	1.2
28th day:													
Mean	127.6	13.8	29.4	82.3	2.18	0.40	261	169	28	161	347	441	2.6
S.D.	14.6	1.8	12.3	11.1	0.47	0.13	64	45	5	62	121	193	1.1
42nd day:													
Mean	122.7	12.6	26.8	81.3	1.81	0.41	255	151	28	151	367	427	2.2
S.D.	17.3	1.4	15.9	12.0	0.52	0.12	78	30	4	64	129	137	0.9
56th day:													
Mean	116.1	10.9	22.3	80.7	2.15	0.46	266	150	31	135	374	378	2.0
S.D.	16.8	1.8	11.9	12.5	0.60	0.16	56	28	6	79	66	98	0.7
84th day:													
Mean	116.6	10.2	21.0	88.4	2.22	0.38	247	130	30	125	343	406	2.0
S.D.	17.0	2.6	13.3	14.5	0.54	0.11	56	33	6	52	90	165	1.2
112th day:													
Mean	127.7	8.7	28.4	88.6	1.84	0.32	236	132	32	120	296	399	1.1
S.D.	25.5	2.6	12.5	18.5	0.83	0.09	38	26	5	48	129	147	0.5

[a]Seventeen healthy women at each stage except 112 days; 12 women at stage 112 days.

From Fomon, 1974.

Human and cow's milk compared. Since most artificial formulas for infants (that is, preparations other than human milk) are based on cow's milk, a comparison of the composition of human and cow's milk is appropriate (see Table 19–4). The water content of these two milks as well as their caloric value is similar. However, there are also some important differences. Cow's milk contains almost four times as much protein, approximately three times as much calcium, and six times as much phosphorus as human milk. Until recently it was stated that breast milk contained 1.1 to 1.2% protein. More modern analysis, not including nonprotein nitrogen, established the protein content to be 0.8 to 0.9%. Cow's milk also contains about five times as much riboflavin as human milk. Human milk, on the other hand, is 1.5 times as high in carbohydrate value as cow's milk. In addition, lactose, vitamin D, vitamin E, and ascorbic acid concentrations are all higher in human than in cow's milk. It should be noted that the composition of human milk varies considerably from one individual to another for certain nutrients, as well as varying with the stage of lactation.

There are also marked differences between human and cow's milk in the composition of their proteins. The amino acid profiles are quite different, with higher levels of cystine and lower concentrations of tyrosine, phenylalanine, and tryptophan in human milk. In addition, human milk contains lactoferrin, an iron-binding protein, in considerable amount, and lysozyme, while cow's milk has only traces of these compounds. On the other hand, cow's milk contains a fairly large amount of β-lactoglobulin, which does not occur at all in human milk.

The lipid components in human and cow's milk also differ (see Table 19–5). Cow's milk is higher in saturated fatty acids, while human milk is higher in unsaturated fatty acids.

In addition to these dissimilarities between human and cow's milk in chemical composition, there are important differences in other properties. The principal protein in cow's milk, casein, forms a relatively firm curd in the stomach even when it is pasteurized and homogenized. This hard curd is not easily digested by the infant's still immature digestive tract. Lactalbumin, the chief protein in human milk, during digestion forms a soft curd that a baby can easily digest and absorb. Another difference between the two types of milk is the high level of lactose in human milk, which is favorable to the absorption of calcium. The feeding of human milk also promotes establishment of a gastrointestinal flora that is advantageous to the infant.

It should be noted that breast milk can also provide a vehicle for the transmission of toxic substances to the infant. In fact, nearly all substances received by a lactating woman will be found in her milk. In some cases, for example, considerable amounts of a drug taken by the mother may be excreted in her milk.

TABLE 19–4 CONTENT PER LITER OF DIFFERENT NUTRIENTS IN HUMAN BREAST MILK, COW'S MILK, EVAPORATED COW'S MILK, AND THREE PROPRIETARY MILKS

				Artificial Formulas		
	Human Breast Milk	*Cow's Milk*	*Evaporated Cow's Milk*	*I (Conventional) Nonfat Milk, Vegetable Oils, Carbohydrate (Lactose)*	*II ("Humanized") Nonfat Milk, Demineralized Whey, Vegetable Oils, and Carbohydrate*	*III ("Milk-free") Soy Flour, Vegetable Oils, Corn Syrup and/or Sucrose*
Energy (kcal)	690	660	1520	700	700	700
Protein (g)	9	35	73	15	15	31
Fat (g)	45	37	82	37	36	26–36
Carbohydrate (g)	68	49	106	70	72	52–77
lactose (g)	68	49	106	70	72	—
Ash (g)	2	7	16	4	3	5–8
Minerals						
Calcium (mg)	340	1170	2750	536	445	1060–1200
Phosphorus (mg)	140	920	2112	454	300	530–800
Sodium (mEq)	7	22	55	11	6	10–22
Potassium (mEq)	13	35	77	19	14	33–41
Chloride (mEq)	11	29	46	12	10	14–16

Magnesium (mg)	40	120	—	40–48	53	—
Sulfur (mg)	140	300	—	130–160	145	—
Iron (mg)	5	5	22	1.5	13	5–8
Iodine (μg)	30	47	—	40–69	69	—
Manganese (μg)	7–15	20–40	—	—	—	—
Copper (mg)	0.4	0.3	—	0.4–0.6	0.4	—
Zinc (mg)	3–5	3–5	—	2–4	3	—
Selenium (μg)	13–50	5–50	—	—	—	—
Vitamins						
A (IU)	1898	1025	1850	1650	2650	1590–2110
Thiamin (μg)	160	440	280	510	710	530
Riboflavin (μg)	360	1750	1900	620	1060	850–1060
Niacin (mg)	1.5	0.9	1	9	9	7–9
Pyridoxine (μg)	100	640	370	410	420	420
Folic acid (μg)	52	55	55	100	32	70
B_{12} (μg)	0.3	4	1–2	2	1	2
C (mg)	43	11	6	52	58	42–53
D (IU)	22	14	420	413	423	420
E (IU)	2	0.4	1	12	9	5–11
K (μg)	15	60	0–160	—	—	90
Examples of products				Enfamil Similac	SMA	Sobee MullSoy

From Hambraeus, 1977.

TABLE 19–5 DISTRIBUTION OF SOME OF THE LIPID COMPONENTS IN HUMAN AND COW'S MILK

	g/100 g Milk Fat in Mature Milk	
	Human	*Cow*
Total fat	3.8	3.7
Fatty acid distribution:		
Saturated fatty acids:		
Butyric	0.4	3.1
Caproic	0.1	1.0
Caprylic	0.3	1.2
Capric	1.7	2.6
Unsaturated fatty acids:		
Linoleic	8.3	1.6
Arachidonic	0.8	1.0

From Macy and Kelly, in Kon and Cowie, 1961.

Breast milk is not produced in maximal amount at the beginning of lactation. The newborn infant undergoes weight diminution after birth, owing partially to water loss on exposure to air after uterine life in the amniotic fluid. The body weight falls from birth for about three days, then increases back to birth weight about 10 days after birth. At the same time, the amount of breast milk produced increases, and growth (body weight) of the infant can be correlated with the quantity available.

INFLUENCE OF NUTRITION ON LACTATION

Studies on the effects of dietary intake on the quantity and quality of lactation in women have been concerned mainly with the relationship of nutritional intake to the composition of milk in regard to its major constitutents. The most striking generalization that can be made is that lactation is remarkably efficient and persistent even under conditions of extreme malnutrition. For example, lactation did occur among mothers subjected to the severe famine of the siege of Leningrad in World War II (see Chapter 7). In the World War II internment camps of Japan, and even at the Belsen concentration camp in Germany, breast feeding took place, although there is some indication that it was not normal.

A number of studies of lactating women, relating their dietary intakes to the composition of their milk, indicated that both the quantity of milk produced and its composition in major nutrients were satisfactory even though the diet was inadequate. The caloric intake of mothers in India who had an extremely poor dietary intake was only 70% of the recommended allowance of the Indian Council on Medical Research. Their protein intake was 40% of the recommended amount, while calcium intake was only about 22%, and vitamin A level 23%. Estimation of the quantity of milk produced by the women indicated that normal amounts were secreted, and in many of the women no weight loss occurred. In those who did lose weight, the amount lost was not very large and extended over nearly a year. The composition of the milk is summarized in Table 19–6 and compared with that from well-fed American women. It can be seen that protein, mineral matter, and calcium content were unaffected by the poor dietary intake of the women. However, there were differences in the concentrations of potassium, magnesium, vitamin A, riboflavin, and vitamin C. There also seemed to be a depression in the fat concentration in the milk of the poorly nourished Indian women. Bantu and Chimbu women who did not receive an adequate diet during lactation also produced milk that was low in fat (Table 19–6). Other studies have also shown a significant correlation between the fat content of a woman's diet and the concentration of fat in her milk.

Protein. The protein concentration of human milk is of importance and has received considerable attention because of the problem of protein calorie malnutrition (see Chapter 19). There is now ample evidence that the protein

TABLE 19–6 COMPOSITION OF HUMAN MILK IN RELATION TO DIETARY ADEQUACY

	Diet			
		Inadequate		
Constituents	*Adequate, U.S.A.*	*Indian*	*Bantu*	*Chimbu*
Solids, %	12.1	12.1	12.8	10.9
Fat, %	3.4	3.4	3.9	2.4
Lactose, %	7.5	7.5	7.1	7.3
Protein, %	1.1	1.1	1.4	1.0
Minerals, %	0.2	0.2	0.2	0.2
Calcium, mg/100 g	34.4	34.2	28.7	
Phosphorus, mg/100 g	14.1	11.9		
Potassium, mg/100 g	51.2	34.7		
Sodium, mg/100 g	17.2	22.1		
Magnesium, mg/100 g	3.5	2.6		
Vitamin A, IU/100 ml	201	70		
Thiamin, μg/100 ml	14.2	15.4		
Riboflavin, μg/100 ml	37.3	17.2		
Vitamin C, mg/100 ml	5.2	2.6		

Adapted from Gopalan and Belavady, 1961.

content of human milk is relatively unchanged by malnutrition of the mother and that therefore it could not influence the development of protein calorie malnutrition in children. The effect of protein supplementation to lactating women on diets with low protein content has also been studied. An increase in the protein intake from 61 to 99 g per day brought about an increase in the yield of milk. At the same time, the concentration of protein in the milk decreased somewhat, so that the overall milk protein produced in 24 hours was unchanged. In other studies, however, women who were existing on 15 to 20 g of protein per day during lactation did show an increased concentration of protein in milk when they were given a dietary protein supplement.

Calcium. As seen in Table 19–6, the calcium content of milk did not change with its intake in the diet even under conditions of extremely low intake. The relationships of calcium in the diet and in the maternal skeleton to the calcium output in milk are similar to those during pregnancy (see Chapter 13). However, the influence of dietary intake on the calcium content of milk is even less significant than that on the calcium content of the fetus in the pregnant state. Thus, although in pregnancy a diet extremely low in calcium will cause a decreased amount of calcification and calcium retention in the fetus, in lactation the amount of calcium in the milk seems to be entirely independent of the amount of calcium in the diet. This means, of course, that under conditions of dietary inadequacy of calcium there is a loss of this element from the maternal skeleton.

Even under conditions of adequate nutrition, it appears that there is some loss of calcium from the maternal skeleton during lactation. Most women are in negative calcium balance while lactating, and it is estimated that the loss of calcium sustained by the mother lactating for six months is about 7 to 8% of the maternal calcium reserve. It is therefore important that an adequate dietary intake of calcium be taken during pregnancy—that is, prior to lactation—as well as after the lactation period is over in order to replenish the calcium stores of the mother's body.

Iron. Relatively little information is available on the influence of dietary iron intake on the iron concentration of human milk, but milk is in general a poor source of iron. In poorly nourished Indian women there was no correlation between their hemoglobin level and the iron concentration of their milk samples.

Iodine. The iodine content of human milk seems to be greatly influenced by the dietary intake of the mother.

Vitamin A. There are numerous indications that vitamin A intake during lactation affects the vitamin A concentration of human milk. In the poorly nourished lactating women of India (see Table 19–6) the vitamin A concentration of the milk was considerably lower than that of American women. In addition, numerous reports (dating back as early as 1883) of xerophthalmia in breast-fed infants whose mothers were inadequately nourished indicate that the dietary intake of the mother was an important factor in the vitamin A content of her milk.

Vitamin D. Vitamin D content of breast milk seems to be little influenced by the maternal diet. Studies in which the dietary intake of vitamin D were compared with the vitamin D concentration of the breast milk did not show any correlation. Even when the mother's intake was high, it appeared that vitamin D was not readily transferred to her milk.

Thiamin. The thiamin content of human milk is also related to the dietary intake of the vitamin by the mother. Many studies have shown that supplementing the mother's diet with thiamin resulted in an increased concentration of thiamin in the milk.

Riboflavin. The riboflavin concentration of milk from poorly nourished Indian women (see Table 19–6) was about half that found in milk from American women. Other studies have also indicated that the riboflavin intake of the mother correlated with the riboflavin concentration of her milk.

Niacin. Relatively few studies are available on the relationship of maternal dietary intake to the niacin content of the milk. In one study, injection of nicotinamide in lactating women caused a rise within two hours in the nicotinamide content of their milk, especially when the original level was low.

Vitamin B_6. In rats, the pyridoxine concentration of the milk could be altered by the amount of the vitamin given the dam.

Ascorbic acid. The ascorbic acid content of human milk seems to be very clearly related to the dietary intake of the lactating woman. Table 19–6 shows that vitamin C concentration was lower in poorly nourished Indian women than in American women. Bantu women who were poorly nourished also showed low ascorbic acid concentration in their milk. The vitamin C level in milk from British women, whose intake of ascorbic acid is in general thought to be lower than that in the United States, was also lower than that of American women. Women who received a diet high in ascorbic acid produced milk with an amount of the vitamin several times the usual level. In a woman with scurvy, the vitamin C content of the breast milk was extremely low.

Thus, in general, the intake of water soluble vitamins by a lactating woman affects their content in breast milk.

Zinc. Little information is available on the influence of maternal diet on the zinc content of milk. In rat experiments, however, a diet extremely deficient in zinc during the lactation period resulted in a marked reduction in the zinc content of the milk (Figure 19–2).

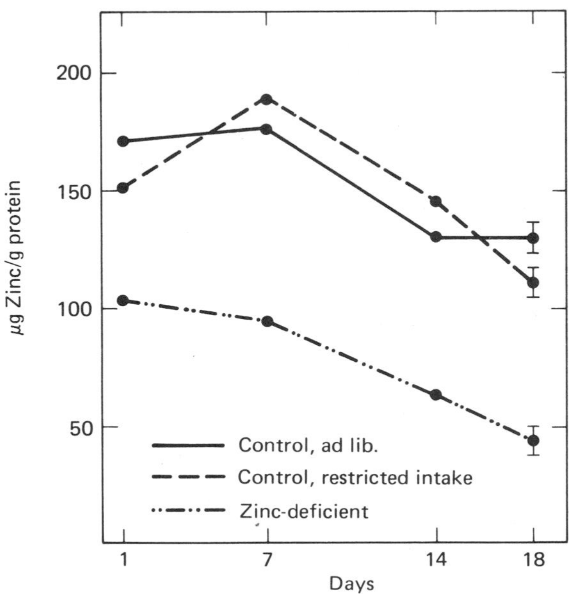

Adapted from Mutch and Hurley, 1974.

Figure 19–2 Rat milk zinc as related to protein concentration during lactation.

Magnesium. No information on the relationship of dietary magnesium intake and magnesium concentration of human milk is available. In rats, a magnesium-deficient diet during lactation caused a low level of magnesium in the milk.

NUTRITIONAL REQUIREMENTS DURING LACTATION

Nutritional requirements are higher during lactation than at any other stage of the life cycle. In addition to the needs for increased nutrients because of the amounts secreted in the milk, nutrients are needed to make up for the energy need involved in the synthesis of the milk and its components. Furthermore, if the nutrient intake is insufficient, losses from the mother's tissues may occur.

The energy requirement for lactation is proportional to the quantity of milk produced. The caloric value of human milk is about 67 to 77 kcal/100 ml, and the efficiency of conversion of maternal caloric value to milk calories is about 80%. Thus approximately 90 kcal are required for each 100 ml of milk. During pregnancy, body fat is stored that is later drawn upon to supply part of the additional energy needed for lactation. According to the

National Research Council, the recommended daily allowance for energy should be increased by 500 kcal/day during the first three months of lactation, with further additions beyond this time.

The recommended dietary allowance for protein during lactation is increased by 20 g per day above the maintenance amount recommended for a woman of a specific age and size. This is based upon a consideration of 70% efficiency of protein utilization to synthesize the additional protein of the milk.

The recommended dietary allowance for vitamin A is also increased above that of the pregnant, as well as the nonpregnant, female in order to provide sufficient vitamin A for the milk. Similarly, for most of the other vitamins and minerals, requirements and recommended dietary allowances are higher than at other stages of life (see Table 18–2).

The recommended dietary allowance for iron is not increased in lactation, since the iron concentration of milk is low. Furthermore, lactating women usually do not menstruate, so loss of iron from the body is minimal.

NUTRITION OF THE INFANT

NUTRITIONAL REQUIREMENTS OF INFANTS

Information on the nutritional requirements of infants for specific nutrients is still very limited. In addition, requirements often vary with age, size, rate of growth, and level of activity, as well as with the composition of the diet and the concentration of other nutrients. Thus, the amounts of specific nutrients that are recommended should not be interpreted too strictly.

Calories. The caloric requirements of the newborn are shown in Table 19–7. It is generally accepted that the basal metabolic need of newborn infants is approximately 48 kcal/kg/day. With additions for physical activity, fecal loss, specific dynamic action, and growth, the total requirement is 92 kcal/kg/day or 42 kcal/lb/day. For the premature newborn, 150 kcal/kg/day would be necessary.

Protein and amino acids. Fomon summarized estimated requirements and advisable intakes of protein for infants and children (see Table 19–8). The protein requirement during early infancy is highly correlated with both body size and rate of gain in body weight. Since caloric intake during ad libitum feeding is generally correlated with these same variables, it is reasonable to express protein requirements in relation to caloric intake.

Estimates of infants' requirements for amino acids are shown in Table 19–9, and a comparison with adult requirements is made. On a body-wieght

TABLE 19–7 APPROXIMATE CALORIC REQUIREMENTS OF PREMATURE AND TERM INFANTS AFTER THE FIRST WEEK OF LIFE

	Daily Caloric Requirements per Kg of Body Weight			
Individual Factors	*Premature Infants*		*Term Infants*	
Basal metabolism	60		50	
Specific dynamic action and activity	10		20	
Total catabolism		70		70
Fecal loss	20		10	
Maintenance		90		80
Weight gain	30		20	
Total	120 (55/lb)		100 (45/lb)	

From Nelson, W. E., Textbook of Pediatrics, *7th ed., W. B. Saunders, 1962, Philadelphia.*

TABLE 19–8 ESTIMATED REQUIREMENTS AND ADVISABLE INTAKES FOR PROTEIN FOR NORMAL FULL-SIZE INFANTS AND CHILDREN

Age	*Requirement*	*Advisable Intake*
Birth to 4 months (g/100 kcal)	1.6	1.9
4 to 12 months (g/100 kcal)	1.4	1.7
12 to 36 months (g/kg/day)	1.2	1.4

From Fomon, 1974.

basis, the infant has much higher requirements than the adult for amino acids, and, because of metabolic differences, certain amino acids are dietary essentials for infants but not for adults.

Other nutrients. The recommended daily dietary allowances for infants and children are summarized in Table 19–10. Infants also need other nutrients besides these. They require essential fatty acids, and in the absence of adequate intake of linoleic acid there is clear evidence of abnormal symptoms. When linoleic acid intake provided less than 0.5 to 1% of the caloric consumption of otherwise normal infants, there were skin lesions typical of fatty acid deficiency (scaly skin) as well as growth impairment.

Other vitamins and minerals are also required by infants. These include vitamin K, folic acid, zinc, copper, manganese, iodine, and fluorine, although no recommended dietary allowances have been developed for these factors.

The question has been raised whether cholesterol is an essential nutrient for the newborn infant. Most mammalian milks are rich sources of cholesterol, and in fact, chemical analyses have shown that serum cholesterol was higher in 6-week-old infants fed human milk than in those fed cow's-milk formula. Studies with experimental animals have suggested that moderate intakes of cholesterol during infancy may be conducive to development of regulatory mechanisms for cholesterol metabolism. Thus, a low intake of cholesterol during infancy, such as is provided by formulas containing vegetable oils, may lead to problems of cholesterol regulation in the adult. This problem is, of course, extremely important, since elevated serum cholesterol in adults has been identified as a major risk factor with respect to atherosclerosis.

Supplementary foods. In recent years the introduction of foods in addition to milk in the infant's dietary has occurred at increasingly early ages. Until about 1920, solid foods were seldom offered to infants before one year of age (see Figure 19–3). At present the introduction of cereal and strained foods generally occurs before the end of the first month, although many experts believe this practice to be undesirable.

It is nevertheless of interest to examine the nutrient intake of infants if their entire food supply is breast milk. In Table 19–11 the daily nutrient intake of infants from the end of the first week of life to the age of six months is compared with the recommended dietary allowances. Through the third

TABLE 19–9 ESSENTIAL AMINO ACID REQUIREMENTS OF INFANTS AND ADULTS, MG/KG/DAY

Amino Acid	*Infant Requirement*	*Adult Requirement*		
		Men	*Women*	*Average*
Histidine	26	—	—	—
Isoleucine	66	10.4	5.2	7.8
Leucine	132	9.9	7.1	8.5
Lysine	101	8.8	3.3	6.1
Methionine	24	—	3.9	3.9
Phenylalanine	57	4.3	3.1	3.7
Cystine	23	—	—	—
Threonine	59	6.5	3.5	5.0
Tryptophan	16	2.9	2.1	2.5
Valine	83	8.8	9.2	9.0

From Fomon, 1974.

TABLE 19–10 RECOMMENDED DIETARY ALLOWANCES FOR INFANTS AND CHILDREN

	Infants		*Children*		
	0.0–0.5	*0.5–1.0*	*1–3*	*4–6*	*7–10*
Weight, kg/lb	6/14	9/20	13/28	20/44	30/66
Height, cm/in	60/24	71/28	86/34	110/44	135/54
Energy, kcal	kg × 117	kg × 108	1300	1800	2400
Protein, g	kg × 2.2	kg × 2.0	23	30	36
Vitamin A activity, IU	1400	2000	2000	2500	3300
Vitamin D, IU	400	400	400	400	400
Vitamin E, IU	4	5	7	9	10
Ascorbic acid, mg	35	35	40	40	40
Folacin, μg	50	50	100	200	300
Niacin, mg	5	8	9	12	16
Riboflavin, mg	0.4	0.6	0.8	1.1	1.2
Thiamin, mg	0.3	0.5	0.7	0.9	1.2
Vitamin B_6, mg	0.3	0.4	0.6	0.9	1.2
Vitamin B_{12}, μg	0.3	0.3	1.0	1.5	2.0
Calcium, mg	360	540	800	800	800
Phosphorus, mg	240	400	800	800	800
Iodine, μg	35	45	60	80	110
Iron, mg	10	15	15	10	10
Magnesium, mg	60	70	150	200	250
Zinc, mg	3	5	10	10	10

From NRC, Recommended Dietary Allowances, 1974.

month of life the amount of milk taken is adequate to meet the requirements. By the sixth month, however, the amounts of calcium, iron, and thiamin are low in relation to the recommended allowance. It is therefore recommended that an infant's diet be supplemented with iron-fortified infant cereals, iron-fortified formula or medicinal iron about the age of four months. Supplementation with vitamin D should begin within the first two weeks, and for the artificially fed infant, supplementation with vitamin C in addition should occur soon after birth.

MODIFICATION OF COW'S MILK FOR INFANT FEEDING: FORMULAS

The basic principle of infant feeding, as of all dietary programs, is that the diet should be adequate but not excessive in calories and all essential

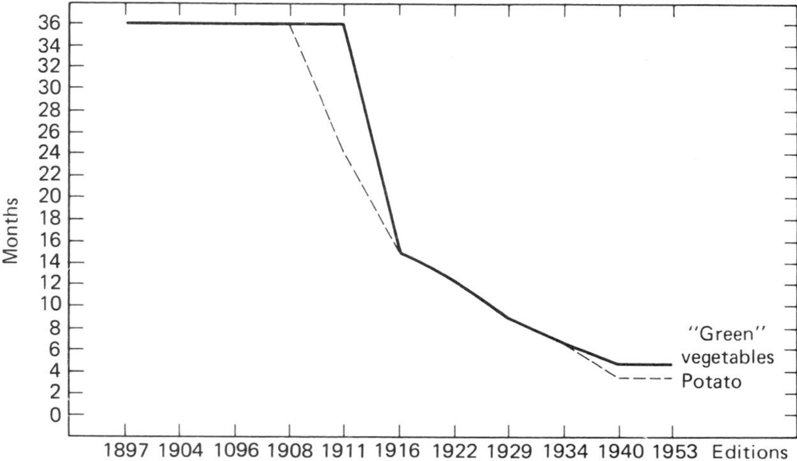

From Adams, S. F., J. Amer. Diet. Assn. **35***: 692–703, 1959.*

Figure 19–3 Earliest age recommendations for introduction of vegetables, as indicated in 11 editions of Holt's *The Diseases of Infancy and Childhood,* published from 1897 until 1953 (5th edition missing). It should be noted that beets are forbidden for ages three to six years until the 6th edition in 1911 ("must be small and fresh"), tomatoes were forbidden until the 8th edition in 1922, and raw vegetables until the 12th edition in 1953.

TABLE 19–11 ESTIMATED DAILY NUTRIENT INTAKE OF HEALTHY BREAST-FED INFANTS COMPARED WITH ESTIMATED DAILY RECOMMENDED ALLOWANCES

	Quantity Taken				*Recommended Allowance,*
Constituent	*End of Week 1*	*During Week 2*	*Weeks 5–13*	*Sixth Month*	*Sixth Month*
Breast milk, ml	400	475	765	935	—
Energy, kcal	232	352	543	664	720
Protein, g	10.8	7.6	9.2	11.2	—
Calcium, mg	120	160	250	310	540
Iron, mg	2	2.1	3.7	4.7	15
Vitamin A, IU	1200	1400	1400	1650	2000
Thiamin, mg	0.06	0.03	0.12	0.15	0.4
Riboflavin, mg	0.12	0.16	0.32	0.40	0.5
Niacin, mg	0.30	0.83	1.32	1.61	6
Ascorbic acid, mg	18	26	33	40	35

Modified from Macy and Kelly, in Kon and Cowie, 1961.

nutrients, including water. There should be a reasonable distribution of calories from protein, fat, and carbohydrate. In addition, there must be easy digestibility and an absence of harmful bacteria.

The differences between cow's milk and human milk necessitate the modification of cow's milk to make it suitable for the infant. Because of the difference in the type of curd formed by cow's milk from that formed by human milk, and because of the higher protein concentration of cow's milk, the milk is diluted with water. This procedure reduces the concentration of protein and thus at the same time decreases the problem of curd formation. Dilution of cow's milk, however, causes an equivalent reduction in the carbohydrate content, which reduces the caloric value. In order to return the caloric content to its original level, carbohydrate is added. Table 19–12

TABLE 19-12 RECOMMENDED NUTRIENT LEVELS OF INFANT FORMULAS (PER 100 KCAL)

Nutrient	*FDA 1971 Regulations: Minimum*	*CON 1976 Recommendations: Minimum*		*CON 1976 Recommendations: Maximum*
Protein (gm)	1.8	1.8		4.5
Fat				
(gm)	1.7	3.3		6.0
(% cal)	15.0	30.0		54.0
Essential fatty acids (linolcate)				
(% cal)	2.0	3.0		—
(mg)	222.0	300.0		—
Vitamins				
A (IU)	250.0	250.0	(75μg)*	750.0 (225μg)*
D (IU)	40.0	40.0		100.0
K (μg)	—	4.0		—
E (IU)	0.3	0.3	(with 0.7 IU/gm linoleic acid)	—
C (ascorbic acid) (mg)	7.8	8.0		—
B_1 (thiamine) (μg)	25.0	40.0		—
B_2 (riboflavin) (μg)	60.0	60.0		—
B_6 (pyridoxine) (μg)	35.0	35.0	(with 15μg/gm of protein in formula)	—
B_{12} (μg)	0.15	0.15		—
Niacin				
(μg)	—	250.0		—
(μg equiv)	800.0	—		—
Folic acid (μg)	4.0	4.0		—
Pantothenic acid (μg)	300.0	300.0		—

TABLE 19-12 (cont.)

Biotin (μg)	—	1.5	—
Choline (mg)	—	7.0	—
Inositol (mg)	—	4.0	—
Minerals			
Calcium (mg)	50.0†	50.0†	—
Phosphorus (mg)	25.0†	25.0†	
Magnesium (mg)	6.0	6.0	—
Iron (mg)	1.0	0.15	—
Iodine (μg)	5.0	5.0	—
Zinc (mg)	—	0.5	—
Copper (μg)	60.0	60.0	—
Manganese (μg)	—	5.0	—
Sodium (mg)	—	20.0 (6 mEq)‡	60.0 (17 mEq)‡
Potassium (mg)	—	80.0 (14 mEq)‡	200.0 (34 mEq)‡
Chloride (mg)	—	55.0 (11 mEq)‡	150.0 (29 mEq)‡

*Retinol equivalents.
†Calcium to phosphorus ratio must be no less than 1.1 nor more than 2.0.
‡Milliequivalent for 670 kcal/liter of formula.

From Committee on Nutrition, Commentary on Breast-Feeding and Infant Formulas, Pediatrics, **57**: *278–285, 1976.*

shows the minimum vitamin and mineral levels that should be provided by an infant-feeding formula. At present by far the largest proportion of infants in the United States are fed commercially prepared milk-based formulas (Figure 19-4). Table 19–4 shows the composition of several commercially prepared infant formulas.

BREAST FEEDING VERSUS BOTTLE FEEDING

The major focus of interest in the differences between human milk and cow's milk relates to their effects on the infant. During the past few decades there has been a marked decline in many countries in the proportion of infants who are breast fed (see Figure 19–4). This change has occurred very rapidly in comparison with the million years during which human infants could only be breast fed. In fact, as Jelliffe has pointed out, from the evolutionary standpoint, lactation developed before placental gestation appeared, since the first mammals laid eggs. The widespread use of cow's milk for feeding infants has therefore "only been in vogue for about 50 years or 5/100,000 of man's existence." Hambraeus has stated that the introduction of infant formula as a breast-milk substitute represents by far "the largest *in vivo* experiment without a control series."

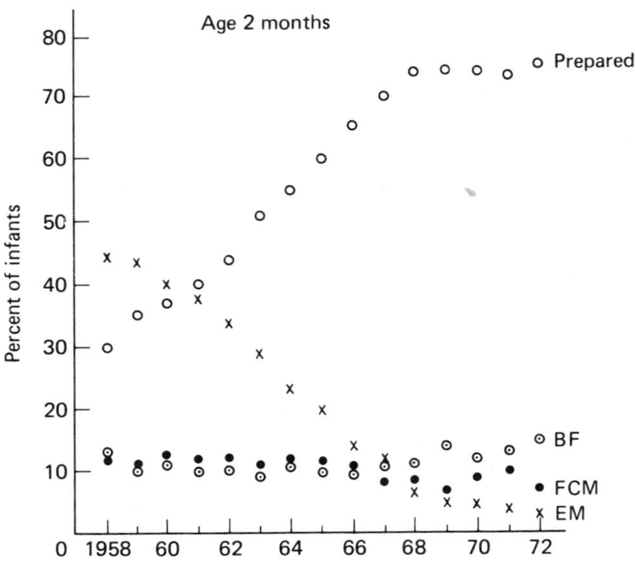

Data of G. A. Martinez, Ross Laboratories, Columbus, Ohio, 1973; in Fomon, 1974.

Figure 19–4 Percent of two-month-old infants in the United States between 1958 and 1972 who were breast fed or received other milks or formulas.

One of the usual criteria for nutritional adequacy, that of growth (usually interpreted as body-weight gain), may be misleading in the case of the young infant. Recent work has shown that bottle-fed infants doubled their birth weights earlier than breast-fed infants. This might be, in part at least, related to the earlier introduction of solid foods that occurred in this group. However, the increases in body weight were not reflected in increases of body length, and thus the infant might be developing either early obesity or a greater susceptibility to obesity. Excessive energy intake by overfeeding milk in bottle-fed infants is probably a factor that does not occur in breast-fed infants, who regulate their caloric intake very well. The mechanism of this regulation is not understood. Concentrating the formula by error or intention may also occur with bottle feeding. Finally, breast-fed infants may spend more time sucking and thus work longer and harder at getting the milk than do bottle-fed infants (see the section on overnutrition in Chapter 20).

The differences between cow's milk and human milk in relation to digestibility have been discussed earlier in this chapter. Another problem with cow's milk is its higher solute load. Human milk has the lowest solute load of all mammalian milks, with low concentrations of sodium and protein. The differences in fatty acid composition of the two milks also lead to differences in body composition of the infant. The subcutaneous fat of infants fed with breast milk is different from that of infants fed cow's-milk-based formula. In normal babies fed cow's milk, there are greater retention and higher serum levels of sodium and urea.

The differences between human breast milk and cow's milk in protein concentration also have some nutritional implications. The low protein content of breast milk implies that the human-milk proteins have very high nutritional quality. The differences in protein composition have another aspect that is important to the infant. Human milk contains significant amounts of immunoglobulins, which provide valuable protection for the infant against infections. In addition to these protective factors, lactoferrin contributes to the resistance observed in breast-fed babies against the infectious gastroenteritis caused by *E. coli*. Another specific milk protein in higher concentration in breast milk than in cow's milk, lysozyme, has a direct bacteriocidal effect. It also has an indirect effect through potentiation of immune antibody activity.

Breast-fed babies are less likely to suffer from rickets than are bottle-fed babies. Recently a previously undetected water-soluble form of vitamin D was found in human milk that is not present in cow's milk.

Breast-fed babies are also more resistant to iron-deficiency anemia than are bottle-fed babies. This is related to the greater bioavailability of iron from human milk. In one study, breast-fed infants absorbed 49% of a test dose of iron in contrast to 10% in cow's-milk-fed babies. In fact, infants fed breast milk during the entire first six to seven months of life developed greater iron stores than did those fed a cow's-milk formula.

Zinc absorption from human milk also seems to be higher than from cow's milk. A zinc-binding complex has been found in human milk that is relatively insignificant in cow's milk, and a role for this substance in zinc absorption has been proposed. Similarly a vitamin B_{12}-binding compound exists in human milk.

It is thus possible that the nutritional value of breast milk for the infant is not entirely expressed by a numerical accounting of its nutrient composition. The current concept is that the nutritional availability of essential nutrients may also be significantly different when breast milk is fed. Research with the rat suggests that breast milk may be especially significant during the early postnatal period until mature mechanisms of intestinal absorption develop. Oliver Wendell Holmes may well have been correct when he stated that "a pair of substantial mammary glands have the advantage over the two hemispheres of the most learned professor's brain in the art of compounding a nutritive fluid for infants."

References and Supplementary Readings

COMMITTEE ON NUTRITION, American Academy of Pediatrics. "Proposed changes in food and drug administration regulations concerning formula products and vitamin-mineral dietary supplements for infants." *Pediatrics* **40**: 916 (1967).

DEVEDAS, R. P., R. G. BAI, AND P. S. NIRMALA. "Studies on human milk." *J. Nutr. Dietet.* **3**: 50–63 (1966).

DUNCAN, J. R., AND L. S. HURLEY. "Intestinal absorption of zinc: a role for a zinc-binding ligand in milk." *Am. J. Physiol.* **235**: E556–E559 (1978).

FOMON, S. J. *Infant Nutrition.* Philadelphia: W. B. Saunders, 1974.

FOMON, S. J. *Nutritional Disorders of Children.* U. S. Department of Health, Education, and Welfare, Public Health Service, Health Services Administration. DHEW Publication No. (HSA) 76–5612 (1976).

GOPALAN, C., AND B. BELAVADY. "Nutrition and lactation." *Fed. Proc.* **20** (Suppl. 7): 177–184 (1961).

HAMBRAEUS, L. "Proprietary milk versus human breast milk in human feeding." *Ped. Clinics N. Amer.* **24**: 17–36 (1977).

HANSEN, S. T., J. HOLM, AND J. LYNGBYE. "Folate binding by human milk protein." Scand. J. Clin. *Lab. Invest.* **37**: 363–367 (1977).

JELLIFFE, D. B. "World trends in infant feeding." *Am. J. Clin. Nutr.* **29**: 1227–1237 (1976).

KOOYMAN, G. L. "Milk analysis of the kangaroo rat, Dipodomys merriami." *Science* **142**: 1467–1468 (1963).

KON, S. K., AND A. T. COWIE. *Milk: The Mammary Gland and Its Secretion*, Vol. II. New York: Academic Press, 1961.

MUTCH, P. B., AND L. S. HURLEY. "Effect of zinc deficiency during lactation on postnatal growth and development of rats." *J. Nutr.* **104**: 828–842 (1974).

NEUMANN, C. G. "Birthweight doubling time: A fresh look." *Pediatrics* **57**: 469–473 (1976).

Recommended Dietary Allowances, 8th ed. Washington, D.C.: Committee on Dietary Allowances, Food and Nutrition Board, National Research Council, National Academy of Sciences. 1974.

SAARINEN, U. M., M. A. SIIMES, AND P. R. DALLMAN. "Iron absorption in infants." *J. Pediatrics* **91**: 36–39 (1977).

THOMSON, A. M., AND A. E. BLACK. "Nutritional aspects of human lactation." *Bull. World Health Organ.* **52**: 163–177 (1966).

20

Malnutrition in infancy and early childhood

CALORIC INTAKE

There is a clear relationship between the caloric intake of infants and their rate of growth. Such a relationship has been demonstrated both in children recovering from marasmus (severe undernutrition, see below) and in normal infants fed milk-based formulas (Table 20–1). Obviously, in the absence of an adequate caloric intake, infants and young children will not grow at the normal rate or at their genetic potential.

It might next be asked: Can the retardation of growth caused by an inadequate intake of calories be recovered? It is well recognized that the phenomenon of "catch-up growth" occurs after illness or after a period of

TABLE 20–1 GAIN IN WEIGHT PER UNIT OF CALORIE INTAKE

Age Interval, Days	Gain in Weight, g/100 kcal			
	Males		Females	
	Mean	S.D.	Mean	S.D.
8–13	8.0	3.7	8.3	3.7
14–27	8.9	1.7	8.1	1.8
28–41	7.6	1.7	6.3	1.5
42–55	6.3	1.7	5.8	1.2
56–83	5.2	1.0	4.8	1.0
84–111	4.2	1.0	3.9	1.2
8–55	7.5	1.1	6.8	1.0
56–111	4.7	0.8	4.4	0.8
8–111	5.9	0.7	5.4	0.8

From Fomon, 1974.

malnutrition, but the full extent of growth recovery is still not certain. A number of factors, such as the timing, degree, and duration of the malnutrition itself, are probably involved.

The phenomenon of catch-up growth has been studied in children with celiac disease. In this condition (which manifests itself during infancy) malabsorption of nutrients causes growth retardation. This sequence can be completely reversed by giving the children gluten-free diets. Under such conditions, catch-up growth of children with celiac disease has been adequate to produce complete recovery as far as growth is concerned.

Studies of hyperactive children treated with amphetamines are also of interest in relation to growth. These drugs are used to treat hyperactivity in children but at the same time they reduce appetite. In the children studied, amphetamines were given during the school year, and growth was accordingly suppressed. During the summer vacation, however, when the drugs were not administered, catch-up growth occurred.

PROTEIN CALORIE MALNUTRITION

The most important nutritional problem of infants and young children on a worldwide basis is that of protein calorie malnutrition (PCM). Although for a variety of reasons the total incidence of malnutrition in the world is difficult to estimate, it is clear that widespread undernutrition exists. Undernutrition aggravates infectious diseases and predisposes children to a severe condition of PCM when seasonal or other food shortages occur. It is difficult to estimate the effect of malnutrition on mortality, since death reports seldom mention this cause. In children whose deaths are attributed to infectious disease malnutrition may often be the underlying or associated cause. Furthermore, relatively little attention has been paid to the more moderate forms of malnutrition that are so important from the public health standpoint.

The Pan American Health Organization sponsored a study of 18 widely separated areas in the Americas to obtain statistics on causes of death in children under five years of age. Malnutrition was found to be an underlying cause in 7% of all deaths in young children and an associated cause in 46%. Thus malnutrition was directly or indirectly responsible for about 53% of all deaths in children under five years of age in the areas studied. In infants under one year of age, about 5% of the deaths were due to kwashiorkor (see below), 26% to marasmus, and 70% to other forms of PCM. In the one- to four-year age group the pattern was different. Kwashiorkor was implicated in 31% of the deaths, marasmus in 18%, and other forms of PCM in about 51%. There were also considerable regional variations. In both age groups these wide variations probably reflected differences in eating habits.

PCM is actually a spectrum of diseases with its extremes seen clinically as marasmus at one extreme and kwashiorkor at the other. Cases with mixed features are termed marasmic kwashiorkor. The less severe forms are characterized by more moderate retardation of growth and development and are referred to as mild and moderate forms of PCM. It is estimated that a considerable number of the several hundred million preschool children in the developing countries are affected to some degree. As Gopalan has stated, "Our assessment of the magnitude of the problem of protein-calorie malnutrition varies depending upon the diagnostic criteria we adopt. For example, in India, on the basis of the incidence of growth failure, we may assess the prevalence at 80%, whereas on the basis of occurrence of kwashiorkor, the prevalence at any point of time can be as low as 1.2%" (in Olson, 1975).

The syndrome of kwashiorkor was first described in 1932 by Dr. Cicely Williams, who gave it its name. Because of the marked differences in appearance of children with kwashiorkor or with marasmus (see Figures 20–1 and 20–2), it was thought for some time that the etiology of the two conditions was markedly different. However, more recent evidence suggests that maras-

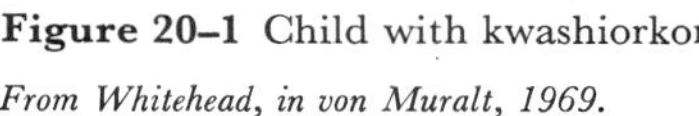

Figure 20–1 Child with kwashiorkor.

From Whitehead, in von Muralt, 1969.

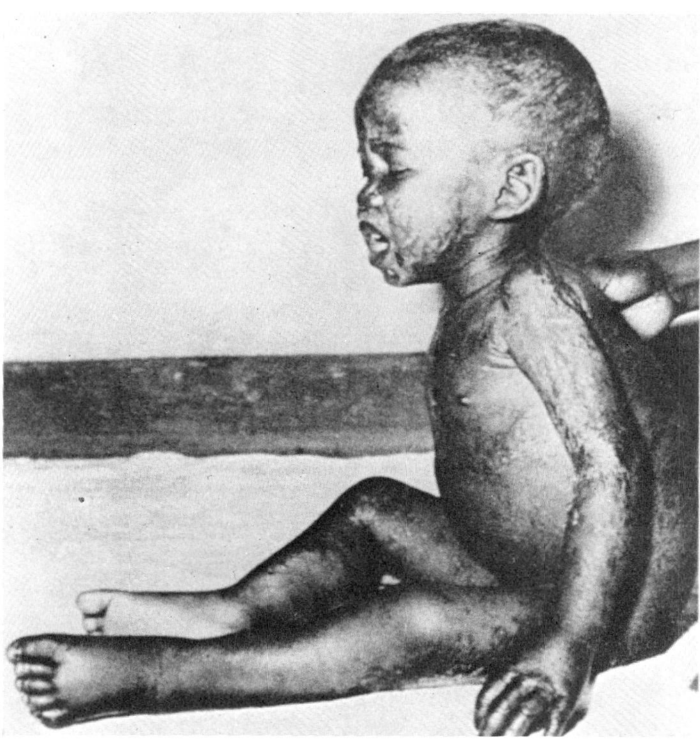

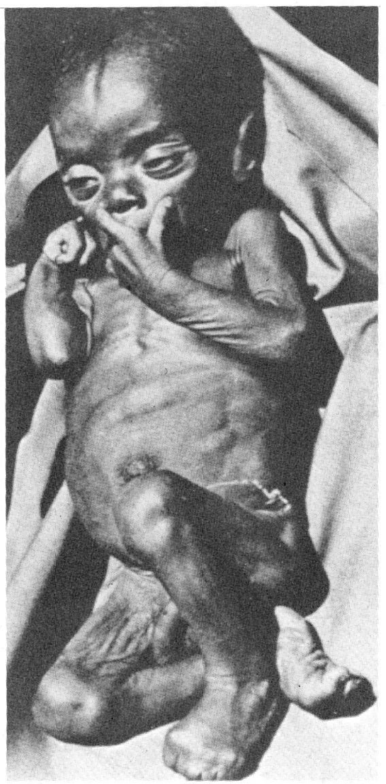

From Whitehead, in von Muralt, 1969.

Figure 20–2 Child with marasmus.

mus and kwashiorkor are the end results of severe degrees of the same type of PCM prevalent in the rest of the community. In a study conducted in India, for example, it was found that the dietary pattern of children who developed kwashiorkor was in no way different from that of children who developed marasmus. All of the children subsisted on the same type of cereal-based diet shown in Table 20–2. Longitudinal studies also confirmed that there were no striking qualitative differences between the dietary patterns or the protein calorie ratios of diets taken by children with marasmus and those with kwashiorkor. The dietary patterns and protein calorie ratios were also similar to those of other undernourished children in the community.

Gopalan has stated that under these conditions marasmic children may develop kwashiorkor (marasmic kwashiorkor), and children with kwashiorkor may show marasmus after their edema is decreased or disappears. Marasmus and kwashiorkor therefore occur in the same community of children. In

TABLE 20–2 PROTEIN AND CALORIE INTAKE OF POOR SOUTH INDIAN CHILDREN

Age Group	Number Surveyed	Mean Weight, kg	Protein Intake		Calorie Intake	
			g/24 h	*g/kg*	*kcal/24 h*	*kcal/kg*
6–12 months	126	6.7	12.5	1.9	550	82
1–2 years	418	7.8	14.0	1.8	610	79
2–3 years	328	9.1	19.8	2.2	860	96
3–4 years	394	10.7	21.2	2.0	910	86
4–5 years	578	12.4	20.0	1.6	900	73

From Gopalan, in von Muralt, 1969.

addition, both of these conditions can be seen in the same child at different times.

Additional evidence from India suggests that the caloric intake is even more deficient than the protein intake in this type of malnutrition in children. When the cumulative frequency distribution of children by intake of protein and calories is considered (see Figure 20–3), it is seen that 92% of the children in this large survey were deficient in calories, whereas only 35% were deficient in protein. Even the children who had an inadequate protein intake would have met their needs for this nutrient if the diet had met their caloric requirements. There was no situation in which the child was adequate with regard to calories and deficient in protein. Thus the major problem, at least in some parts of the world, appears to be calories rather than protein.

Figure 20–3 Cumulative frequency (percentage) distribution of preschool children (Hyderabad region) by intake of proteins (——) and calories (---). The abscissa is the nutrient intake expressed as a percentage of requirements suggested by an ICMR expert group, 1968, based on actual body weights.

From Gopalan, in Olson, 1975.

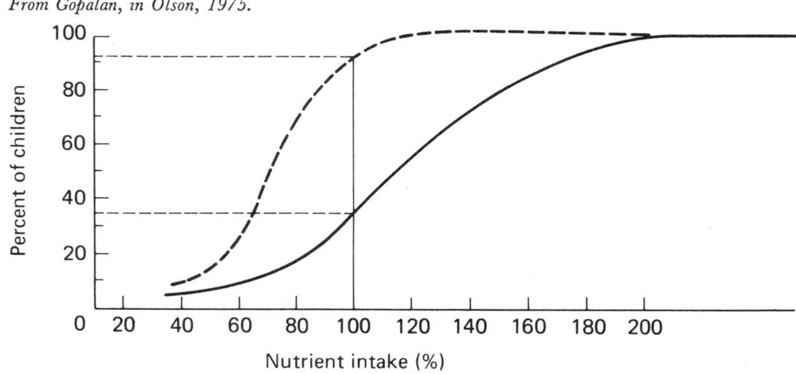

The diets of these children are deficient not only in calories and in protein but also in some minerals and vitamins (see Table 20–3). (This aspect of PCM will be further discussed below.) In southern India the diets of the children were low in riboflavin, vitamin C, iron, and calcium, and extremely low in vitamin A. Because of the multiple nature of PCM, it has been suggested that this term be replaced by *calorie protein deficiency* or by *chronic starvation*.

ETIOLOGY OF PCM

The classical development of malnutrition in young children is related to the weaning period. Traditionally, in the regions where PCM is prevalent, children are breast fed for about two years and at weaning are given a low-protein diet, chiefly of vegetable origin and insufficient in caloric value. Gastroenteritis occurs, initially from poor sanitary conditions, and as malnutrition progresses, attacks of diarrhea occur more frequently. During such episodes the diet is commonly limited to starch and water or to carbohydrates and water, and laxatives may be given. By the second or third year of life the child may be irritable, anorexic, emaciated, with edema, skin lesions, depigmented hair, and marked growth retardation. One author (Pena Chaviarria in Caddell, 1969) described these children as follows: "They are indifferent to their surroundings and remain immobile for hours with open eyes and expressionless features, suggesting a mask rather than a human face. This immobility is often accompained by a monotonous wailing without tears and the children refuse all food and whimper at the least touch."

TABLE 20–3 VITAMIN AND MINERAL INTAKE OF PRESCHOOL CHILDREN[a]

Nutrient	*Units*	*Average Intake*	*Recommended Allowance (ICMR, 1968)*[b]
Thiamin	mg/kcal	0.53	0.5
Riboflavin	mg/kcal	0.30	0.55
Niacin equivalents	mg/kcal	9.90	6.6
Ascorbic acid	mg/day	4.4	30–50
Vitamin A (Retinol)	μg/day	61	250–300
Iron	mg/day	5.9	15–20
Calcium	mg/day	193	400–500

[a]Based on diet survey in the Hyderabad region.

[b]ICMR Special Report Series No. 60, C. Gopalan and B.S. Narasinga Ras.

From Gopalan, in Olson, 1975.

The peak incidence of the classical picture of PCM, with kwashiorkor as the major severe form, is in the second and third years of life in many parts of Africa. In the Caribbean region, however, PCM occurs at much younger ages. Jelliffe has characterized the main features of the pattern of PCM in the Caribbean as follows:

1. Severe syndromes occur mostly in the first year of life. For example, in Trinidad, the major incidence of kwashiorkor was between the ages of five and seven months. It was due essentially to the very early weaning of children from the breast, after which they were fed largely on carbohydrates. Infantile kwashiorkor in these cases is rather different from the classical picture seen in the second and third years of life. In particular, marked hair changes are common, skin lesions are not as frequent, and enlargement of the liver is seen in the majority of cases. The possible permanent effects of infantile kwashiorkor are important because of the possibility that damage may occur to the central nervous system, which is still vulnerable at this age.
2. Marasmus, frequently associated with diarrhea, is more common than kwashiorkor. This is the most common cause of admission to hospitals and the most frequent cause of death in young children.
3. Mild to moderate PCM is extremely common.

The most important reason, of course, for the development of PCM in mild or severe forms is the absence of food intake adequate in quantity and quality for the young child. However, the alarming change in the onset of these conditions to younger and younger ages is also related to cultural changes that are occurring as westernization, urbanization, and industrial development increase. Jelliffe and Jelliffe have summarized these trends dramatically. They see the dominant change in the pattern of child nutrition as a decline in breast feeding, a rise in attempted bottle feeding with cow's milk, and a tendency to purchase expensive processed infant foods.

> In part, but in part only, it (*the trend toward abandonment of breast feeding*) may reflect the difficulties of continuing breast feeding in urban employment. In addition, however, it is due to socio-cultural pressures generated by imitation of 'economic superiors', as well as locally unethical and inappropriate advertising by milk firms, and poor advice from friends, neighbors, and sometimes, unfortunately, poorly educated health and nutrition personnel. Too often the end-result is an early decline of lactation . . . .
>
> As an alternative, the mother attempts to feed her baby on one of the processed milks, usually the most widely advertised and hence the most expensive. The money available only permits the purchase of totally inadequate amounts, and her home surroundings and education make the preparation of clean feedings improbable (if not impossible). Thus the baby is starved . . . with a heavy dose of contaminating bacteria.

Jelliffe and Jelliffe have pointed out that similar nutritional problems were widespread in Europe and North America among the urban poor, even quite recently. These authors have summarized the risk factors related to the development of PCM (see Tables 20–4 and 20–5).

TABLE 20–4 SOME BIOLOGIC AT-RISK FACTORS IN THE PROTEIN CALORIE MALNUTRITION OF CHILDHOOD

Young Child

Twins. Low birth weight. Some congenital abnormalities (e.g., cleft palate).
Close-spaced (< 2 years). Large family size. Birth order.
Transitional period (after second year).
Age range of maximal mortality.
Growth failure (weight curve; other anthropometric indices).
Signs of malnutrition.
Infections (measles; diarrhea; whooping cough; "nonimmunized").
Family history (previous weanling deaths; previous malnutrition).

Mother

Maternal illness and malnutrition (e.g., maternal height).
M. presence. M. age (young or old). M. infections (malaria and low birth weight). M. death. M. intelligence/competence. (M. = maternal)

From Jelliffe and Jelliffe, 1973.

TABLE 20–5 SOME ENVIRONMENTAL AT-RISK FACTORS IN THE PROTEIN CALORIE MALNUTRITION OF CHILDHOOD

Cultural

Weaning practices (age; suddenness; separation; associated traumatic practices).
Weaning food.
Child feeder.
Mother working.
Sex of child.
Traditional practices with infections. Newly urbanized.

Socioeconomic

Economic level (relation to protein supply for young children in each economy, expecially urban).
Educational considerations (literacy; language for immigrants).
Incomplete family (absence or inadequate support by father; death or temporary or permanent absence of mother).
Abandoned children.
Alcoholism.

Geographic-Climatic

Seasonal (especial relation to weaning).
Geographically distant.

Miscellaneous

Nonattenders at health services.

From Jelliffe and Jelliffe, 1973.

Although breast milk alone will not provide sufficient nutrition after six months of age (see Chapter 19), infants who are breast fed, even in extremely poor communities where PCM is endemic, show growth normal or equal to U. S. standards for the first six months of life. At this time, and even later when they are given additional foods, the calories and protein that are provided in a sterile condition by breast milk may be an important or critical additional factor in the prevention of malnutrition. The importance of breast feeding as a preventive measure against PCM as well as the use of induced lactation and the possibility of its induction have been stressed by Brown.

It should be clear from this discussion that the problem of protein calorie malnutrition in young children and its prevention is not a simple one. It is related to a large number of biological and socioeconomic as well as political factors that are interrelated in an extremely complex fashion. Cravioto has prepared a diagram illustrating the interrelationships among some of these factors (see Figure 8–12).

MICRONUTRIENT DEFICIENCIES COMMONLY ASSOCIATED WITH PCM

Vitamins. The findings of several studies are consistent with the idea that protein calorie malnutrition in early childhood is actually total undernutrition with deficiencies of many nutrients. Preschool children in the Hyderabad region of India had deficiencies of certain minerals and vitamins in their dietary intake (see Table 20–3). Likewise, studies in Thailand have shown similar findings with relation to water-soluble vitamins. For example, 50% of Thai children with PCM showed ocular evidence of vitamin A deficiency. Clinical signs of thiamin deficiency were minimal, but 58% of children with kwashiorkor and 32% of children with marasmic kwashiorkor or marasmus showed evidence of riboflavin deficiency. On the other hand, there was little evidence of deficiencies of folic acid, vitamin B_{12}, vitamin B_6, niacin, or vitamin C in children with PCM in Thailand.

In the Dominican Republic, where PCM is widespread, a nutritional survey showed that per capita intake of many nutrients was considerably below the recommendations by the Institute of Nutrition of Central America and Panama (INCAP). In this area, growth of children was definitely and markedly retarded and a high percentage of children under five years of age had low levels of serum albumin. Almost 40% of those below the age of three showed some evidence of thiamin deficiency (low urinary thiamin), and 35% of this age group had a marginal level of riboflavin excretion (Figure 20–4).

Although the degree of adequacy or deficiency of certain of the B vitamins appears to vary in PCM in different parts of the world, there seems to

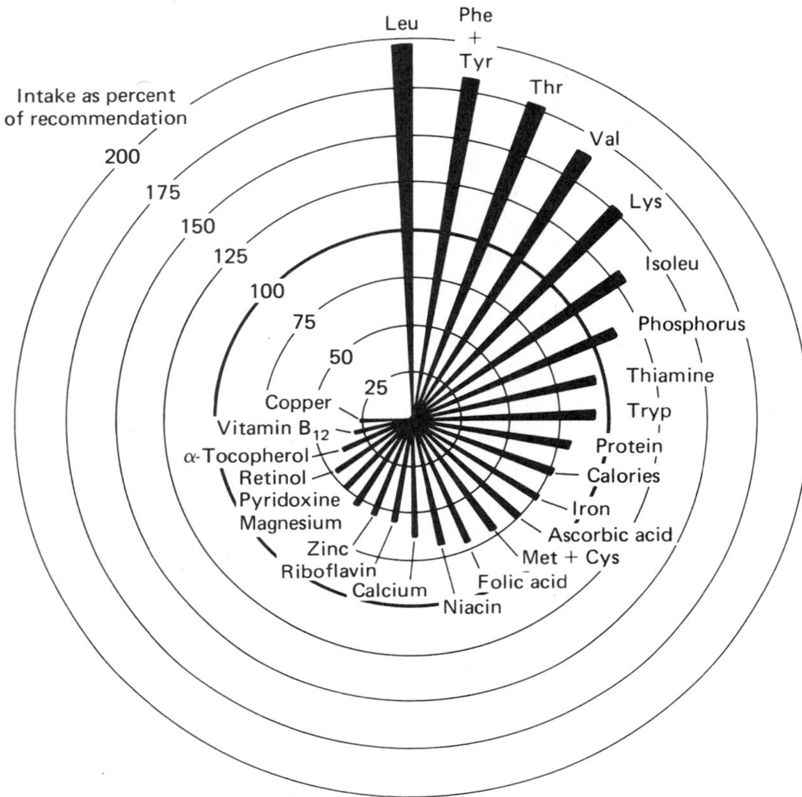

From Sebrell, in Olson, 1975.

Figure 20–4 Average daily per capita nutrient intakes in the Dominican Republic as percent of recommended allowance. The length of each bar represents the average per capita daily intake as measured by analysis of traditionally cooked composite diets or by dietary survey data expressed as percent of INCAP recommendation.

be agreement that PCM is generally accompanied by vitamin A deficiency. With severe vitamin A deficiency, xerophthalmia occurs, leading eventually to blindness, loss of life, or both. Xerophthalmia is characteristically a disease of infants and young children and is usually associated with a severe form of PCM. It is the commonest cause of blindness in these age groups. The incidence of vitamin A deficiency with PCM, however, varies from one region to another. In Indonesia about three-fourths of all cases of kwashiorkor also have xerophthalmia, but in Uganda, West Africa, and the West Indies not more than 1% have eye lesions. The variation, of course, depends upon the differences in carotene intake in these parts of the world. Children with severe PCM but no clinical signs of vitamin A deficiency often have low serum and liver levels of the vitamin.

There is some evidence that vitamins D, E, and K may also be deficient in children with PCM and that they are more susceptible to rickets (Figure 20–5).

Mineral elements: potassium. Children with PCM have in general a low level of whole-body potassium. The decreased body potassium is thought to reflect the children's malnutrition, which causes a reduction in the mass of those tissues that ordinarily contain most of the body potassium. This idea was developed from studies that showed the deficit in whole-body potassium in malnourished children to be considerably greater (23%) than the deficit in muscle potassium (12%).

Magnesium. Children with PCM also show evidence of magnesium deficiency. Balance studies indicate that after apparent recovery from PCM there is still considerable retention of magnesium. Even two to three weeks of therapy with magnesium in malnourished children produced no increase in muscle concentration of the element, although its level in serum had returned to normal. The magnesium deficiency of malnourished children is usually the result of chronic diarrhea. In some cases magnesium depletion occurs so rapidly that symptomatic hypomagnesemia is seen.

The state of magnesium nutrition was measured in a group of hospitalized malnourished children in Thailand. On admission to the hospital, the plasma magnesium levels in these PCM patients were normal or low normal. However, while they were being treated, they developed significant hypomagnesemia, indicating low magnesium reserves. Symptoms such as anorexia, neuromuscular hyperirritability, and electrocardiographic changes, which are known to occur in magnesium deficiency, could be correlated with the plasma magnesium values. It appeared that an important factor was the lack of balance between magnesium and the elements calcium, sodium, and potassium that resulted from their treatment, a therapy that restored cations other than magnesium and provided nutrients for protein

Figure 20–5 Prevalence of rickets in Northern Thai children with PCM.

From Damrongsak, in Olson, 1975.

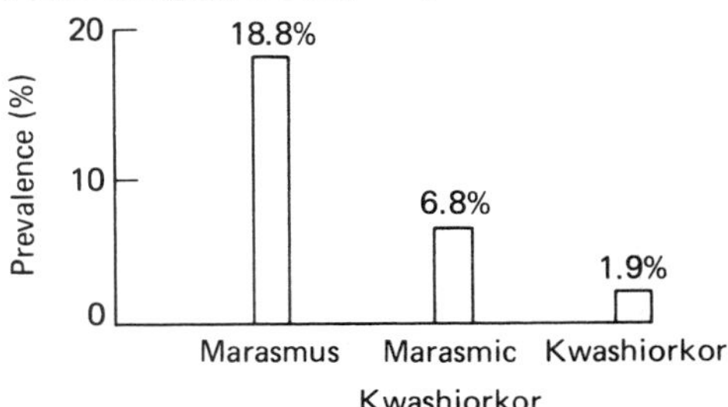

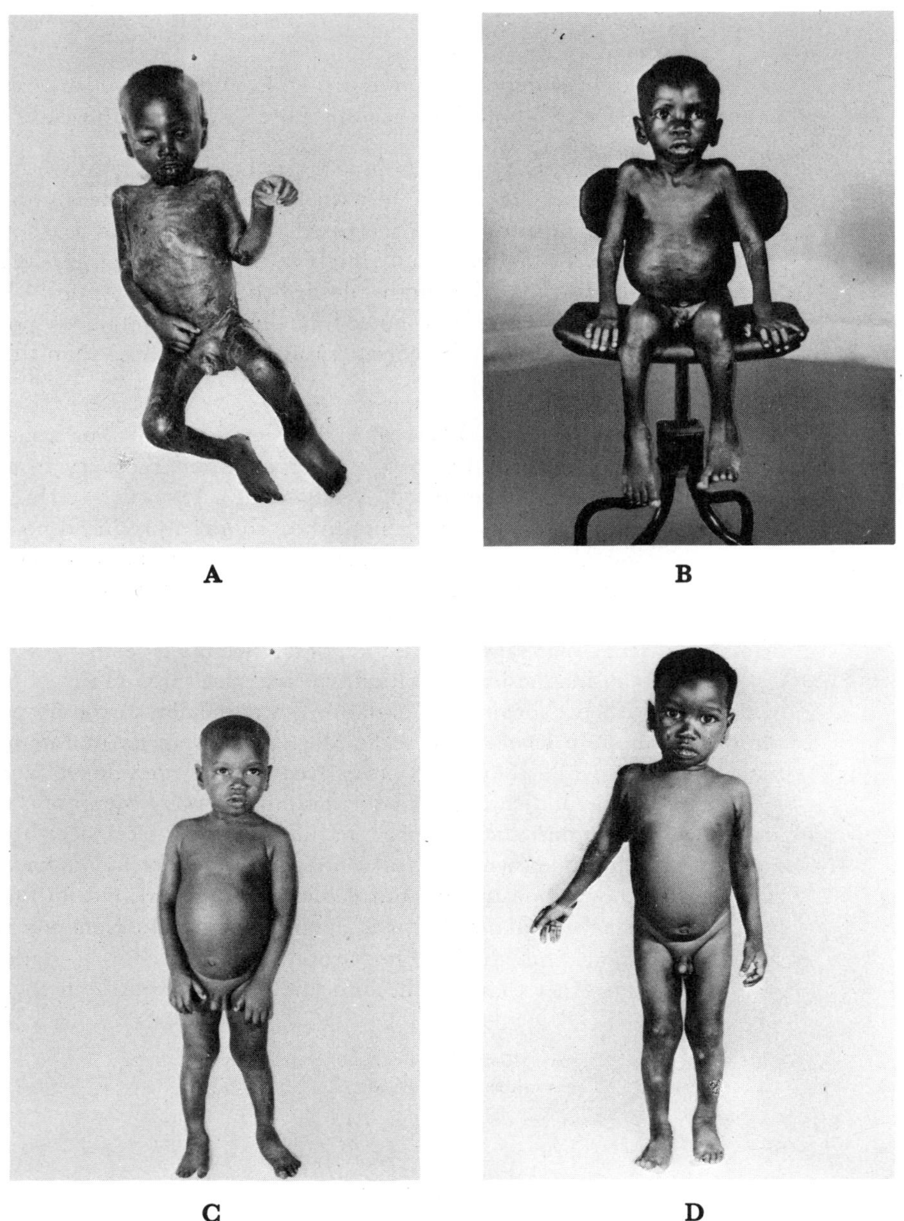

From Caddell, 1969.

Figure 20–6 (a) Nigerian child is shown here on the fourth day of therapy that included magnesium. He weighed 7.8 kg. (b) At three weeks he weighed 9.3 kg. (c) At two months his posture reflected poor muscle tone. He now weighed 11.25 kg. (d) At seven months he weighed 14.54 kg and liked to run.

anabolism. In severely malnourished Nigerian children, magnesium supplementation improved the rate and extent of recovery from severe PCM (see Figure 20–6).

Sodium. Metabolism of sodium may also be deranged in children with PCM. Many reports show either normal or low values for plasma sodium. In children with edema, however, the total body content of this element is increased.

Trace elements. Certain trace element deficiencies are also associated with PCM. Infants fed milk exclusively for a prolonged period following recovery from PCM have developed a copper-responsive anemia, leucopenia, thinning of bone cortices, and pathological fractures, all of which are signs of copper deficiency. Serum concentrations of copper have been found to be low in children with PCM, and evidence of chromium deficiency has also been observed. Selenium in whole blood and plasma was decreased as well. In one study of trace elements in kwashiorkor in children in South Africa, serum iron, zinc, manganese, molybdenum, nickel, and copper were all low.

One of the consistent effects of PCM in young children is anemia. This anemia is related to low intakes of iron and protein, but it is a very complex condition because of the multiple vitamin and mineral deficiency states that are frequently associated with PCM.

PROTEIN INTAKE IN THE UNITED STATES

Several surveys in the United States have investigated the protein intake of children between one and three years of age (see Table 20–6). Less than 4% of the children in this age group received less than 20 g of protein per day. Even the children receiving 10 to 20 g of protein per day were undoubtedly getting more than the estimated 1.2 g/kg/day required for this age group. It appears that protein deficiency is uncommon in young children in the United States.

LACTOSE INTOLERANCE

In almost all mammals the activity of intestinal lactase, necessary for the digestion of lactose, the sugar of milk, declines after weaning. This is true for most humans as well as other mammals, except mainly for some ethnic groups of white European descent. If milk in fairly large quantities is ingested by a young child who is lactose intolerant, or by an individual after lactase has decreased in activity, severe gastrointestinal disturbance may

TABLE 20–6 INTAKES OF PROTEIN BY CHILDREN 12 TO 36 MONTHS OF AGE IN THE UNITED STATES

Age (Months)	*Survey*[a]	*Number of Children*	*Intake of Protein (g/day)* < 10	10–19	20–29	> 29
			(Percent of Children)			
12–24	10-State	693	< 1	3	9	88
	PNS	632	0	2	14	84
	USDA	93	0	1	9	90
	NCRS	497				> 90
24–36	10-State	708	< 1	3	9	87
	PNS	681	0	1	7	92
	USDA	105	0	4	6	90
	NCRS	551				> 90

[a] 10-State is Ten-State Nutrition Survey, 1968–1970 (Center for Disease Control, 1972); PNS is Preschool Nutrition Survey (Owen et al., *Pediatrics* 53: 597, 1974); USDA is U.S. Department of Agriculture Survey of low-income families (Eagles and Steele, DHEW/HSMHA Publ. No. 725605. Maternal and Child Health Serv. 1972); and NCRS is North Central Regional Survey (Fryer et al., *J. Amer. Diet. Assn.*, 59: 228, 1971).

From Fomon, 1974.

result, with diarrhea and gas. The prevalence of lactose intolerance and malabsorption among the world's population should be remembered not only in the general feeding of children but especially in the treatment of those with PCM.

VITAMINS

VITAMIN A

Deficiency. Vitamin A deficiency is extremely prevalent in developing countries where malnutrition of infants occurs in high incidence (see above). In developed countries, however, this deficiency is quite rare, since intake of dairy products and yellow and green vegetables is relatively large (Table 20–7). The amount of fat in the diet also assures adequate absorption of the vitamin and its precursors.

Hypervitaminosis A. Excessive intake of vitamin A is toxic, and many cases of hypervitaminosis A have been reported in children. The acute form of vitamin A toxicity is shown by bulging fontanelles, vomiting, irritability, and insomnia, all probably related to the associated increased intracranial pressure. In chronic hypervitaminosis A, which is more prevalent than the acute form, there is anorexia, desquamation of the skin, fissures of the lips, localized subcutaneous and bone tenderness, demonstrable changes in the long bones seen in X-rays, and increased concentration of vitamin A in the serum.

According to Fomon, the daily ingestion of 20,000 IU of vitamin A per day for one or two months is likely to be toxic. Since the normal, otherwise adequate, diet of infants in the United States provides a sufficient amount of vitamin A, it is not necessary to supplement infants and young children with the vitamin. In a statement on the subject by the Nutrition Committee of the Canadian Pediatrics Society, the recommendation was made that physicians should not prescribe vitamin A supplements containing more than 25,000 IU per dose. The Committee on Nutrition of the American Academy of Pediatrics has advised against the use of preparations providing more than 6000 IU per dose.

In one dramatic report, a 30-month-old boy taken to a New Haven, Connecticut, hospital was shown to have chronic hypervitaminosis A. He had anorexia, lethargy, stiff neck, inability to walk, increased head size, patchy alopecia, and an exfoliative pruritic rash. His mother was a health faddist and had fed her children a variety of "health" foods and vitamins for about a year. The daily diet had apparently included estimated minima of at least 57,000 IU of vitamin A, 1000 IU of vitamin D, 200 IU of vitamin

TABLE 20–7 PERCENTAGE OF CHILDREN 12 TO 36 MONTHS OF AGE RECEIVING VARIOUS INTAKES OF VITAMIN A

		Intake of Vitamin A (IU/day)		
Survey[a]	*Number of Subjects*	*< 1000*	*1000–1999*	*> 1999*
		(Percent of Children)		
PNS:				
Unsupplemented	600	7	26	67
Supplemented	713	< 0.05	2	98
USDA	198	16	24	61
10-State	1401	9	29	62

[a]PNS is Preschool Nutrition Survey (Owen et al., *Pediatrics* 53: 597, 1974) with intakes listed separately for infants reported to be receiving or not to be receiving vitamin supplements; USDA is U.S. Department of Agriculture survey of low-income families (Eagles and Steele, DHEW/HSMHA Publ. No. 725605. Maternal and Child Health Serv. 1972); 10-State is Ten-State Nutrition Survey, 1968–1970 (Center for Disease Control, 1972).

From Fomon, 1974.

E, 480 mg of vitamin C, 1600 mg of calcium, and 750 mg of phosphate. The child's serum calcium level was initially very high (13.5 mg/100 ml), but fell to normal (10.0 mg/100 ml) after the calcium and vitamin D supplements were stopped. The serum vitamin A concentration was markedly elevated on admission to the hospital; it fell ten days later. Radiographic examination showed widening of the cranial sutures and enlargement of the cranial vault relative to the size of the facial bones. The child's clinical condition improved rapidly when all vitamin supplements were stopped, and by the end of the week he was able to walk. Two months later X-rays showed healing of the bone lesions.

The 12-month-old sister of this boy was also hypervitaminotic with respect to vitamin A. She had been given a daily intake of 25,000 IU of vitamin A over a period of nine months and was brought to the hospital because of irritability and vomiting. She also had exfoliated dermatitis, bulging fontanelles, elevation of serum vitamin A, and increased cerebral spinal fluid pressure. Five days after the supplementation with vitamin A was stopped, her symptoms were gone.

VITAMIN D

Deficiency. Vitamin D deficiency results in rickets. Although both the cause of rickets and its prevention are very well understood, there are still many cases of this deficiency disease in infants and children in the United States.

Hypervitaminosis D. Like vitamin A, vitamin D taken to excess can cause serious toxicity. Because of its role in the promotion of calcium absorption from the gut, too much vitamin D produces hypercalcemia. Associated with hypercalcemia is calcification of soft tissues, which is especially serious in the kidney.

There is some suggestion that excessive amounts of vitamin D may be a factor in the development of infantile idiopathic hypercalcemia. In the severe form of this condition there is vomiting, growth retardation, bony changes, mental retardation, elevated concentration of calcium in the serum, and in some cases aortic stenosis or progressive renal failure and hypertension. Intakes of more than the 400 IU of vitamin D recommended per day should be avoided.

VITAMIN E

Vitamin E deficiency can be a problem in infants or children with chronic steatorrhea (fatty stools), infants of low birth weight, or infants with low intakes of the vitamin. It is of especial concern for premature infants in whom hemolytic anemia responsive to vitamin E has occurred.

VITAMIN K

Vitamin K is especially important during the first few days of life. Since breast milk is low in vitamin K, many infants, especially those who are breast fed, develop a mild deficiency of the vitamin shortly after birth. This is manifested by bleeding and is termed "hemorrhagic disease of the newborn." The Committee on Nutrition of the American Academy of Pediatrics has recommended that every newborn infant should receive a parenteral dose of vitamin K soon after birth.

VITAMIN C

The deficiency disease associated with ascorbic acid is scurvy. Infants are especially susceptible to this disease. Figure 20–7 shows the age incidence of infantile scurvy in 1965. In infants, in addition to capillary fragility, irritability, and tenderness of the joints, there are bony abnormalities as well. In two surveys in the United States it was shown that about a third of the children between one and three years of age received low intakes of vitamin C, less than 15 mg/day. Thus, a significant proportion of American small children were not being given recommended amounts of this vitamin. However, scurvy is now quite rare in the United States.

B VITAMINS

Thiamin deficiency occurs in breast-fed infants whose mothers have a deficient intake of the vitamin, but in the United States and Canada it has almost never been reported. Riboflavin deficiency is not a problem in these countries either, and the same is true of niacin.

Figure 20–7 Age incidence of scurvy.

From Grewar, Clin. Pediatr. 4, 82–89, 1965.

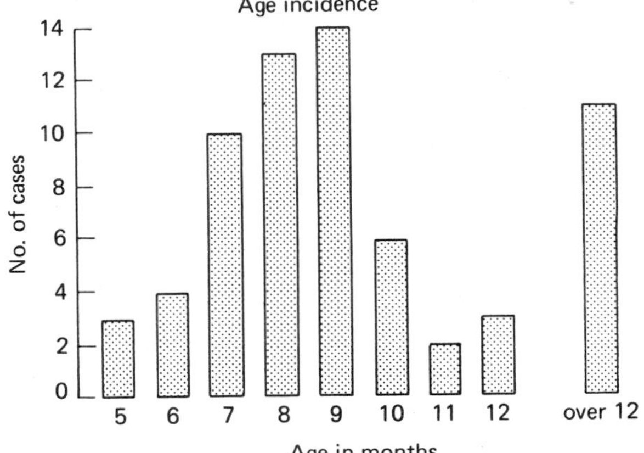

Vitamin B_6 deficiency, on the other hand, has occurred in infants through an improperly prepared commercial formula. Heat processing destroyed some of the vitamin B_6 and made the amount inadequate for normal nutrition of the infants. Convulsive seizures and other manifestations of vitamin B_6 deficiency occurred, such as abnormal electroencephalograms and abnormal tryptophan load tests. These disappeared after pyridoxine was given.

Vitamin requirements are much higher than normal in infants who have vitamin-responsive inborn errors of metabolism. In these hereditary vitamin-dependency diseases, there is an aberrant metabolic state that responds to vitamins at continuous and pharmacological dose levels.

MINERALS

MAJOR MINERALS

Calcium. The importance of calcium for normal development and calcification of the skeleton in infants and children is well known. Calcium is also, of course, necessary for normal function of the nervous system. When serum calcium falls below a certain narrow range, convulsions may result. Shortly after birth the infant's serum concentration of calcium falls, even in the healthy newborn, but this fall is more marked in premature infants. After an infant is fed, the serum calcium rises. Serum calcium is higher in breast-fed babies than in those fed cow's-milk formulas that actually contain higher concentrations of minerals. Beyond the immediate newborn period, the late type of neonatal hypocalcemia may occur in infants fed formulas with a high intake of phosphorus. Under these conditions, where there is a low calcium-to-phosphorus ratio, the resulting hyperphosphatemia produces hypocalcemia.

Magnesium. Magnesium and the effects of its deficiency have been discussed in relation to PCM (see above). Clinically, magnesium deficiency usually occurs as part of complex malnutrition. Magnesium depletion might develop under conditions of prolonged losses of body fluids such as in diarrhea without magnesium replacement. It may also appear in a young child experiencing rapid growth and getting a diet in which magnesium is a limiting factor.

Caddell and her associates have developed a load test for the evaluation of magnesium status in children. In this 24-hour test, the retention of more than a certain percentage of a parenteral dose of magnesium is indicative of magnesium depletion. Premature infants and those born to mothers with an inadequate intake of magnesium apparently have poorer magnesium reserves than full-term infants born to well-nourished mothers. Caddell has also suggested a possible link between magnesium deficiency and the sudden-infant-death syndrome.

Sodium. Considerable concern has been voiced about the intake of sodium by infants and young children. Animal experiments have indicated that hypertension develops more readily in animals given a diet high in salt during the early part of their lives. Infants receive an adequate intake of sodium from the milk they consume, and the addition of salt to infant food is a questionable practice. Similar reservations and concerns have been expressed regarding the amount of sodium added to commercial foods for infants.

TRACE ELEMENTS

Iron. The consequence of iron deficiency is primarily anemia, which has been defined for children from six months to six years of age by the World Health Organization Scientific Group on Nutritional Anemias as a hemoglobin concentration less than 11.0 g/100 ml. Anemia actually is a late manifestation of iron deficiency. Stages of iron deficiency are, first, iron depletion, or hyposiderosis, characterized in adults by total or partial depletion of bone-marrow iron stores; second, iron deficiency without anemia, or sideropenia. In this stage the iron stores of the marrow are absent and, in addition, erythropoiesis is impaired due to low levels of circulating iron bound to transferrin. The third stage of iron deficiency is anemia.

Iron-deficiency anemia is quite prevalent in the United States and occurs with higher frequency in infants of low-income families than in other economic groups. Figure 20–8 shows the percentage of children of various ages with concentrations of hemoglobin less than 11.0 g/100 ml. Although this figure shows data from only one study, numerous other investigations are in general agreement with these findings, including the Ten-State Nutrition Survey of the United States. In this latter survey, for example, it was found that 44% of children below the age of two had hemoglobin levels less than 11.0 g/100 ml. Data on the intake of iron as well as hemoglobin determinations show that more than two-thirds of American children appear to receive intakes less than 9 mg iron per day, and more than 40% get less than 6 mg per day.

Thus, it seems apparent that the iron intake of a large proportion of children in the United States is inadequate to meet their needs. The higher incidence of anemia among infants of families of low economic level may be due partly to the greater incidence of low birth weight in this group. The low birth weight may indicate that the nutritional status of the mother during pregnancy was not optimal and that therefore the iron stores of the infant may be low at birth (see Chapter 19).

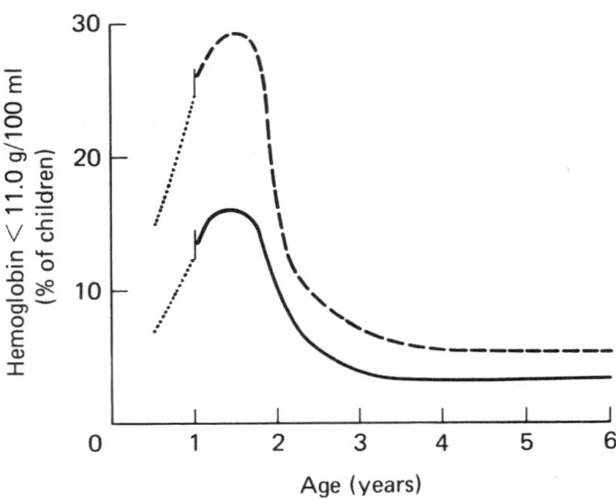

From Fomon, 1974.

Figure 20–8 Percent of children with hemoglobin concentrations less than 11.0 g/100 ml at various ages among the lowest-income group (upper curve) and other income groups combined (lower curve).

The normal newborn has a high body content of iron as compared with other age groups and a hemoglobin level of 14 to 20 g/100 ml. During the newborn period the hemoglobin falls to a mean value of 11 g/100 ml in full-term infants and 9 g/100 ml in premature infants, reaching its lowest point at approximately 6 to 8 weeks, the so-called "physiological anemia of the newborn." This fall in hemoglobin is due to decreased hemoglobin production, relatively increased erythrocyte destruction, and hemodilution from an increase in blood volume during growth. The American Medical Association committee on iron deficiency has stated that "during infancy (3 to 24 months), because of the rapid rate of growth, iron requirements in proportion to food intake exceed those of any other period of life." If iron intake is not adequate after the period when the 6- to 8-week-old infant is experiencing a low level of hemoglobin, then a second period of anemia due to iron deficiency will develop (see Figure 20–9).

Copper. At birth, normal infants have relatively large hepatic stores of copper, which enable them to cope with the low level of copper in milk. Copper deficiency is known to occur in infants secondary to conditions that influence absorption of the element—for example, severe malnutrition, chronic diarrhea, cystic fibrosis of the pancreas and celiac disease, or under conditions of increased intestinal loss, such as protein-losing enteropathy (malabsorption syndrome). Anemia, neutropenia, and bone changes resembling those of scurvy are signs of copper deficiency along with hypocupremia (see also PCM above). Copper deficiency has also been found during prolonged parenteral feeding of infants when copper was not included in the solution, and in premature babies as well. A genetic disease involving copper metabolism has been recognized and is called Menkes' kinky (or steely) hair syndrome (see Chapter 14).

Zinc. Although zinc has been known to be a biologically functional element since 1869, because of the element's ubiquity, zinc deficiency was for many years considered to be improbable in humans. Discovery of the condition in people of the Middle East brought about revised concepts. This work, carried out in the 1960s, demonstrated that zinc deficiency could occur even under natural conditions. This syndrome, affecting an estimated 3% of the adolescents in rural areas of Egypt and Iran, also occurs in other countries, including Turkey, Morocco, Portugal, and Panama. Its major feature is hypogonadal dwarfism: short stature and absent or retarded sexual development. Young people, in their early twenties, have the body size and physical appearance of prepuberal children. Bone age is grossly retarded, and epiphyses (see Chapter 21) often remain open long past the normal age of closure. An important etologic factor in the development of zinc deficiency under these conditions is the type of diet consumed, which consists largely of unleavened coarse whole wheat bread. Although its total content of zinc is not very low, its high concentration of phytate and fiber prevent good absorption.

Zinc deficiency has also been found to occur in the United States. In Denver, approximately 5% of a group of otherwise healthy children over the age of four years from middle-income families, were found to have low hair zinc levels, with low growth rates, poor appetite, and diminished taste

Figure 20–9 Mean hemoglobin levels in the first two years of life.

From Burman, 1971.

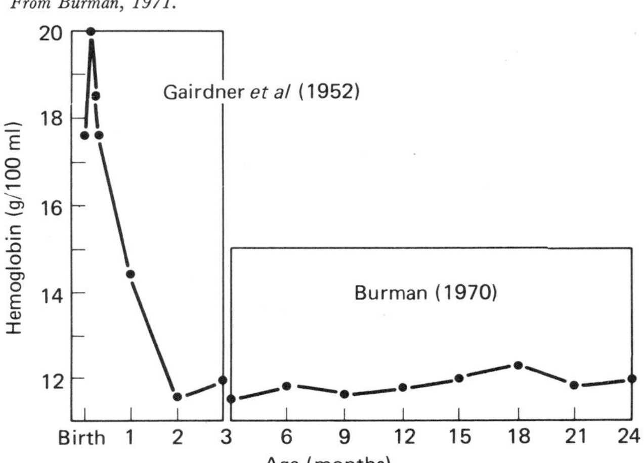

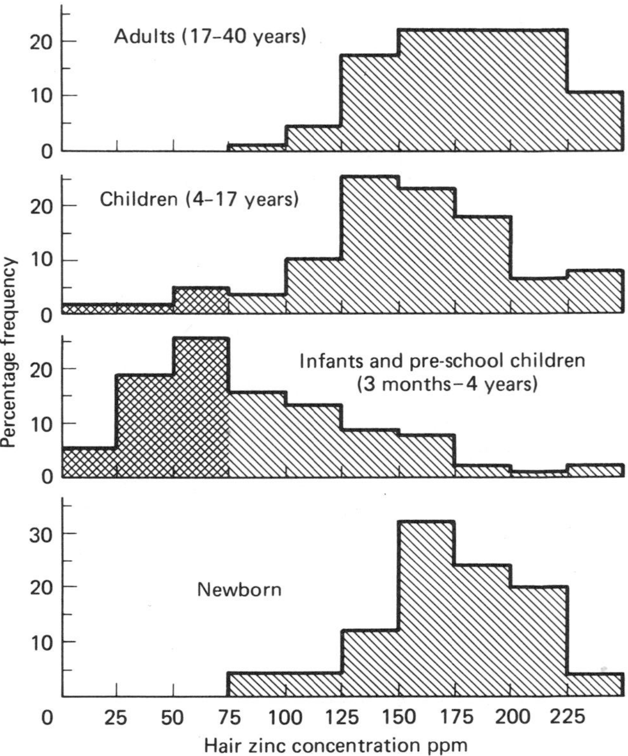

From Hambidge et al., 1972.

Figure 20–10 Concentrations of zinc in hair (88 adults; 132 children aged 4 to 17 years; 93 subjects aged three months to four years; and 25 neonates). Checkered area indicates percentage of subjects with levels of zinc in hair less than 75 ppm.

acuity (Figure 20–10). Supplementation with zinc was beneficial. In children from low-income families, 30% of a group whose heights were below the third percentile showed laboratory evidence of zinc depletion.

Hambidge has shown that zinc levels of hair decline markedly during the first year of life in infants in the United States but not in some other countries. An experimental investigation also demonstrated that male (but not female) infants fed a zinc-supplemented formula grew better than did those fed the usual formula (see Figure 20–11). These findings may be related to a lack in these children of the zinc-binding ligand (ZBL) found in human milk but very low in cow's milk (see Chapter 19). If efficient absorption of zinc in the neonatal period is aided by the ZBL, the high frequency of bottle feeding in the United States could contribute to the apparent prevalence of marginal zinc deficiency in infants.

Iodine. Iodine is an essential element for infants as it is at other stages of the life cycle. The effects of iodine deficiency during development and related problems are discussed in Chapter 14.

Fluoride. Fluoride is essential for the maintenance of strong, caries-free teeth. There is no question that the incidence of decayed, missing, and filled teeth is related to the concentration of fluoride in the drinking water. A level of 1 ppm of fluoride in the water is the recommended amount. Unfortunately, less than half the population of the United States receives this level of fluoride, either from naturally or artifically fluoridated water supplies. The fluoride content of food is extremely low, so that the amount in the water is most important. In the absence of fluoridated water, supplementation of infants and children with fluoride is recommended.

OVERNUTRITION

OBESITY

Obesity, which is defined as an excessive accumulation of adipose tissue, is the most significant problem of overnutrition. It appears likely that childhood obesity is important as a forerunner of adult obesity, although this concept is not yet proven. Approximately 80% of all overweight children remain obese, or are obese as adults. Two peaks for the onset of juvenile obesity seem to occur, between birth and four years of age, and between seven and 11 years of age.

The increased amount of adipose tissue in obese individuals can develop

Figure 20–11 Growth increments from birth to six months of age for the male infants. Control infants ($n = 8$) are indicated by the *shaded blocks*, test infants ($n = 14$) by the *open blocks* (Zn supplemented).

From Walravens and Hambidge, 1976.

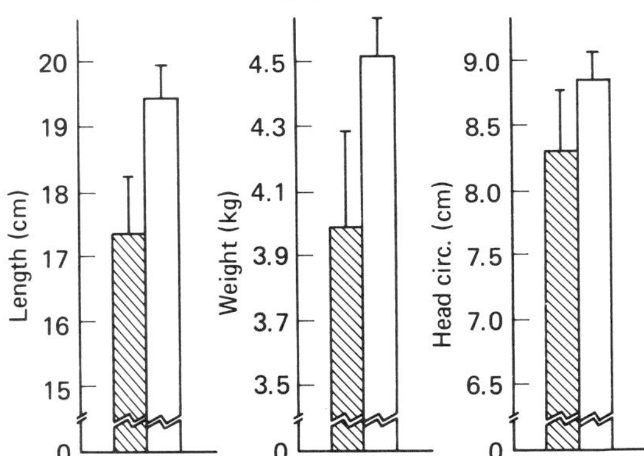

through an increase in the *number* of adipose cells or in their *size*, or both. In grossly obese subjects, the enlargement of fat depots is due mainly to an increase in the number of cells of adipose tissue (adipocytes). In moderately obese individuals cellular enlargement plays a more prominent role. Weight reduction results in a smaller cell size without any change in cell number.

It appears that once the adult cell number has been achieved, it cannot be altered by nutritional means. Hirsch and Knittle classified the number of adipocytes in individuals according to the age at which onset of obesity occurred. Their classification shows that the majority of individuals with an early age of onset had the highest cell number, and those whose obesity developed at later ages (after 20 years) had the lowest cell number. However, all obese persons had higher numbers of adipocytes than did nonobese individuals (see Figure 20–12). In contrast, when adults were made obese experimentally, no increase in adipose cell number occurred, although the cell size was increased. Adult rats made obese with high-fat diets did show an increase in the number of fat cells as well as in their size.

In experimental animals it has also been shown that nutritional manipulation before the time of weaning—that is, in early life—does affect the number of adipose cells even through adulthood. Rats that had been underfed during their preweaning period were smaller in total size than animals that had a very large food intake during the same period. In addition, both the number and the size of the fat cells were lower in the previously underfed animals, even when they had become ad libitum fed adults. These studies suggest that the early nutrition of humans as well as of animals may be

Figure 20–12 Adipose cellularity of 20 obese subjects shown in groupings as to age of onset.

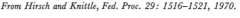

From Hirsch and Knittle, Fed. Proc. 29: 1516–1521, 1970.

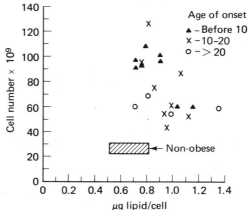

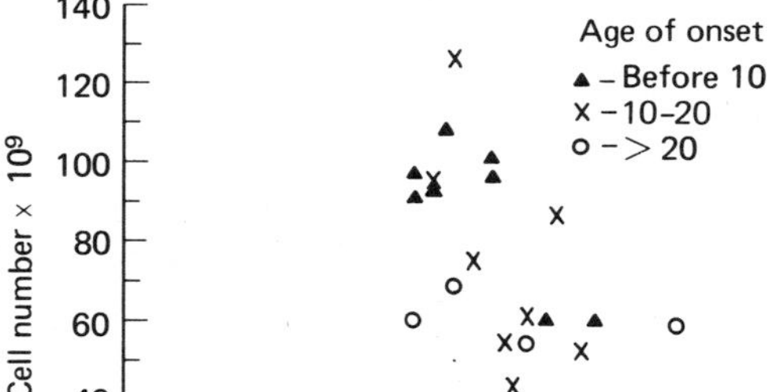

crucial in the development of obesity by affecting the cellularity of the adipose tissue.

As yet, insufficient information is available to establish the validity of this theory or the optimal nutritional treatment based upon it. However, if the concept is correct, then it may be extremely inadvisable to provide infants with more food than meets their caloric requirements. In this connection the differences between the growth of formula-fed and breast-fed infants become pertinent (see Chapter 19). Bottle-fed infants gain more rapidly in weight and length during the first few months of life than do breast-fed babies. Furthermore, bottle-fed babies generally gain more weight for a specified gain in length than do breast-fed infants. Fomon considers that the higher weight gain of bottle-fed babies reflects the consequences of overfeeding. Thus overfeeding might contribute to subsequent obesity by development of a large number of fat cells or through establishment of a habit of overeating.

The breast-fed baby, of course, regulates its own food intake, and the mother does not know how much milk the infant has actually taken. The bottle-fed baby, however, may be encouraged to eat more than would be the case if he were allowed to eat at his own level. It seems, therefore, that formula feeding is more likely to produce overfeeding than is nursing at the breast. Breast feeding may thus be a means of preventing at least one factor in the development of obesity.

Similar concerns have been raised regarding the introduction of supplementary foods (in addition to milk) at very early ages. It is estimated that most infants in the United States currently receive commercially prepared infant foods before the end of the first month. Since infants can meet all of their nutritional requirements from breast milk or formula without the addition of supplementary foods during the first six months of life, there appears to be little nutritional advantage in the practice. Furthermore, the early introduction of solid foods may encourage overfeeding and the establishment of poor food habits.

NURSING-BOTTLE SYNDROME

Although the nursing-bottle syndrome is not strictly in the category of overnutrition, it may be classified as such since it involves the giving of nutritional material in excess of the infant's nutritional needs. The nursing-bottle syndrome is characterized by rampant dental caries, decay of all the upper teeth and, in some instances, some of the lower posterior teeth. It never involves the lower anterior (front) teeth. This syndrome is caused by direct contact of the teeth with sugar, syrup, honey-sweetened water, milk, or fruit juice drunk from a nursing bottle. Such bottles containing sweetened liquids are usually used as pacifiers at bedtime by children beyond the usual bottle feeding age.

Caries results from the contact of the sweetened liquid with the teeth. Usually the child is lying down while using the nursing bottle. His tongue extends slightly out of his mouth and covers the lower front teeth. The liquid is thus in contact with all of the upper teeth and the lower back teeth but not the lower front teeth, which are protected by the tongue. As the child falls asleep, the sugary beverage tends to pool around the teeth, making continuous contact with the bacterial plaque on the teeth during the hours of sleep. The sugar is then fermented to organic acids, which continue to demineralize the teeth until they decay.

The consequences of such rampant caries in young children are obvious, involving possible malocclusion of the permanent teeth and development of speech impediments as well as loss of the teeth themselves. The destruction of the teeth in this syndrome is usually extensive, and often the entire crown may be destroyed. A sugar-sweetened beverage should never be used in this way, and if a pacifier is not appropriate or if the nursing bottle is necessary, then plain milk or fluoridated water should be used.

References and Supplementary Readings

ALTON-MACKEY, M. G., AND B. L. WALKER. "The physical and neuromotor development of progeny of female rats fed graded levels of pyridoxine during lactation." *Am. J. Clin. Nutr.* **31**: 76–81 (1978).

BROWN, R. E. "Breast feeding in modern times." *Am. J. Clin. Nutr.* **26**: 556–562 (1973).

BURGER, F. J., AND Z. A. HOGEWIND. "Changes in trace elements in kwashiorkor." *S. A. Med. J.* **48**: 502–504 (1974).

BURMAN, D. "Iron requirements in infancy." *British J. Haematol.* **20**: 243–247 (1971).

CADDELL, J. L. "Magnesium deficiency in protein-calorie malnutrition: A follow-up study." *N. Y. Acad. Sci.* **162**: 874–890 (1969).

CADDELL, J. L. "Magnesium deprivation in sudden unexpected infant death." *Lancet* **II**: 258–262 (1972).

CADDELL, J. L. "Magnesium in the nutrition of the child." *Clin. Pediatrics* **13**: 263–272 (1974).

CADDELL, J. L., P. A. BYRNE, R. A. TRISKA, AND A. E. MCELFRESH. "The magnesium load test: III. Correlations of clinical and laboratory data in infants from one to six months of age." *Clin. Pediatrics* **14**: 478–484 (1975).

COMMITTEE ON NUTRITIONAL MISINFORMATION, National Academy of Sciences. *Hazards of Overuse of Vitamin D.* Washington, D.C., 1974.

FOMON, S. J. *Infant Nutrition.* Philadelphia: W. B. Saunders, 1974.

JELLIFFE, D. B., AND E. F. P. JELLIFFE. "The urban avalanche and child nutrition: I and II." *J. Am. Diet. Assoc.* **57**: 111–118 (1970).

JELLIFFE, D. B., AND E. F. P. JELLIFFE. "The at-risk concept as related to young child nutrition programs." *Clin. Pediatrics* **12**: 65–67 (1973).

HAMBIDGE, K. M., C. HAMBIDGE, M. JACOBS, AND J. D. BAUM. "Low levels of zinc in hair, anorexia, poor growth and hypogeusia in children." *Ped. Res.* **6**: 868–874 (1972).

HAMBIDGE, K. M., AND P. WALRAVENS. "Trace elements in nutrition." *Practice of Pediatrics* **1**, Chap. 29: 1–40 (1975).

HURLEY, L. S., J. R. DUNCAN, M. V. SLOAN, AND C. D. ECKHERT. "Zinc-binding ligands in milk and intestine: A role in neonatal nutrition?" *Proc. Natl. Acad. Sci. USA* **74**: 3547–3549 (1977).

LINDER, M. C., AND H. N. MUNRO. "Iron and copper metabolism during development." *Enzyme* **15**: 111–138 (1973).

MARTORELL, R., C. YARBROUGH, A. LECHTIG, H. DELGADO, AND R. E. KLEIN. "Genetic-environmental interactions in physical growth." *Acta Paediatr. Scand.* **66**: 579–584 (1977).

OLSON, R. E., ed. *Protein-Calorie Malnutrition.* The Nutrition Foundation. London: Academic Press, 1975.

SCRIVER, C. R. "Vitamin-responsive inborn errors of metabolism: Relevance to perinatal pharmacology and metabolism." In: J. DANCIS AND J. C. HWANG, eds., *Perinatal Pharmacology: Problems and Priorities*, pp. 161–175 New York: Raven Press, 1974.

SIEGEL, N. J., AND T. J. SPACKMAN. "Chronic hypervitaminosis A with intracranial hypertension and low cerebrospinal fluid concentration of protein." *Clin. Pediatrics* **11**: 580–584 (1972).

STERN, J. S., AND M. R. C. GREENWOOD. "A review of development of adipose cellularity in man and animals." *Fed. Proc.* **33**: 1952–1955 (1974).

STERN, J. S., AND P. R. JOHNSON. "Size and number of adipocytes and their implications." in H. Katyen and R. Mahler, eds., *Advances in Modern Nutr., Vol. II, Diabetes, Obesity, and Vascular Disease, Part I*, New York: Hemisphere Press, 1978, pp. 303–340.

THEUER, R. C. "Iron undernutrition in infancy." *Clin. Pediatrics* **13**: 522–531 (1974).

VON MURALT, A., ed. *Protein-Calorie Malnutrition.* Berlin: Springer-Verlag, 1969.

WALRAVENS, P. A., AND K. M. HAMBIDGE. "Growth of infants fed a zinc supplemented formula." *Am. J. Clin. Nutr.* **29**: 1114–1121 (1976).

WILLIAMS, C. D. "The story of kwashiorkor." *Courier* **13**: 361 (1931). Reprinted in: A Special Number Marking the Eightieth Year of Cicely D. Williams, *Nutr. Rev.* **31**: 330–384 (November 1973).

21

Adolescence

CHANGES OCCURRING DURING ADOLESCENCE

INCREASED RATE OF GROWTH

Adolescence is marked by a great increase in growth. An individual's growth when recorded on an *absolute* basis shows a continuous curve. Tanner cites one of the earliest records of such a growth curve, the changes in height of a young man from his birth in 1759 until he was 18 years old (Figure 21–1A). However, if the same changes in height are recorded not as absolute growth, but as *gain per year* (Figure 21–1B), it is seen that the rate of growth is not continuous. The rate of growth, or gain per year, decreases rapidly from the time of birth to four years of age, then plateaus to nine years, declines slightly, and after about 12 years of age increases sharply and then declines. This peak in the rate of growth is called the "adolescent growth spurt."

There is a significant and important difference in the growth patterns of boys and girls. If the mean growth rate of a group of boys is examined, it is seen that the boys have a peak velocity (adolescent growth spurt) between 14 and 15 years of age, while a group of girls will have a peak velocity between 12 and 13 years of age. The adolescent growth spurt occurs about two years earlier in girls than in boys (see Figure 21–2). The difference in size between adult men and women is to a large extent the result of this difference in the adolescent growth spurt.

It is important to note, however, that there are differences between mean curves of growth rates and individual growth-rate curves. The actual time at which the adolescent growth spurt begins varies considerably from one child to another. The mean or average curve, however, flattens out the peak; this phenomenon explains the plateaus in the mean curve shown in Figure 21–2. The mean of the growth-rate curve actually characterizes the average velocity curve very poorly, since it smooths out the growth spurt (Figure 21–3).

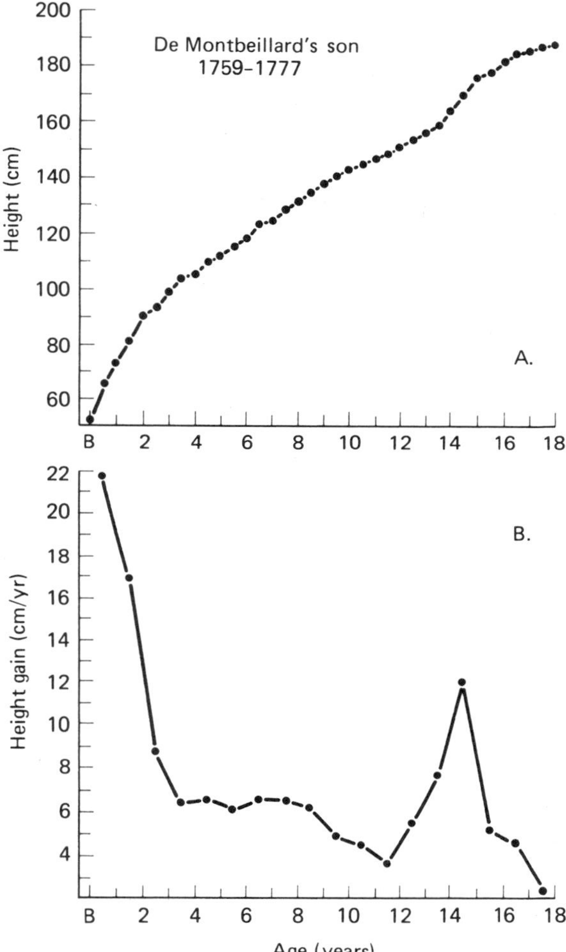

From Tanner, 1962.

Figure 21–1 Growth in height of de Montbeillard's son from birth to 18 years, 1759–1777. A. Distance curve, height attained at each age. B. Velocity curve, increments in height from year to year.

Every muscular and skeletal dimension of the body takes part in the adolescent growth spurt. Even the head diameter accelerates somewhat and is involved in the overall peak of growth rate. The length of the foot is the first of the skeletal dimensions below the head to stop growing. The familiar case of the puppy with big feet who eventually "grows into" his feet is an illustration. There seems to be a gradient of growth peaks in which the foot stops growing first, then the calf, then the thigh. In the arms, similarly, the

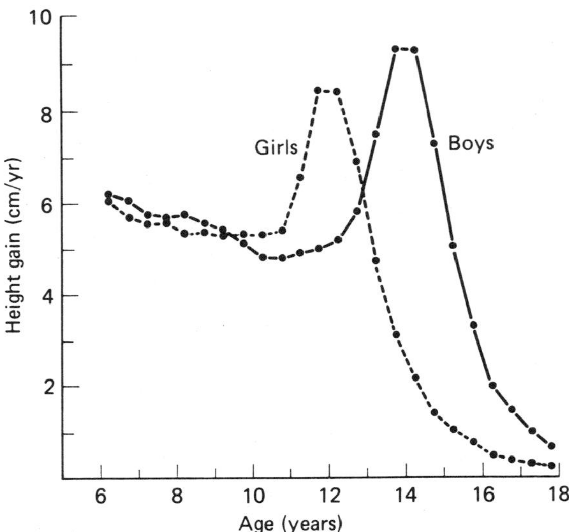

From Tanner, 1962.

Figure 21–2 Adolescent spurt in height growth for girls and boys. The curves are from subjects who have their peak velocities during the modal years 12–13 for girls and 14–15 for boys. (Actual mean increments, each plotted at center of its $\frac{1}{2}$-year period.)

forearm stops growing six months before the upper arm. Thus the peripheral parts of the limbs seem to be more advanced than the proximal. There is also a fairly regular order in which various dimensions of the body accelerate in general. Length of the legs reaches its peak before the rest of the body, which is why gangling adolescents have long-legged proportions. Approximately four months after leg-length peak, hip width and chest spread reach their maximum rates.

The two constituents of stature or height are leg length and trunk length, and their peaks of growth rate are separated by about a year. The peak of growth rate for stature velocity as a whole lies between the peaks for leg length and for trunk length, and the shape of the individual stature curve is subject to the same smoothing effect as shown in Figure 21-3. The height spurt is due to an increase more in the length of the trunk than in the length of the leg, and the ratio of trunk length to leg length increases during adolescence.

In addition to growth in height and weight, other morphological changes occur during adolescence. The cartilages of the wrist grow and ossify more rapidly, the heart and abdominal organs grow faster, and in particular the reproductive organs enlarge. Figure 21–4 shows growth of

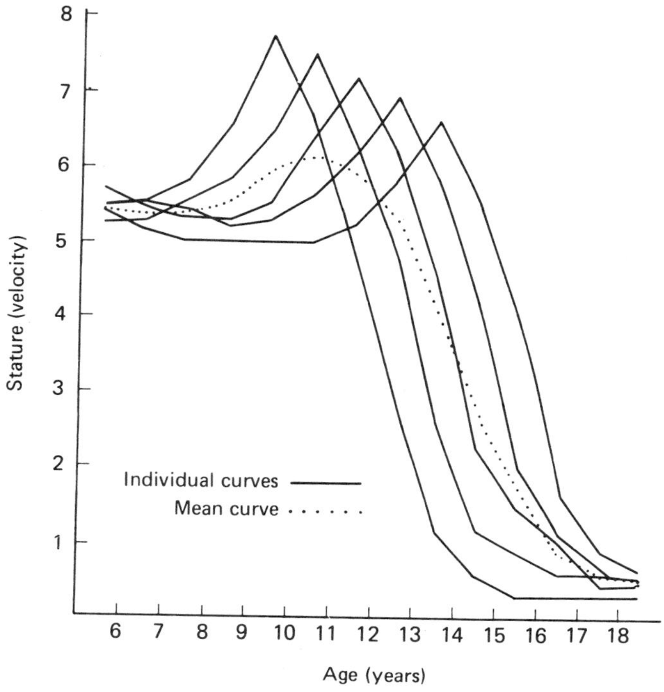

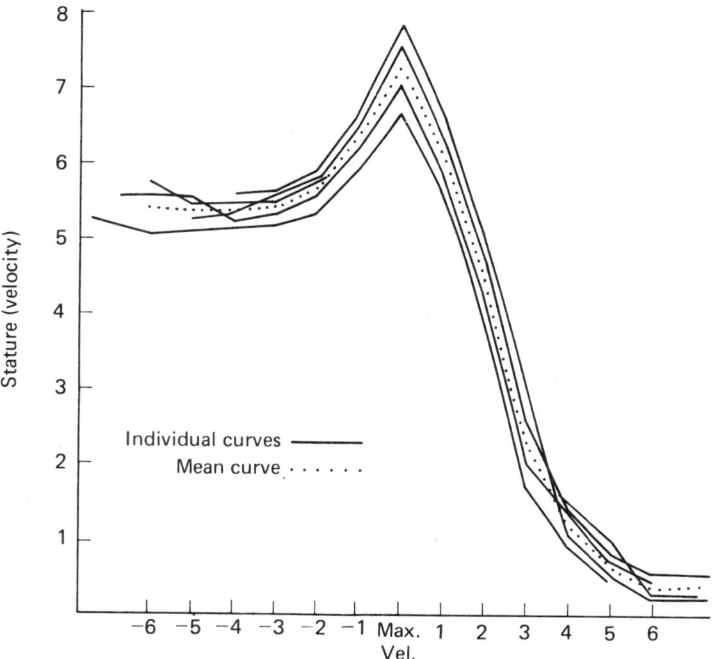

From Tanner, 1962.

Figure 21–3 Relation between individual and mean velocities during the adolescent spurt. On the left, the height curves are plotted against chronological age; on the right, they are plotted according to their time of maximum velocity.

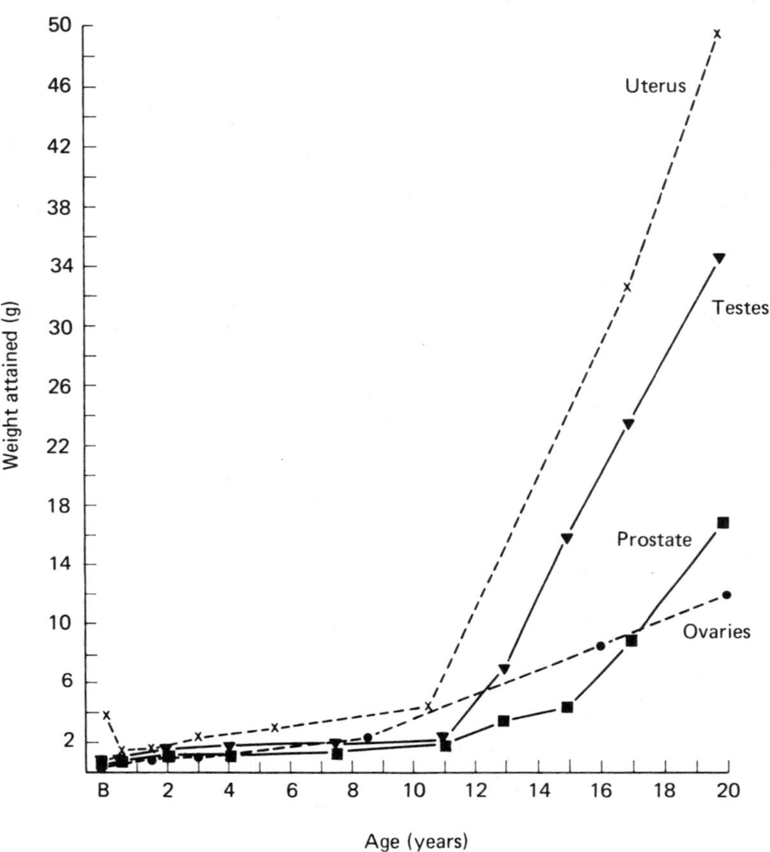

From Tanner, 1962.

Figure 21–4 Growth in weight of the testes, prostate, ovaries, and uterus. Distance curves; weight attained.

the reproductive organs in relation to age. The female organs begin to enlarge markedly earlier than do the male organs.

The head also changes in its overall growth and proportions during adolescence, and there are profound facial changes, which are related to differences in proportional growth of the various components. The head increases in length, breadth, and circumference. These dimensions are about 96% of the adult value by age ten, but acceleration in head length, circumference, and breadth can be seen (Figure 21–5). Increments are small, less than 2 mm/year at the maximum rate, but acceleration is nevertheless evident. The peak velocity for facial measurements is usually reached a few months after the peak in growth rate for stature. The growth spurt is largest in the mandible, the lower jaw. The significance of this growth spurt in the mandible is apparent when it is recognized that between 12 and 20 years of age, only 6 to 7% of growth remains to be completed in the cranial base, but there is still 25% of mature growth to be achieved in the height of the mandible in boys.

SUBCUTANEOUS FAT

Changes in subcutaneous fat also occur during adolescence. In boys, a year or more before the height spurt starts, subcutaneous fat increases in quantity. This increase lasts for about two years; then, while the general growth spurt is occurring, there is a thinning of subcutaneous fat in the limbs. In postadolescence, subcutaneous fat increases in the trunk, so that the level is the same as in preadolescence, but in the arms and legs the thinning of the fat persists for several years. In girls there is somewhat more subcutaneous fat at all ages, particularly after age five or six, when the thickness

Figure 21–5 Velocity curves of head length and breadth for boys with peak velocity in stature between ages $14\frac{1}{4}$ and $15\frac{3}{4}$. Mixed longitudinal data; actual increments.

From Tanner, 1962.

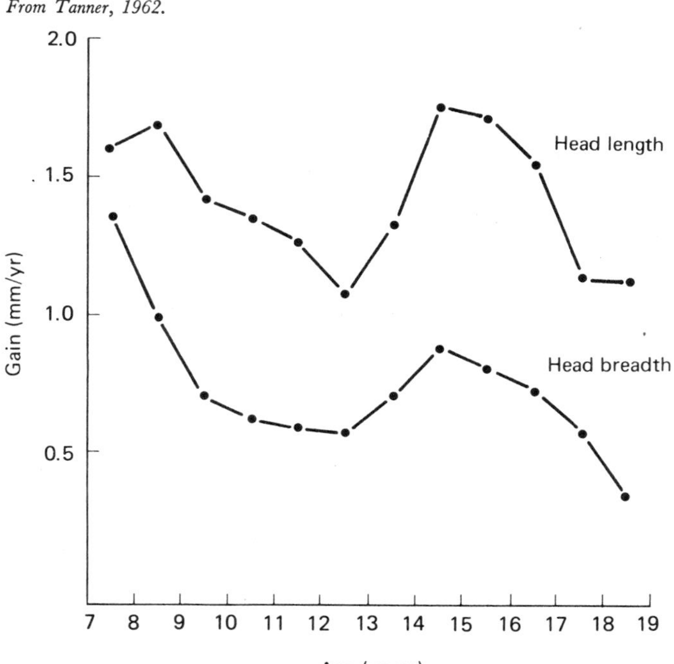

of the subcutaneous fat layer begins to increase steadily in both limbs and trunk, continuing to increase in the trunk during the adolescent spurt.

POSTADOLESCENT GROWTH

Growth does not entirely cease at the end of the adolescent period. In man, the epiphyses of the long bones close completely and become calcified. After this closure, the long bones can no longer increase in length, and further growth of the arms and legs is impossible. There is a definite sequence of closure of the epiphyses. The earliest to close are those at the elbow; those of the knee close about a year later. The medial end of the clavicle is usually last; it is not closed in men until about age 24 or 25.

Bones that do not grow by the enlargement and subsequent ossification of the epiphyseal plate or growth cartilage, as do the long bones, but rather by surface deposition of the calcium phosphate bone salt (the other major form of bone growth), may respond to stimulation and continue to grow. An example is seen in acromegaly, a pituitary disease involving an excessive amount of growth hormone. After epiphyseal closure, acromegaly can affect only those bones that continue to grow by surface deposition, such as the bones of the face, which therefore become massive in the adult form of the disease. If the long bones are affected, as happens before epiphyseal closure, the individual becomes a giant.

Despite the closure of epiphyses of the long bones, however, there are small increments of growth in stature even after adolescence. In one study in which a number of persons were followed for nine years, it was found that stature increased about one-half centimeter from the age of 20 to 29, remained stationary to age 45, and then decreased. The increase in height was due to an increase in the growth of trunk length. In contrast, the head and face measurements increased steadily by 2 to 4% from 20 to 60 years of age.

FACTORS AFFECTING RATE OF GROWTH AND AGE AT PUBERTY

The rate of growth of individuals and the age at which puberty occurs are affected by a number of factors.

ADULT PHYSIQUE

There are, in general, differences in the adult physique between individuals who mature early and those who mature late. These differences can be seen both before adolescence and after it is completed. Boys and girls

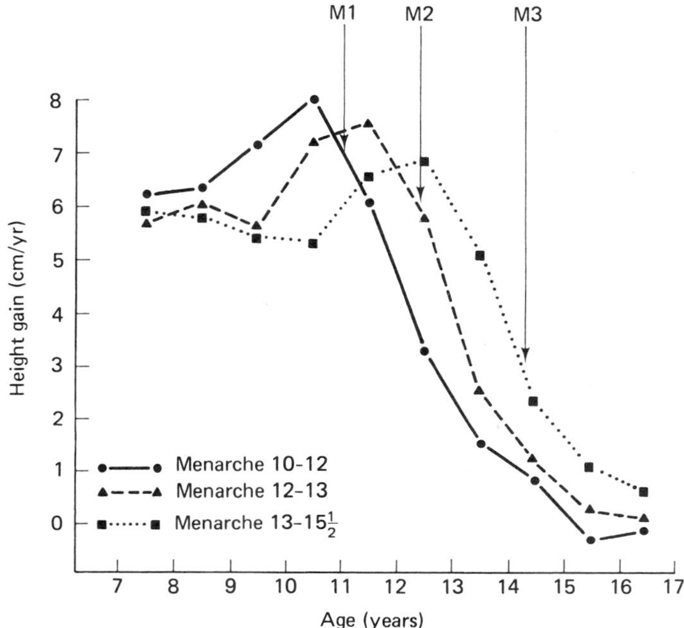

From Tanner, 1962.

Figure 21–6 Relation of peak velocities in height for early, average, and late maturing girls; and of time elapsing between peak velocity and menarche for the three groups. M_1, M_2, M_3, average time of menarche for each group.

who are tall before puberty usually begin adolescence earlier than those who are short. Linear people, that is, those who are tall for their body weight, in general develop late. Only a small part of this linearity is caused by the delay in adolescence that allows more growth of the legs before epiphyseal closure, since there are differences in physique between late and early maturers even before the growth spurt takes place. As early as two years of age, those who at puberty will be late maturers weigh less for their height than do early maturers. Figure 21–6 shows the growth spurts of three groups of girls in relation to the menarche (onset of menstruation). In those whose menarche occurred earlier, the growth spurt was also early.

NUTRITION

Nutrition, of course, influences the rate of growth. This has been demonstrated in numerous nutritional studies involving experimental animals as well as humans (see Chapter 20).

CLIMATE AND RACE

Neither climate nor race influences the rate of growth and the onset of puberty as much as does nutrition. In animals, growth and development appear to be slowed by cold, but such temperature effects in the wild are probably due to nutritional deficiency from a food supply inadequate for the higher metabolic rate produced by cold. In man, climate has only a minor effect. For example, the age at menarche of Nigerian upper-class girls was 14.3 years, while that of Alaskan Eskimo girls was 14.4 years. In a study of girls from India, the age at menarche was inversely related to their socioeconomic class as indicated by the father's occupation. Girls from the highest socioeconomic class had the lowest ages at menarche.

The effect of race is difficult to separate from those of nutrition and socioeconomic factors. For example, a study was made of the difference between girls of Japanese ancestry born and reared in California and those born in California and reared in Japan. The girls born and reared in California started menstruating one and a half years earlier than did those born in California and reared in Japan. In addition, their skeletal age was advanced by one to two years. The California-Japanese were also taller and heavier than those reared in Japan, but their leg length remained shorter than average for Americans. Thus, body proportions were unaltered although growth was increased.

GENETIC CONTROL OF RATE OF DEVELOPMENT

The genetic control of rate of development is a fundamental control. Evidence to support this concept comes from two sources, age at menarche and skeletal maturation. There is a high correlation between the ages of menarche in related women (Table 21–1). In identical twins, the time of menarche differed by only 2.8 months. Nonidentical twins were the same as other sisters, while the age of menarche in unrelated women differed con-

TABLE 21–1 DIFFERENCE IN AGE AT MENARCHE OF RELATED AND UNRELATED WOMEN

Relationship	*No. of Pairs*	*Difference, Months*
Identical twins	51	2.8
Nonidentical twins	47	12.0
Sisters	145	12.9
Unrelated women	120	18.6

Adapted from Tanner, 1962.

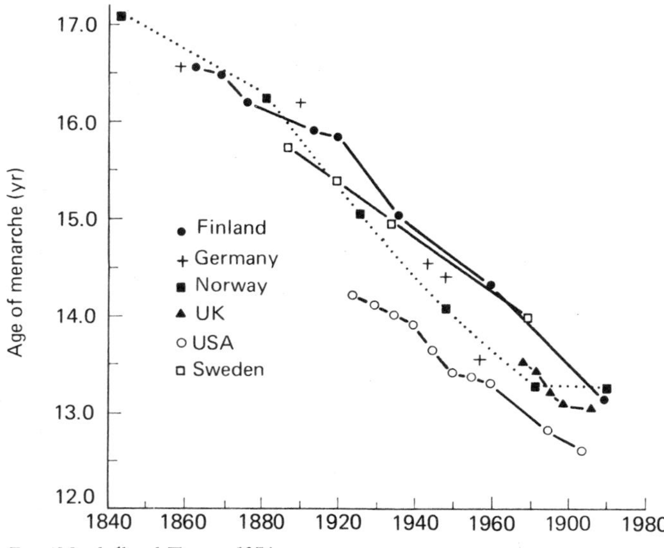

From Marshall and Tanner, 1974.

Figure 21–7 Secular trend in age of menarche.

siderably. There was also a correlation between the age of menarche of mothers and daughters.

SECULAR TREND IN AGE AT PUBERTY

The age at menarche has declined steadily in many countries for more than a century (Figure 21–7). Although the cause of this secular trend is not fully understood, improved nutrition is undoubtedly one of the important factors. This trend is seen also in the onset of puberty in boys. Frisch has proposed the hypothesis that a critical body weight triggers menarche. According to this investigator, both recent and historical evidence indicates that the mean weight of menarche of Caucasian girls has been about 46 kg for over a century. This intriguing hypothesis is not fully accepted as yet and remains to be further tested.

SUMMARY

The factors most important in affecting the rate of growth and the onset of puberty are:

1. adult physique,
2. genetic factors,
3. nutritional effects.

NUTRITIONAL NEEDS DURING ADOLESCENCE

TEENAGERS' DIET

Because of the very rapid growth rate that is characteristic of adolescence, it is obvious that nutritional requirements are high during this period. However, in response to the question, "What do teenagers actually eat?" very little definite information is available. In 1950, summaries of nutritional surveys of the United States indicated that teenage girls were the poorest age and sex group in relation to meeting their nutritional needs. It was found that teenagers, both boys and girls, had low blood levels of hemoglobin, vitamin A, and vitamin C, and low levels of urinary riboflavin. Table 21–2 shows the percentage of low and deficient hemoglobin values in this population.

In an earlier study in Iowa it was observed that in teenagers the average consumption of almost every nutrient was adequate, but iron intake of girls was substantially less than the recommended amount. In some individuals the intake of calcium fell below the recommended level. A longitudinal study of 127 teenagers showed that even though mean intake of all nutrients except iron and calcium met or exceeded the recommended dietary allowances, 15% of the girls failed to meet two-thirds of the allowances for vitamins A and C. Among the boys, 10% failed to meet this level for vitamin A, and 30% for vitamin C. There were no really low protein intakes, but approximately half of the girls were low in iron and calcium intake. Even though roughly 10% of both boys and girls consumed less than two-thirds the allowance for calories, obesity was quite common and was due in part to physical inactivity.

Thus iron, vitamin A, vitamin C, and calcium appear to be the nutrients most often inadequate in teenagers' diets. However, there is no information

TABLE 21–2 PERCENTAGE OF DEFICIENT HEMOGLOBIN VALUES

Age	*White*	*Black*	*Spanish-American*	*Deficient Hemoglobin, g/100 ml*
All, 6–12	13.9	35.2	9.8	< 11.4
Males, 13–16	5.0	19.0	11.2	< 12
Females, 13–16	6.2	26.6	10.9	< 11.4
Females, 17–44	16.0	39.4	22.9	< 12

From Ten-State Nutrition Survey in the United States, 1968–1970: Preliminary Report to the Congress. Atlanta, Public Health Service Center for Disease Control, 1971.

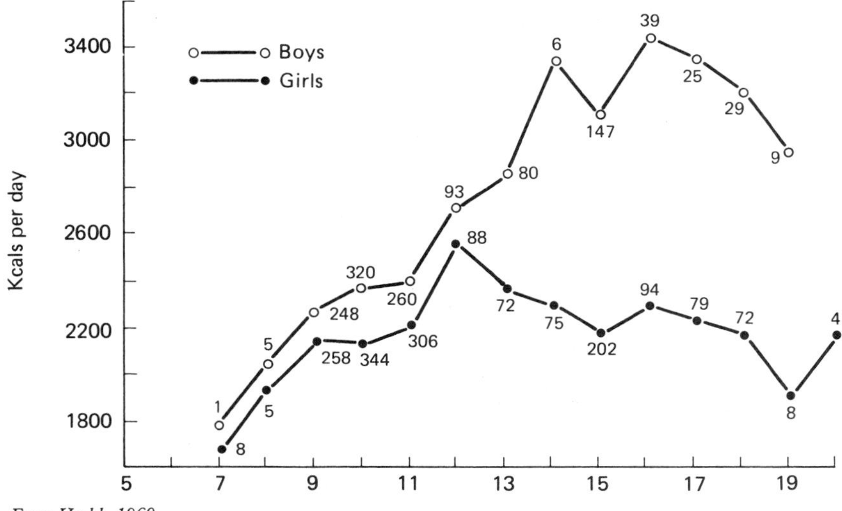

From Heald, 1969.

Figure 21–8 Average daily caloric intake in children and adolescents. Numbers refer to number of cases.

available in regard to trace elements and certain vitamins such as B_6 and pantothenic acid.

An interesting aspect of teenagers' diets is that their eating patterns appear to be unorthodox or random. In a sample of this age group in California, lunch was the meal most often omitted. About a third of all the subjects in this study and 90% of the black teenagers showed highly irregular eating practices. However, those with regular structured meals, usually augmented by snacks, tended to have better nutrient intake than the irregular eaters.

Heald and his co-workers have summarized data from a large number of studies on the intake of calories, protein, and fat in children and adolescents in the United States. Figure 21–8 shows the caloric intake of boys and girls from age seven to age 19. The peak caloric demands of girls appear to occur at the time of menarche and are followed by a slow decline. In boys, the caloric intake seems to parallel the adolescent growth spurt, increasing until the age of 16, and then decreasing to age 19. The protein intake during this age period is shown in Figure 21–9. In girls, the peak of protein intake occurs at age 12, and there is a secondary rise at age 17. These intakes of protein for both boys and girls are in general above the RDA for this age group.

The daily fat intake of children and adolescents is summarized in Figure 21–10. There is a general upward trend in the fat intake of boys from age

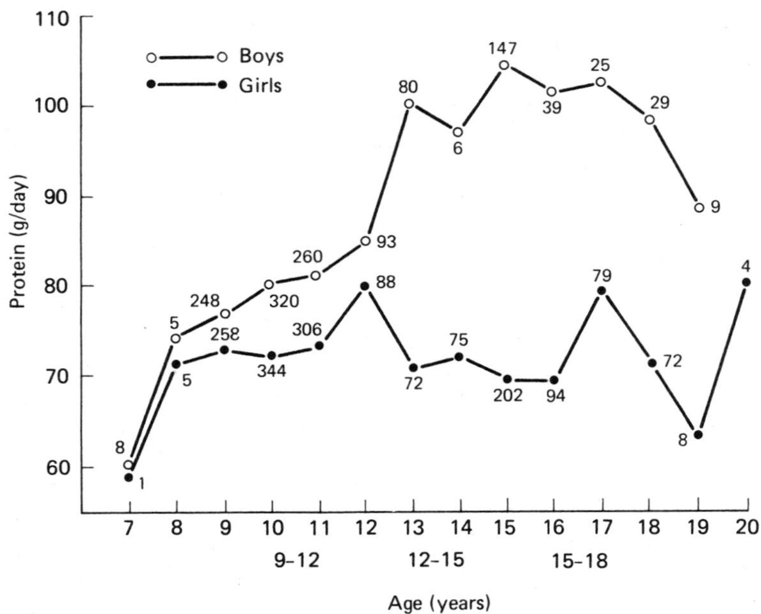

From Heald, 1969.

Figure 21–9 Average daily protein intake in children and adolescents. Numbers refer to number of cases.

Figure 21–10 Average daily fat intake of children and adolescents. Numbers refer to number of cases.

From Heald, 1969.

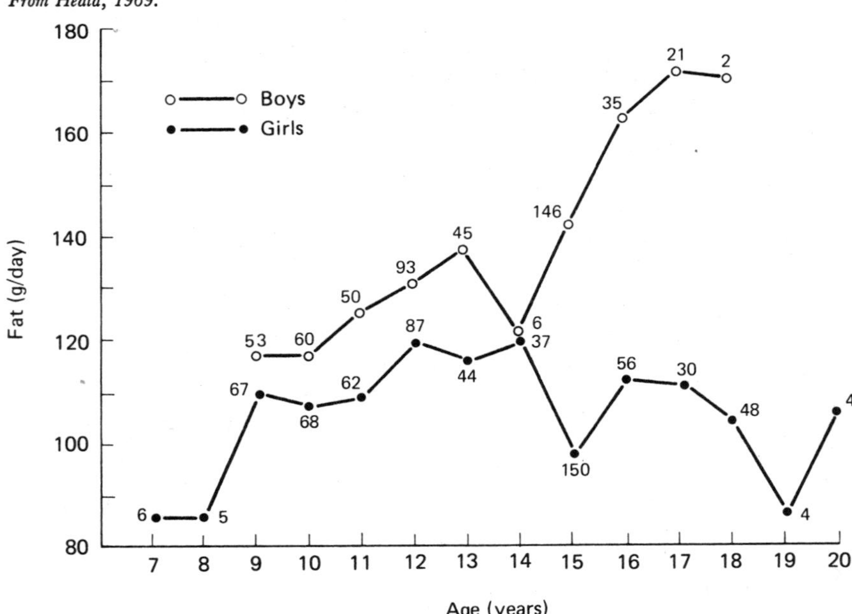

nine through age 18, with a considerable increase in consumption during adolescence. Girls show a steady increase in fat intake from age eight through 12, but this levels off and then declines during late adolescence.

Obesity, as indicated above, is one of the major problems of adolescent nutrition. In one report, the incidence of obesity in this age group was estimated as 13% of adolescent girls and 10% of adolescent boys. The possible etiology of obesity was discussed in Chapter 19.

The nutritional needs of adolescents are still far from being understood. As Hegsted has said,

> The best summary that one can make about the calorie, fat, protein and amino acid needs of adolescents is that there are so few factual data available for this age group that nearly everything we presumably know is obtained by extrapolation and then conclude that extrapolation is a very dangerous business. We need actual data. However, I do not want to leave the impression that the final solutions will necessarily come simply from a large expansion of studies with adolescents. The limitations in studies on human subjects of any age are very great and the greatest deficit in knowledge is at the fundamental level. When we understand those factors and mechanisms which modify and govern the utilization of calories, those which govern the circulating level of plasma cholesterol and lipoproteins, those which control the efficiency of utilization of proteins and amino acids, etc., then we will know how to deal logically with the difficult problems that should be solved. Many of these answers are more likely to come from fundamental investigations with experimental animals and the application of imaginative biochemistry. Studies with human subjects are more likely to define the problems rather than provide the answers.

RECOMMENDED DIETARY ALLOWANCES

The recommended dietary allowances for adolescents are summarized in Table 21–3.

PREGNANCY IN ADOLESCENCE

Pregnancy during adolescence represents a special problem in nutritional requirements. The teenage girl who has the additional nutritional requirements of pregnancy imposed upon her still-growing and developing body is at risk in terms of her own health as well as that of her baby.

PREGNANT ADOLESCENTS AS A HIGH-RISK GROUP

Because of the increased nutritional needs related to the rapid growth of adolescence as well as the additional requirements for pregnancy itself, we can raise the question as to whether pregnancy during adolescence imposes a special risk for the complications of pregnancy. One line of evi-

TABLE 21–3 RECOMMENDED DIETARY ALLOWANCES FOR ADOLESCENTS

Nutrient	Boys 11–14	Boys 15–18	Girls 11–14	Girls 15–18
Calories, kcal	2800	3000	2400	2100
Protein, g	44	54	44	48
Vitamin A, IU	5000	5000	4000	4000
Vitamin D, IU	400	400	400	400
Vitamin E, IU	12	15	12	12
Ascorbic acid, mg	45	45	45	45
Folacin, mg	0.4	0.4	0.4	0.4
Vitamin B_{12}, μg	3	3	3	3
Niacin, mg	18	20	16	14
Riboflavin, mg	1.5	1.8	1.3	1.4
Thiamin, mg	1.4	1.5	1.2	1.1
Vitamin B_6, mg	1.6	2.0	1.6	2.0
Calcium, g	1.2	1.2	1.2	1.2
Phosphorus, g	1.2	1.2	1.2	1.2
Iodine, μg	130	150	115	115
Iron, mg	18	18	18	18
Magnesium, mg	350	400	300	300
Zinc, mg	15	15	15	15

From Food and Nutrition Board, NRC, NAS, 1974.

TABLE 21–4 PERCENTAGE DISTRIBUTION OF LIVE BIRTHS BY BIRTH WEIGHT UNDER 2500 g AND BY AGE OF MOTHER AND COLOR: UNITED STATES, 1965

Age of Mother, years	Birth Weight 2500 g or Less, %	Color: White, %	Color: Nonwhite, %
Total	8.3	7.2	13.8
Under 15	18.7	13.0	21.3
15–19	10.5	8.5	16.4
20–24	7.9	6.9	13.3
25–29	7.3	6.5	12.2
30–34	7.9	7.0	12.8
35–39	8.9	8.0	13.4
40–44	9.0	8.3	12.5
45–49	8.7	8.5	9.8

From U. S. Department of Health, Eduction, and Welfare Statistics, 1967.

dence is the high incidence of low birth weight in very young mothers (see Table 21–4). As maternal age increases, the proportion of low-birth-weight infants decreases up to age 40, with the lowest rate occurring in the 25- to 29-year age group. Mortality rates of infants are also much higher for mothers under 15 years of age than for older mothers (Table 21–5), especially during the first month of life.

The most consistent high-risk characteristic of adolescent pregnancy is toxemia. When other variables correlated with poor nutrition, such as nonwhite race and poverty, are added, the incidence of toxemia is even higher. Anemia, another problem common in the pregnant adolescent, is associated with the amount of prenatal care received. Fetal pelvic disproportion and prolonged labor are other complications of teenage pregnancy. The pregnant adolescent is also at greater risk of having a baby with congenital malformations, especially of the central nervous system (see Table 21–6).

The psychological aspects of teenage pregnancy may also have an effect on the nutritional status of the mother and perhaps of her infant. Many teenage pregnancies are unwanted and involve unmarried mothers. Such births, or the teenage pregnancy of a very young marriage, often lead to the vicious circle of the "adolescent trap" (Figure 21–11). Thus, as with many problems of nutrition in humans, it is difficult to separate nutritional factors

TABLE 21–5 MORTALITY OF WHITE AND NONWHITE INFANTS BY AGE OF MOTHER AND AGE AT DEATH: UNITED STATES, 1960 BIRTH COHORT

Age of Mother, years	*Neonatal*[a] *(under 28 days)*			*Postneonatal*[a] *(28 days–11 months)*			*Infant*[a] *(under 1 year)*		
	Total	*White*	*Non-white*	*Total*	*White*	*Non-white*	*Total*	*White*	*Non-white*
Total	18.4	16.9	26.7	6.7	5.3	14.7	25.1	22.2	41.4
Under 15	41.2	32.1	46.5	17.6	15.5	18.8	58.7	47.5	65.3
15–19	22.7	20.4	30.9	10.1	7.7	18.6	32.8	28.1	49.5
20–24	17.3	15.9	25.3	6.9	5.5	14.8	24.2	21.4	40.2
25–29	16.6	15.3	24.2	5.8	4.6	13.1	22.4	20.0	37.3
30–34	18.3	17.0	26.4	5.3	4.2	12.0	23.7	21.2	38.4
35–39	19.7	18.4	27.3	5.8	4.5	13.9	25.5	22.9	41.2
40–44	23.1	22.0	29.4	7.5	6.1	15.4	30.6	28.1	44.7
45 and over	31.3	31.8	28.9	9.8	7.1	21.6	41.1	38.9	50.5

[a]Rate per 1000 live births.

From U. S. Department of Health, Education, and Welfare Statistics, 1967.

TABLE 21–6 INCIDENCE OF BABIES DYING WITH SELECTED NEURAL TUBE DEFECTS BY AGE OF MOTHER[a]

	Age of Mother, years		
Abnormality	*< 20*	*25–30*	*40+*
Anencephalus	3.5	2.0	3.3
Spina bifida	1.7	0.9	1.5
Occipital meningocele	0.35	0.2	0.35
Hydrocephalus	0.28	0.32	0.70

[a]Rates are per 1000 live births.

From Butler and Alberman, Perinatal Problems, *Wilkiams & Willins Co., Baltimore, 1969, in Ballard and Gold, 1971.*

Figure 21–11 The adolescent trap.

From Ballard and Gold, 1971.

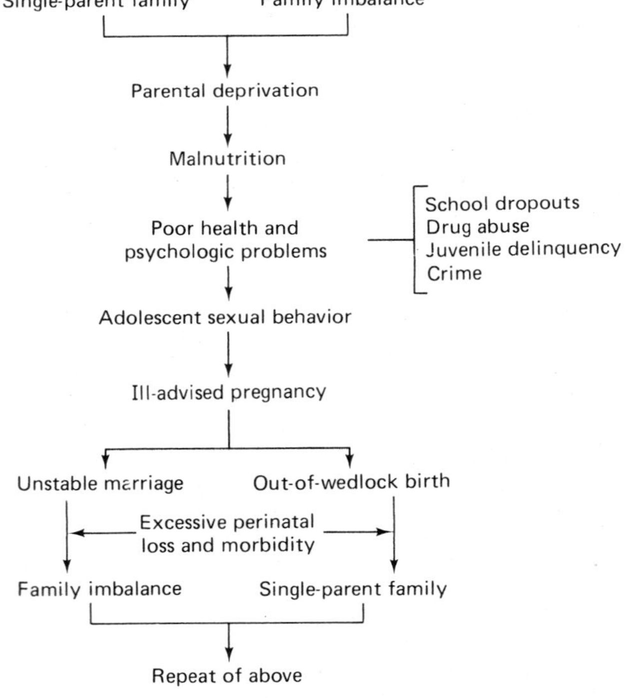

from the complex web of psychological, social, and economic correlates that are involved.

DIET OF PREGNANT TEENAGERS

Very few studies have been made of the actual dietary intake of pregnant teenagers. However, the limited data available indicate that the diets of pregnant adolescents are not adequate. In one well-controlled study of 18 pregnant teenagers in San Francisco, the nutrients most poorly supplied by the diet during and after pregnancy were calcium, iron, vitamin A, and calories. The infants weighed less than a matched control group, and five of them were not in good condition. In a larger study of 142 teenage pregnancies, the young women showed considerable evidence of nutritional deficiency. Low levels of hemoglobin, vitamin B_6, niacin, folate, vitamin A, thiamin, and vitamin B_{12} were seen in from 13 to 58% of the patients. Folate intake in pregnant teenagers has also been found to be less than one-third of the recommended level, with average blood values for whole-blood folate below suggested standards.

References and Supplementary Readings

Ballard, W. M., and E. M. Gold. "Medical and health aspects of reproduction in the adolescent." *Clin. Obstet. Gynec.* **14**: 338–366 (1971).

Committee on Maternal Nutrition, Food and Nutrition Board, National Research Council. "Relation of nutrition to pregnancy in adolescence." In: *Maternal Nutrition and the Course of Pregnancy.* Washington, D.C.: National Academy of Sciences, 1970.

Food and Nutrition Board, National Research Council, National Academy of Sciences. *Recommended Dietary Allowances,* 8th ed. Washington, D.C., 1974.

Frisch, R. E. "Weight at menarche: Similarity for well-nourished and undernourished girls at differing ages, and evidence for historical constancy." *Ped.* **50**: 445–450 (1972).

Frisch, R. E. "Population, food intake, and fertility." *Science* **199**: 22–30 (1978).

Hampton, M. C., R. L. Huenemann, L. R. Shapiro, and B. W. Mitchell. "Caloric and nutrient intakes of teenagers." *J. Am. Diet. Assoc.* **50**: 385–396 (1967).

Heald, F. P., ed. *Adolescent Nutrition and Growth.* New York: Appleton-Century-Crofts, 1969.

Hodges, R. E., and W. A. Krehl. "Nutritional status of teenagers in Iowa." *Am. J. Clin. Nutr.* **17**: 200–210 (1965).

Huenemann, R. L. "A review of teenage nutrition in the United States." *Health Services Rep.* **87**: 823–829 (1972).

Kaminetzky, H. A., A. Langer, H. Baker, O. Frank, A. D. Thomson, E. D. Munves, A. Opper, F. C. Behrle, and B. Glista. "The effect of nutrition in teen-age gravidas on pregnancy and the status of the neonate. I. A nutritional profile." *Am. J. Obstet. Gynec.* **115**: 639–644 (1973).

KING, J. C., S. H. COHENOUR, D. H. CALLOWAY, AND H. N. JACOBSON. "Assessment of nutritional status of teenage pregnant girls. I. Nutrient intake and pregnancy." *Am. J. Clin. Nutr.* **25**: 916–925 (1972).

MARSHALL, W. A., AND J. M. TANNER. "Puberty." In J. A. Davis and J. Dobbing, eds. *Scientific Foundations of Pediatrics.* London: Heinemann Medical Books, 1974, pp. 124–151.

McKIGNEY, J. I., AND H. N. MUNRO, eds. *Nutrient Requirements in Adolescence.* Cambridge, Mass.: The MIT Press, 1976.

MORGAN, A. F. "Nutritional status U.S.A." *Calif. Ag. Exp. Station Bull.* 769 (1959).

TANNER, J. M. *Growth at Adolescence*, 2nd ed. Oxford: Blackwell Scientific Publications, 1962.

VAN DE MARK, M. S., AND A. C. WRIGHT. "Hemoglobin and folate levels of pregnant teenagers." *J. Am. Diet. Assoc.* **61**: 511–516 (1972).

Index